Practical Differential Diagnosis for CT and MRI

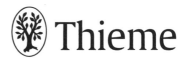

Practical Differential Diagnosis for CT and MRI

Eugene C. Lin, MD
Clinical Assistant Professor
Department of Radiology
University of Washington
Attending Radiologist
Virginia Mason Medical Center
Seattle, WA

Edward J. Escott, MD
Assistant Professor
Department of Radiology,
 Division of Neuroradiology
University of Pittsburgh Medical
 Center
Pittsburgh, PA

Kavita D. Garg, MD
Professor
Department of Radiology
Anschutz Centers for
 Advanced Medicine
University of Colorado Health
 Sciences Center
Aurora, CO

Andrew G. Bleicher, MD
Assistant Professor
Department of Radiology,
 Division of Neuroradiology
University of Pittsburgh
 Medical Center
Pittsburgh, PA

David Alexander, MD
Radiology Fellow
University of Washington
Seattle, WA

Thieme
New York • Stuttgart

Thieme Medical Publishers, Inc.
333 Seventh Ave.
New York, NY 10001

Executive Editor: Timothy Hiscock
Editorial Assistant: David Price
Vice-President, Production and Electronic Publishing: Anne T. Vinnicombe
Vice-President, International Marketing and Sales: Cornelia Schulze
Production Editor: Torsten Scheihagen
Chief Financial Officer: Peter van Woerden
President: Brian D. Scanlan
Compositor: Thomson Digital
Printer: Maple-Vail Book Manufacturing Group

Library of Congress Cataloging-in-Publication Data

Practical differential diagnosis for CT and MRI / Eugene Lin . . . [et al.].
    p. ; cm.
 Includes bibliographic references and index.
 ISBN 978-1-58890-655-7 (alk. paper)
 1. Diagnosis, Differential—Handbooks, manuals, etc. 2. Tomography—Handbooks, manuals, etc.
 3. Magnetic resonance imaging—Handbooks, manuals, etc. I. Lin, Eugene.
 [DNLM: 1. Magnetic Resonance Imaging—methods—Handbooks. 2. Tomography,
X-Ray Computed—methods—Handbooks. 3. Diagnosis, Differential—Handbooks. WN 39 P8947 2008]
 RC71.5.P73 2008
 616.07'57—dc22   2008014877

Important note: Medical knowledge is ever-changing. As new research and clinical experience broaden our knowledge, changes in treatment and drug therapy may be required. The authors and editors of the material herein have consulted sources believed to be reliable in their efforts to provide information that is complete and in accord with the standards accepted at the time of publication. However, in view of the possibility of human error by the authors, editors, or publisher of the work herein or changes in medical knowledge, neither the authors, editors, nor publisher, nor any other party who has been involved in the preparation of this work, warrants that the information contained herein is in every respect accurate or complete, and they are not responsible for any errors or omissions or for the results obtained from use of such information. Readers are encouraged to confirm the information contained herein with other sources. For example, readers are advised to check the product information sheet included in the package of each drug they plan to administer to be certain that the information contained in this publication is accurate and that changes have not been made in the recommended dose or in the contraindications for administration. This recommendation is of particular importance in connection with new or infrequently used drugs.

Some of the product names, patents, and registered designs referred to in this book are in fact registered trademarks or proprietary names even though specific reference to this fact is not always made in the text. Therefore, the appearance of a name without designation as proprietary is not to be construed as a representation by the publisher that it is in the public domain.

Printed in the United States

5 4 3 2 1

TMP ISBN 978–1–58890–655–7

To Satish, Samita and Sandip for their love, support and patience. Thank you to my residents, fellows and clinical colleagues for a lifetime of professional joy.

— *Kavita D. Garg, MD*

I would like to thank Patty Smith for her help preparing references.

— *Edward J. Escott, MD*

I would like to thank Bonnie Marston for help in preparing the manuscript. I would also like to thank my colleagues in the radiology department at Virginia Mason Medical Center. In particular, Dr. Neal Conti for reviewing the manuscript and providing many helpful comments.

— *Eugene Lin, MD*

With gratitude to all who have helped me reach this stage, with appreciation of my family and their continued support, with hopes for a shared future of growth and happiness.

— *Andrew G. Bleicher, MD*

Contents

BRAIN
Edward J. Escott, MD
Andrew G. Bleicher, MD
Jawad Tsay, MD
Melissa Kang, MD
Parvez Masood, MD
Sunayna Bakaya, MD

HEAD AND NECK
Edward J. Escott, MD
Sunayna Bakaya, MD
Andrew G. Bleicher, MD
Mohsin Rahman, MD
Melissa Kang, MD

CHEST
Kavita Garg, MD

ABDOMEN
Eugene Lin, MD
David Alexander, MD

PELVIS
Eugene Lin, MD

MUSCULOSKELETAL
Eugene Lin, MD

SPINE
Edward J. Escott, MD
Andrew G. Bleicher, MD

Preface

This text, *Practical Differential Diagnosis for CT and MRI*, is intended to be just that: a concise guide to the common diagnostic considerations for findings that one may encounter while interpreting CT or MRI scans. It is meant to be a handy reference for both residents and practicing radiologists. The text is meant to be used while interpreting studies at the workstation (or viewbox), to provide not only the list of differential diagnoses of an imaging finding, but also the features that will help one differentiate the common entities which may have similar imaging findings. The text is organized in a way that we hope will facilitate easy access to this information during a busy workday. We hope this book will serve as a useful aid in your day-to-day work, and a reference to which you will turn often.

Edward Escott, MD
Eugene Lin, MD

List of Contributors

Eugene C. Lin, M.D.
Clinical Assistant Professor
Department of Radiology
University of Washington
Attending Radiologist
Virginia Mason Medical Center
Seattle, Washington

Edward J. Escott, M.D.
Assistant Professor
Department of Radiology, Division
  of Neuroradiology
University of Pittsburgh Medical Center
Pittsburgh, Pennsylvania

Kavita D. Garg, M.D.
Professor
Department of Radiology, Section
  of Thoracic & Body Imaging
University of Colorado at Denver
  and Health Sciences Center
Anschutz Centers for Advanced
  Medicine
Aurora, Colorado

Andrew G. Bleicher, M.D.
Assistant Professor
Department of Radiology, Division
  of Neuroradiology
University of Pittsburgh Medical Center
Pittsburgh, Pennsylvania

David Alexander, M.D.
Radiology Fellow
University of Washington
Seattle, Washington

Sunayna Bakaya, M.D.
Fellow
Department of Radiology, Body Imaging
Hospital of the University of Pennsylvania
Philadelphia, Pennsylvania

Neal Conti, M.D.
Department of Radiology
Virginia Mason Medical Center
Seattle, Washington

Melissa Kang, M.D.
Fellow
Department of Radiology, Section
  of Neuroradiology
University of Pittsburgh Medical Center
Pittsburgh, Pennsylvania

Parvez Masood, M.D.
Associate Staff
Diagnostic Radiology
Cleveland Clinic
Cleveland, Ohio

Mohsin Rahman, M.D.
Visiting Clinical Assistant Professor
Department of Radiology, Section
  of Neuroradiology
University of Pittsburgh Medical Center
Pittsburgh, Pennsylvania

Jawad Tsay, M.D.
Assistant Professor
Department of Radiology, Section
  of Neuroradiology
University of Pittsburgh Medical Center
Pittsburgh, Pennsylvania

I Brain

1

Peripherally Enhancing Cystic Brain Lesions

The main differential consideration between peripherally enhancing parenchymal lesions is cystic/necrotic neoplasm (primary or metastatic) versus abscess. Neoplasms include high-grade necrotic gliomas such as glioblastomas and anaplastic astrocytomas, and lower-grade neoplasms such as hemangioblastoma, pilocytic astrocytoma, and ganglioglioma, as well as metastases. Occasionally, demyelinating lesions or evolving hematoma can have a similar appearance. Some of these lesions have distinguishing features such as a mural nodule (hemangioblastoma or pilocytic astrocytoma), but others may look similar on conventional imaging, with peripheral enhancement and surrounding reaction or edema (low density on computed tomography or hyperintensity on T2-weighted magnetic resonance (MR) imaging. A variety of differentiating features has been described based on characteristics of the wall, the enhancement found, and the surrounding reaction (**Table 1.1**). Recently, newer imaging techniques such as diffusion weighted imaging, MR perfusion imaging, and MR spectroscopy have also been shown to help in differentiating these lesions.

Table 1.1 Differentiating Features between Peripherally Enhancing Neoplasm and an Abscess

	Neoplasm	Abscess
Enhancement of Wall	Nodular	Smooth
Surrounding Edema	Variable; may be less extensive for primary tumors, but more extensive for metastases	Relatively extensive for lesion size
Rim Thickness	>5 mm	≤5 mm with thinning of medial wall (more pronounced on CT than MRI)
Rim Signal T1WI Pre-contrast	Intermediate	Isointense to hyperintense (thought to be due to free radicals)
Rim Signal on T2WI	Intermediate	Isointense to hypointense (thought to be due to free radicals)
Signal of Contents on MRI	Slightly hyperintense to CSF on T1WI Similar to mildly hyperintense to GM or CSF on T2WI	Slightly hyperintense to CSF on T1WI Similar to hyperintense to GM or CSF on T2WI

(Continued on page 4)

Table 1.1 *(Continued)* Differentiating Features between Peripherally Enhancing Neoplasm and an Abscess

	Neoplasm	Abscess
Daughter/Satellite Lesions	More common in abscess	Occasional
Perfusion Imaging	Generally greater in high-grade neoplasms Increased rCBV when compared with normal WM	Generally lower rCBV in rim when compared with normal WM
Diffusion Weighted Imaging	Low signal on DWI, high ADC	High signal on DWI, low ADC (but can overlap tumor; not toxoplasmosis/cysticercosis variable)
Proton MR Spectroscopy	Elevated lactate and Cho peaks	Elevated lactate and cytosolic amino acids (leucine, isoleucine, valine with or without succinate (2.4 ppm), and acetate (if succinate is elevated with respect to acetate and DWI signal is intermediate to low then consider cysticercosis)

Abbreviations: ADC, apparent diffusion coefficient; Cho, choline; CSF, cerebrospinal fluid; CT, computed tomography; DWI, diffusion weighted imaging; GM, gray matter; MRI, magnetic resonance imaging; rCBV, regional cerebral blood volume; T1WI, T1-weighted MRI; T2WI, T2-weighted MRI; WM, white matter.

Additional Readings

1. Agarwal M, Chawla S, Husain N, Jaggi RS, Husain M, Gupta RK. Higher succinate than acetate levels differentiate cerebral degenerating cysticerci from anaerobic abscesses on in-vivo proton MR spectroscopy. Neuroradiology 2004;46(3):211–215
2. Chong-Han CH, Cortez SC, Tung GA. Diffusion-weighted MRI of cerebral toxoplasma abscess. AJR Am J Roentgenol 2003;181(6):1711–1714
3. Falcone S, Post MJ. Encephalitis, cerebritis, and brain abscess: pathophysiology and imaging findings. Neuroimaging Clin N Am 2000;10(2): 333–353
4. Guzman R, Barth A, Lovblad KO, et al. Use of diffusion-weighted magnetic resonance imaging in differentiating purulent brain processes from cystic brain tumors. J Neurosurg 2002;97(5): 1101–1107
5. Haimes AB, Zimmerman RD, Morgello S, et al. MR imaging of brain abscesses. AJR Am J Roentgenol 1989;152(5):1073–1085
6. Holmes TM, Petrella JR, Provenzale JM. Distinction between cerebral abscesses and high-grade neoplasms by dynamic susceptibility contrast perfusion MRI. AJR Am J Roentgenol 2004;183(5):1247–1252
7. Lai PH, Ho JT, Chen WL, et al. Brain abscess and necrotic brain tumor: discrimination with proton MR spectroscopy and diffusion-weighted imaging. AJNR Am J Neuroradiol 2002;23(8):1369–1377
8. Mishra AM, Gupta RK, Jaggi RS, et al. Role of diffusion-weighted imaging and in vivo proton magnetic resonance spectroscopy in the differential diagnosis of ring-enhancing intracranial cystic mass lesions. J Comput Assist Tomogr 2004;28(4):540–547

2

Metastases versus Primary Brain Neoplasms

Brain metastasis is the most common neoplastic condition affecting the brain parenchyma. A major differential diagnostic consideration would be a primary high-grade brain neoplasm, which may be indistinguishable. Some features, however, can aid in differentiating these lesions (**Table 2.1**). Abscesses can also be difficult to differentiate from cystic or necrotic neoplasm and diffusion-weighted imaging can be useful. Abscesses have true restricted diffusion, although hemorrhagic metastasis may also have a similar appearance (see Chapter 1 for further discussion).

The most frequent primary brain tumors in adults are gliomas and primary central nervous system (CNS) lymphomas. Gliomas are classified according to aggressiveness from low-grade glioma to anaplastic astrocytoma and glioblastoma multiforme (characterized by necrosis and hemorrhage).

The differential diagnosis for lesions with imaging features of an aggressive glioma includes metastasis, radiation necrosis, and evolving hematoma. Positron emission tomography (increased fluorodeoxyglucose [FDG] uptake in neoplasm), magnetic resonance spectroscopy (the choline [Cho]/creatine [Cr] and Cho/N-acetyl aspartate [NAA] ratios are significantly higher, and the NAA/Cr ratios significantly lower, in tumor than in radiation injury), and thallium-201 scan (increased uptake in neoplasm) may help in differentiating between neoplasms and radiation necrosis or evolving hematoma (benign).

Table 2.1 Differentiating Features between Metastases and Gliomas

	Metastasis	High-grade Glioma	Low-grade Glioma
Shape	Generally spherical	Irregular and geographic	Variable
Pattern of Enhancement	Variable; peripheral nodular enhancement in a larger cavitating lesion to heterogeneous or homogeneous enhancement in a smaller or solid lesion, or ring enhancement	Nodular and thick enhancement of wall if lesion is cystic/necrotic to heterogeneous enhancement in a solid lesion	None (generally)**
Surrounding Edema*	Extensive	Variable; may be relatively little for lesion size to extensive	None to very minimal edema

(Continued on page 6)

Table 2.1 *(Continued)* Differentiating Features between Metastases and Gliomas

	Metastasis	High-grade Glioma	Low-grade Glioma
Signal of Contents on MRI if Cystic or Necrotic	If nonhemorrhagic – T2WI: High T1WI: Low No restricted diffusion If hemorrhagic – Signal of blood products If solid – T1WI: Intermediate to low T2WI: Intermediate to high	Heterogeneous signal of blood products and necrotic material with peripheral enhancement Solid components – T1WI: Intermediate to low T2WI: Intermediate to high	Generally solid** T2WI: High T1WI: Low Mass effect Minimal to no peripheral edema
Daughter/Satellite Lesions	None Metastases are often multiple.	Occasional[†] May be multifocal	None May be multifocal
Perfusion Imaging	Increased rCBV when compared with normal WM	Increased rCBV when compared with normal WM Generally greater in high-grade neoplasms	Normal to slightly higher rCBV than surrounding brain tissue
Proton MR Spectroscopy	Elevated lactate and Cho peaks Decreased NAA	Elevated lactate and Cho peaks Decreased NAA	Elevated lactate and Cho peaks Decreased NAA[††] May have elevated MI

Abbreviations: CBV, regional cerebral blood volume; Cho, choline; Cr, creatine; FLAIR, fluid-attenuated inversion recovery; NAA, *N*-acetyl aspartate; MRI, magnetic resonance imaging; MI, myo-inositol; T1WI, T1-weighted MRI; T2WI, T2-weighted MRI; WM, white matter.

*It should be noted that the "edema" seen on T2WI and FLAIR images surrounding an enhancing glioma often will also be comprised of nonenhancing tumor as well as edema.

**Some low-grade neoplasms such as pleomorphic xanthoastrocytoma (PXA), pilocytic astrocytoma (PA), ganglioglioma (GG), and dysembryoplastic neuroepithelial tumor (DNET) can have cystic areas, and PA, PXA, and GG can commonly have enhancement.

[†]Due to extension along WM tracts and cross over from corpus callosum and transependymal spread

[††]Cho/Cr and Cho/NAA less than higher-grade neoplasms

Additional Readings

1. Al-Okaili RN, Krejza J, Wang S, Woo JH, Melhem ER. Advanced MR imaging techniques in the diagnosis of intraaxial brain tumors in adults. Radiographics 2006; 26(Suppl 1):S173–S189

2. Behin A, Hoang-Xuan K, Carpentier AF, Delattre JY. Primary brain tumours in adults. Lancet 2003; 361(9354):323–331

3. Chang SC, Lai PH, Chen WL, et al. Diffusion-weighted MRI features of brain abscess and cystic or necrotic brain tumors: comparison with conventional MRI. Clin Imaging 2002;26(4):227–236

4. Holmes TM, Petrella JR, Provenzale JM. Distinction between cerebral abscesses and high-grade neoplasms by dynamic susceptibility contrast perfusion MRI. AJR Am J Roentgenol 2004;183(5):1247–1252

5. Rees JH, Smirniotopoulos JG, Jones RV, Wong K. Glioblastoma multiforme: radiologic-pathologic correlation. Radiographics 1996;16(6):1413–1438 quiz 1462–3

6. Ricci PE. Imaging of adult brain tumors. Neuroimaging Clin N Am 1999;9(4):651–669

7. Tamura M, Shibasaki T, Zama A, et al. Assessment of malignancy of glioma by positron emission tomography with 18F-fluorodeoxyglucose and single photon emission computed tomography with thallium-201 chloride. Neuroradiology 1998;40(4):210–215

8. Weybright P, Sundgren PC, Maly P, et al. Differentiation between brain tumor recurrence and radiation injury using MR spectroscopy. AJR Am J Roentgenol 2005; 185(6):1471–1476

3

Intraventricular Neoplasms

Overall, intraventricular neoplasms are more common in children than they are in adults, where they are relatively uncommon. There are differences in the presentation and etiology of these lesions between the adult and pediatric population. For example, ependymomas constitute almost one third of all brain tumors in patients younger than 3 years and are more common in the 4th ventricle in pediatric patients, whereas they are frequently extraventricular and supratentorial within the adult population. However, choroid plexus papillomas present more commonly in children's lateral ventricles, but in the 4th ventricle in adults. Choroid plexus carcinomas, which represent 26 to 35%

of choroid plexus tumors, are more common in children, but are rare brain neoplasms. Both papillomas and carcinomas can seed the subarachnoid space. Subependymomas are rarely seen in children; they occur in middle-aged and older adults, and are more commonly found in the 4th ventricle as opposed to the lateral ventricle. In the lateral ventricles, they usually have no or little enhancement, which when present is heterogeneous. In the 4th ventricle, they can enhance more intensely and calcify more commonly. Differentiating features for these tumors can be found in **Table 3.1**.

Central neurocytomas are rare tumors, generally found in young adults. They usually occur

Table 3.1 Differentiating Features between Ependymoma, Subependymoma, and Choroid Plexus Tumors

	Ependymoma	Subependymoma	Choroid Plexus Papilloma	Choroid Plexus Carcinoma
Location	4th v > supratentorial When supratentorial more commonly extraventricular	4th v > lateral vs (commonly in the frontal horn/ body)	Lateral vs (more common in children) 4th v (more common in adults)	Same as CPP May more commonly involve/invade 3rd v than CPP
CT	Isodense to hypodense Occasionally hyperdense (may be higher grade) Heterogeneous	Hypodense to isodense Well-defined, lobulated Heterogeneous	Isodense to hyperdense No brain invasion May engulf glomus	More heterogeneous with necrosis and brain invasion

Table 3.1 *(Continued)* Differentiating Features between Ependymoma, Subependymoma, and Choroid Plexus Tumors

	Ependymoma	Subependymoma	Choroid Plexus Papilloma	Choroid Plexus Carcinoma
Calcifications	Common - punctuate foci of calcifications to large calcifications	Relatively common in 4th v tumors, but not lateral v tumors	Fairly common and may be scattered punctuate calcifications to extensive calcifications	Same as papilloma
Cysts	Supratentorial > infratentorial	Small cysts can occur.	Some	Same as papilloma
Enhancement	Variable and heterogeneous Soft tissue component usually intense	Mild & focal or absent, but may be intense particularly on MRI 4th v > lateral v	Intense Dilated feeding vessels	Intense MRI shows prominent flow voids and dilated feeding vessels
T1WI	4th v: heterogeneous isointense to GM Supratentorial: hypointense to isointense	Heterogeneous – hypointense to isointense to WM	Hypointense to isointense to normal brain	Heterogeneous
T2WI	4th v: heterogeneous Supratentorial: hyperintense to GM	Hyperintense to WM Heterogeneous	Variable SI, flow voids	Heterogeneous More vasogenic edema than papilloma
Other	4th ventricular lesions commonly extend through foramen of Magendie &/or Luschka	Does not invade adjacent brain Most common nonenhancing lateral v mass Little surrounding parenchymal reaction or mass effect	Often associated with hydrocephalus May extend out to CP angle; rarely multifocal or extraventricular	Screen spine with MRI to exclude drop metastases FDG-avid

Abbreviations: CP, cerebellopontine; CPP, choroid plexus papilloma; FDG, fluorodeoxyglucose; GM, gray matter; MRI, magnetic resonance imaging; SI, signal intensity; T1WI, T1 weighted MRI; T2WI, T2 weighted MRI; v, ventricle; vs, ventricles; WM, white matter.

in the bodies of the lateral ventricles either arising from the septum or from the superolateral wall of the ventricle, where they may present with symptoms related to obstruction. They can extend into the 3rd ventricle, but very rarely arise within the 3rd or 4th ventricle. Intraventricular meningiomas account for 0.5 to 3% of intracranial meningiomas and are generally located at the trigone, with most presenting in individuals from 40 to 60 years of age with a gender predilection reported as 1:1 or with a female predominance of 2:1. Less commonly, they can arise in the 3rd ventricle, and only rarely arise from the 4th (77.8% lateral, 15.6% 3rd, 6.6% 4th). Meningioma is the most common atrial mass in the adult population. Differentiating features for these neoplasms can be found in **Table 3.2**.

Intraventricular metastases are relatively uncommon, presenting mainly in older individuals. They are most common to the lateral ventricles and choroid plexus, where renal cell carcinoma and lung carcinoma are most common. Metastases generally enhance with contrast. Colloid cysts, although not truly neoplasms, are the most common 3rd ventricular mass and occur in the anterosuperior 3rd ventricle between the forniceal columns near the foramen of Monro. The imaging appearance is variable, but they are commonly hyperdense on computed tomography, hyperintense on T1-weighted magnetic resonance (MR) images, and hypointense on T2-weighted MR images. If they enhance with contrast, generally only the capsule does. Subependymal giant cell astrocytomas arise in the lateral ventricles near the foramen of Monro, usually, if not exclusively, in patients with tuberous sclerosis and generally in children, adolescents, and young adults. They are enhancing isoattenuating to hypoattenuating masses on CT, hypointense on T1-weighted images and heterogeneously hypointense on T2-weighted MR images. They may have cysts, calcification, or hemorrhage. In neonates, the signal intensity characteristics can be reversed on MR imaging (MRI).

Table 3.2 Differentiating Features between Central Neurocytoma and Meningioma

	Central Neurocytoma	Meningioma
Location	Most in anterior half of the lateral v near foramen of Monro	Most commonly in trigone of lateral v 3rd, 4th v uncommon
CT	Isodense to mildly hyperdense Circumscribed, lobulated	Hyperdense Well defined
Calcifications	50–69%	50%
Cysts	Up to 85%	Occasional
Enhancement	Moderate, heterogeneous	Intense, generally homogeneous
T1WI	Isointense to hypointense (occasionally mildly hyperintense) Heterogeneous	Hypointense to isointense
T2WI	Isointense to hyperintense Heterogeneous	Isointense to hyperintense
Other	Hypermetabolic: Increased CBF, CBV, FDG uptake on PET MRS: Increased choline, decreased NAA, increased Ch/Cr and Ch/NAA ratios; lactate peak and unidentified peak at 3.55 ppm which may be a specific marker May have flow voids	MRS: Decreased NAA and CR, elevated alanine (doublet @ 1.47 ppm)

Abbreviations: CBF, cerebral blood flow; CBV, cerebral blood velocity; Ch, choline; Cr, creatine; CR, creatine, CT, computed tomography; FDG, fluorodeoxyglucose; lateral vs, lateral ventricles; MRS, magnetic resonance spectroscopy; NAA, *N*-acetyl aspartate; PET, positron emission tomography; ppm, parts per million; T1WI, T1-weighted magnetic resonance imaging; T2WI, T2-weighted magnetic resonance imaging; v, ventricle; vs, ventricles; WM, white matter.

Types of Lateral Ventricle Tumors

- Meningioma
- Central neurocytoma
- Subependymal giant cell astrocytoma
- Ependymoma and subependymoma
- Choroid plexus papilloma
- Metastases
- Lymphoma

Types of Third Ventricle Tumors/Masses

- Colloid cyst
- Meningioma (rare)

- Metastases (rare)
- Extension of hypothalamic/chiasmatic glioma
- Large Massa intermedia
- Extension of craniopharyngioma

Types of Fourth Ventricular Tumors

- Ependymoma
- Choroid plexus papilloma
- Medulloblastoma
- Exophytic brainstem glioma
- Subependymoma
- Metastases

Additional Readings

1. Armington WG, Osborn AG, Cubberley DA, et al. Supratentorial ependymoma: CT appearance. Radiology 1985;157(2):367–372
2. Koeller KK, Sandberg GD. From the archives of the AFIP. Cerebral intraventricular neoplasms: radiologic-pathologic correlation. Radiographics 2002;22(6):1473–1505
3. Majos C, Coll S, Aguilera C, Acebes JJ, Pons LC. Intraventricular mass lesions of the brain. Eur Radiol 2000;10(6):951–961
4. Majos C, Cucurella G, Aguilera C, Coll S, Pons LC. Intraventricular meningiomas: MR imaging and MR spectroscopic findings in two cases. AJNR Am J Neuroradiol 1999;20(5):882–885
5. Rath TJ, Sundgren PC, Brahma B, Lieberman AP, Chandler WF, Gebarski SS. Massive symptomatic subependymoma of the lateral ventricles: case report and review of the literature. Neuroradiology 2005; 47(3):183–188
6. Strojan P, Popovic M, Surlan K, Jereb B. Choroid plexus tumors: a review of 28-year experience. Neoplasma 2004;51(4):306–312

4

Tumefactive Demyelination

Multiple sclerosis (MS) is the most common of the demyelinating diseases of the central nervous system and thorough descriptions of its usual imaging manifestations abound. Standard unenhanced or enhanced computed tomography (CT) does little more than to aid in the identification of gross white matter changes, and volume loss in advanced cases, while excluding emergent diagnoses such as hemorrhage in a patient with relatively acute neurological deficit(s). The typical periventricular linear lesions as well as frequent corpus callosum involvement are best identified on magnetic resonance imaging (MRI), specifically the sagittal fluid-attenuated inversion recovery (FLAIR) pulse sequence, with assessment of the brainstem and visual pathways best accomplished by dedicated MRI. MS has a predilection for these sites as well as the subcortical U-fibers, and occasionally the cortex and spinal cord. The periventricular lesions occur perpendicular to

the ventricles along perimedullary veins (Dawson's fingers). Acute and chronic lesions are hyperintense on T2-weighted MR images (T2WI). Acute lesions may be isointense or hypointense on T1-weighted MR images (T1WI) and enhance, with enhancement beginning as a solid nodule and then enhancement becoming peripheral. Chronic lesions also may be hypointense- to isointense on T1WI, with hypointense lesions termed *black holes*.

Tumefactive demyelination, part of the spectrum of demyelinating disease, poses a diagnostic conundrum by mimicking a high-grade neoplasm. Whether tumefactive demyelination is another manifestation of MS or represents a distinct entity is apparently a matter of contention. Certain features on standard as well as advanced MRI can potentially promote the diagnosis of tumefactive demyelination and obviate the need for biopsy (**Table 4.1**). The signal intensity is similar to MS lesions

Table 4.1 Differentiating Features between Tumefactive Demyelination and a High-grade Neoplasm

	Tumefactive Demyelination	**High-grade Neoplasm**
Size	>2 cm with less mass effect and edema than would be expected for a neoplasm	>2 cm with mass effect and edema as expected for size
Location	Supratentorial WM with relative sparing of cortex	Supratentorial WM; may involve GM
Enhancement	Approximately 50% enhance Most commonly Incomplete, irregular ring with open portion of ring on GM side May be complete ring or solid	Complete, irregular ring ± Satellite foci of enhancement

Table 4.1 *(Continued)* Differentiating Features between Tumefactive Demyelination and a High-grade Neoplasm

	Tumefactive Demyelination	High-grade Neoplasm
Necrosis/Cystic Degeneration	May be present	Commonly present
Vessels	Structures thought to represent central dilated veins have been noted on dynamic T2WI and on post-contrast T1WI	Displaced
Perfusion	No frank angiogenesis with inflammation causing decreased perfusion in most cases Mean rCBV compared with contralateral parenchyma decreased Vast majority of cases below rCBV value of 1.5 with none >1.8	Angiogenesis causing marked increase in perfusion Mean rCBV of 6.5 Vast majority of cases above rCBV of 1.6 with none below 1.5
Diffusion	Mildly increased apparent diffusion coefficient	Mildly increased apparent diffusion coefficient
Hemorrhage	Uncommon	Not uncommon
Spectroscopy	Decreased NAA ± Elevated Cho May have lipid and lactate peaks	Decreased NAA Elevated Cho May have lipid and lactate peaks

Abbreviations: Cho, choline; GM, gray matter; NAA, *N*-acetyl aspartate, rCBV, relative cerebral blood volume; T1WI, T1-weighted magnetic resonance images; T2WI, T2-weighted magnetic resonance images; WM, white matter.

elsewhere, and these lesions are often low in density on CT, with lesion margins usually well defined. In addition, one should attempt to identify any additional findings that would be consistent with MS. Undoubtedly, the clinical course of the patient would have to be considered as well as follow-up imaging obtained to ensure the correct diagnosis.

Additional Readings

1 Cha S, Pierce S, Knopp EA, et al. Dynamic contrast-enhanced T2*-weighted MR imaging of tumefactive demyelinating lesions. AJNR Am J Neuroradiol 2001; 22 (6): 1109–1116

2 Ge Y. Multiple sclerosis: the role of MR imaging. AJNR Am J Neuroradiol 2006; 27 (6): 1165–1176

3 Given CA II, Stevens BS, Lee C. The MRI appearance of tumefactive demyelinating lesions. AJR Am J Roentgenol 2004; 182 (1): 195–199

4 Gonzalez-Toledo E, Kelley RE, Minagar A. Role of magnetic resonance spectroscopy in diagnosis and management of multiple sclerosis. Neurol Res 2006; 28 (3): 280–283

5 Saindane AM, Cha S, Law M, Xue X, Knopp EA, Zagzag D. Proton MR spectroscopy of tumefactive demyelinating lesions. AJNR Am J Neuroradiol 2002; 23 (8): 1378–1386

6 Tan HM, Chan LL, Chuah KL, Goh NS, Tang KK. Monophasic, solitary tumefactive demyelinating lesion: neuroimaging features and neuropathological diagnosis. Br J Radiol 2004; 77 (914): 153–156

5

Posterior Fossa Neoplasms in Children

The majority of posterior fossa neoplasms in children are intraaxial with pilocytic astrocytomas and medulloblastomas as the most common types. These two tumors combined account for roughly two thirds to three quarters of posterior fossa neoplasms in children. Ependymomas are the third most common posterior fossa tumor, accounting for up to 10%. Medulloblastomas are also categorized as primitive neuroectodermal tumors (PNET).

Pilocytic astrocytomas are typically well-delineated, cystic tumors arising in the cerebellar hemispheres or less frequently, the vermis.

Medulloblastomas are often well-circumcised, homogeneous, hyperdense vermian masses projecting into the 4th ventricle. Ependymomas are frequently calcified, isodense 4th ventricular masses with a tendency to spread through the foramina of the 4th ventricle. There are features that can aid in the differentiation of these tumors (**Table 5.1**). In addition to conventional imaging, techniques such as apparent diffusion coefficient (ADC) measurement can serve to differentiate these tumors. A study evaluating the efficacy of ADC in differentiating cerebellar tumors did not find any overlap between the major tumor

Table 5.1 Differentiating Features between Ependymoma, Medulloblastoma, and Pilocytic Astrocytoma

	Ependymoma	Medulloblastoma	Pilocytic Astrocytoma
Age/Sex	1st decade, M = F	5 – 15, M > F	2nd decade, M = F
Non-contrast CT	Isodense	Hyperdense	Nodule: Hypodense to isodense Cyst: Hypodense
Contrast CT	Minimal to mild, but can be avid	Moderate to avid	Avid for nodule Minimal to no cyst wall enhancement
T1WI (Pre-contrast)	Hypointense/isointense/ heterogeneous	Hypointense/isointense	Nodule: Isointense/ hypointense Cyst: Fluid signal
T2WI	Hyperintense/ heterogeneous Associated calcification often markedly hypointense	Hypointense/isointense (most common) Can be hyperintense	Nodule: Hyperintense to brain Nodule: Isointense to CSF in up to 50% of cases Cyst: Fluid signal
T1WI (Post-contrast)	Usually avid enhancement	Usually avid enhancement Heterogeneous	Nodule: Avid enhancement Cyst wall: Usually none to mild enhancement
Surrounding Edema	None to mild	Marginal	Mild for size of tumor

Table 5.1 *(Continued)* Differentiating Features between Ependymoma, Medulloblastoma, and Pilocytic Astrocytoma

	Ependymoma	Medulloblastoma	Pilocytic Astrocytoma
Location	Arises from ependymal lining and fills 4th ventricle	Cerebellar vermis projecting into 4th ventricle	Hemispheric
Cyst(s)	Up to 20%	Up to 59%	Up to 90%
Calcification	Up to 80%	Up to 20%	Up to 5%
Hemorrhage	Up to 10%	<1%	<1%
Foraminal Spread*	Frequent	Uncommon	No
Hydrocephalus	Frequent	Frequent	Frequent
Subarachnoid Seeding	Up to 10%	Up to 50%	<1%
Apparent Diffusion Coefficient[†]	$1.00 - 1.30 \times 10^{-3}$ mm^2/s	$<0.9 \times 10^{-3}$ mm^2/s (decreased[††])	$>1.4 \times 10^{-3}$ mm^2/s (increased[††])
Diffusion Weighted Imaging[†]	Mildly restricted to mildly facilitated	Restricted	Facilitated
MR Spectroscopy	NAA decreased Cho elevated May have elevated lipid, lactate Cr:Cho higher than for astrocytomas and medulloblastomas	NAA decreased Cho elevated Cr decreased May have elevated lipid, lactate NAA:Cho lower than for ependymoma and astrocytomas	NAA decreased Cho elevated May have elevated lipid, lactate

Abbreviations: CBF, cerebralbloodflow; CSF, cerebrospinal fluid; Cho, choline; Cr, creatine; CT, computed tomography; F, female; FDG, fluorodeoxyglucose; M, male; MR, magnetic resonance; NAA, *N*-acetyl aspartate; T1WI, T1-weighted MR imaging; T2WI, T2-weighted MR imaging.

* Foramen of Luschka and Magendie

[†] Of solid enhancing portion of tumor

[††] Compared with normal cerebellum

types (pilocytic astrocytoma, ependymoma, medulloblastoma). Magnetic resonance (MR) spectroscopy has also shown promise in differentiating neoplasms, and when combined with hemodynamic imaging, also may aid in differentiating neoplasm from normal tissue, treated tumor, and areas of necrosis, and may be helpful in evaluating tumor response to therapy as well.

For additional discussion of pilocytic astrocytoma, please see Chapter 6.

Differential Diagnosis of Posterior Fossa Masses in Children

Intraaxial masses are the overwhelming majority of posterior fossa masses found in children. With regard to extraaxial masses, neoplasms are rare, but cysts and malformations not uncommon.

Types of Intraaxial Masses

- Cerebellar astrocytomas (usually pilocytic)
- Brainstem astrocytomas (usually fibrillary, infiltrative, and aggressive and located in the pons; tectal may be less aggressive, and diencephalic are usually low-grade fibrillary or pilocytic)
- Medulloblastoma
- Ependymoma
- Choroid plexus papilloma/carcinoma (more commonly found in the lateral ventricle in children)
- Lymphoma

- Teratoma
- Hemangioblastoma
- Metastasis (rare)
- Lhermitte–Duclos (cerebellar gangliocytoma)
- Atypical teratoid/rhabdoid tumor

Types of Extraaxial Masses

- Arachnoid cyst
- Dermoid
- Epidermoid
- Neurenteric cyst
- Dandy–Walker spectrum
- Teratoma
- Schwannoma
- Meningioma
- Metastasis
- Skull base tumors

Additional Readings

1. Arai K, Sato N, Aoki J, et al. MR signal of the solid portion of pilocytic astrocytoma on T2-weighted images: is it useful for differentiation from medulloblastoma? Neuroradiology 2006;48(4):233–237
2. Chen CJ, Tseng YC, Hsu HL, Jung SM. Imaging predictors of intracranial ependymomas. J Comput Assist Tomogr 2004;28(3):407–413
3. Erdem E, Zimmerman RA, Haselgrove JC, Bilaniuk LT, Hunter JV. Diffusion-weighted imaging and fluid attenuated inversion recovery imaging in the evaluation of primitive neuroectodermal tumors. Neuroradiology 2001;43(11):927–933
4. Koeller KK, Rushing EJ. From the archives of the AFIP: medulloblastoma: a comprehensive review with radiologic-pathologic correlation. Radiographics 2003;23(6):1613–1637
5. Koeller KK, Rushing EJ. From the archives of the AFIP: pilocytic astrocytoma: radiologic-pathologic correlation. Radiographics 2004;24(6):1693–1708
6. Koeller KK, Sandberg GD. From the archives of the AFIP. Cerebral intraventricular neoplasms: radiologic-

pathologic correlation. Radiographics 2002;22(6):1473–1505
7. Lee YY, Van Tassel P, Bruner JM, Moser RP, Share JC. Juvenile pilocytic astrocytomas: CT and MR characteristics. AJR Am J Roentgenol 1989;152(6):1263–1270
8. Quadery FA, Okamoto K. Diffusion-weighted MRI of hemangioblastomas and other cerebellar tumors. Neuroradiology 2003;45(4):212–219
9. Rumboldt Z, Camacho DL, Lake D, Welsh CT, Castillo M. Apparent diffusion coefficients for differentiation of cerebellar tumors in children. AJNR Am J Neuroradiol 2006;27(6):1362–1369
10. Tzika AA, Vajapeyam S, Barnes PD. Multivoxel proton MR spectroscopy and hemodynamic MR imaging of childhood brain tumors: preliminary observations. AJNR Am J Neuroradiol 1997;18(2):203–218
11. Wang Z, Sutton LN, Cnaan A, et al. Proton MR spectroscopy of pediatric cerebellar tumors. AJNR Am J Neuroradiol 1995;16(9):1821–1833

6

Posterior Fossa Cystic Neoplasms

The "cyst with a mural nodule" morphology is suggestive of a less-aggressive etiology such as a pilocytic astrocytoma, ganglioglioma, pleomorphic xanthoastrocytoma (PXA), or hemangioblastoma. Metastases can be cystic; however, other neoplasms such as medulloblastoma are rarely predominantly cystic. Infectious etiologies such as cysticercosis can also cause cysts in the cerebellum. Ganglioglioma and PXA are more common in the supratentorial brain. However, within the posterior fossa, the configuration of a cyst and mural nodule narrows the differential consideration mainly to juvenile pilocytic astrocytoma (JPA) or hemangioblastoma (**Table 6.1**). (See Chapters 1 and 5 as supplements to this chapter.)

Table 6.1 Differentiating Features between Cerebellar Juvenile Pilocytic Astrocytoma and Hemangioblastoma

	Juvenile Pilocytic Astrocytoma	**Hemangioblastoma**
CT	Hypoattenuating cystic component with hypoattenuating to isoattenuating mural nodule with avid contrast enhancement	Hypoattenuating cyst and isodense nodule with avid contrast enhancement
T1WI	Well-demarcated lesion Solid component: Isointense to hypointense relative to normal brain Cystic component follows fluid signal intensity.	Well-demarcated lesion Nodule peripherally located near pial surface and isointense to gray matter on T1WI Cyst: Isointense or slightly hyperintense on T1WI compared with CSF
T2WI	Nodule: Hyperintense to normal brain with minimal surrounding T2WI signal Cyst: Follows fluid signal	Nodule: Hyperintense Cyst: High signal intensity
Vascularity/ Enhancement	Avid enhancement of mural nodule No reported abnormal flow voids	Avid enhancement of solid components Peripheral in location due to vascular supply from pia mater with nodule located near pial surface May see abnormal vessels or flow voids associated with enhancing mural nodule

(Continued on page 18)

Table 6.1 *(Continued)* Differentiating Features between Cerebellar Juvenile Pilocytic Astrocytoma and Hemangioblastoma

	Juvenile Pilocytic Astrocytoma	Hemangioblastoma
Diffusion/ADC	Low signal on DWI and high on ADC map	Low signal on DWI and high signal on ADC map
Calcifications/ Blood	Rarely calcifies Rarely hemorrhage into the nodule or within the subarachnoid space	May hemorrhage into cyst leading to hematocrit levels If hemorrhage into nodule appearance depends on age of hemorrhage

Abbreviations: ADC, apparent diffusion coefficient; CSF, cerebrospinal fluid; CT, computed tomography; DWI, diffusion weighted imaging; T1WI, T1-weighted magnetic resonance imaging; T2WI, T2-weighted magnetic resonance imaging.

Hemangioblastoma

A hemangioblastoma is a benign neoplasm of endothelial origin. Hemangioblastomas account for 1.1 to 2.4% of all central nervous system (CNS) tumors and 7.3% of posterior fossa tumors. They are the most common primary posterior fossa tumor in adults. Hemangioblastomas usually occur in the posterior fossa (usually cerebellar hemisphere followed by the vermis) or the spinal cord. Hemangioblastomas of the CNS can present as a sporadic lesion or as a manifestation of von Hippel-Lindau syndrome (VHL). Spinal and retinal hemangioblastomas are more prevalent in patients with VHL. Otherwise, hemangioblastomas usually occur in the posterior fossa and supratentorial hemangioblastomas are exceptionally rare. The cyst wall is usually composed of neuroglial cells and never has tumor involvement. Cerebellar hemangioblastomas are described in four radiographic types. Type 1 (5%) is a simple cyst without a macroscopic nodule, type 2 is a cyst with a mural nodule (60%), type 3 is a solid tumor (26%), and type 4 is a solid tumor with small internal cysts (9%).

The nidus of the tumor always abuts the pia mater, from which the tumor receives its vascular supply. The tumors are therefore usually superficial in location. Abnormal tumor vessels usually appear as serpentine areas of signal void at the periphery of the mass. The association of the peripheral cyst in the posterior fossa and mural nodule supplied by enlarged vessels is virtually pathognomonic for a hemangioblastoma.

Juvenile Pilocytic Astrocytoma

JPA is the most common pediatric cerebellar neoplasm and pediatric glioma; most present before 20 years of age. It appears well circumscribed, yet occasionally it infiltrates surrounding brain. The nodule component intensely enhances (occasionally more than highly malignant astrocytoma), yet it is not a high-grade neoplasm.

There are four predominant imaging patterns of JPA: (1) mass with a nonenhancing cyst and intensely enhancing nodule (21%), (2) mass with an enhancing cyst wall and an intensely enhancing nodule (46%), (3) necrotic mass with a neutral nonenhancing zone (16%), and (4) predominantly solid mass with minimal to no cyst-like component (17%). Cyst wall enhancement occurs occasionally and is not indicative of tumor involvement. The most frequent location is the cerebellum, optic nerves, or chiasm and the region around the 3rd ventricle, with 82% of lesions located around the ventricular system. Lesions in the optic nerve and chiasm can be associated with neurofibromatosis type I (NF-1). Lesions within the cerebellum are more likely to be cystic, whereas those involving the optic chiasm and around the 3rd ventricle tend to be solid.

Additional Readings

1. Koeller KK, Rushing EJ. From the archives of the AFIP: pilocytic astrocytoma: radiologic-pathologic correlation. Radiographics 2004;24(6):1693–1708
2. Lee SR, Sanches J, Mark AS, Dillon WP, Norman D, Newton TH. Posterior fossa hemangioblastomas: MR imaging. Radiology 1989;171(2):463–468
3. Lee YY, Van Tassel P, Bruner JM, Moser RP, Share JC. Juvenile pilocytic astrocytomas: CT and MR characteristics. AJR Am J Roentgenol 1989;152(6):1263–1270
4. Rees JH, Smirniotopoulos JG, Jones RV, Wong K. Glioblastoma multiforme: radiologic-pathologic correlation. Radiographics 1996;16(6):1413–1438 quiz 1462–3
5. Slater A, Moore NR, Huson SM. The natural history of cerebellar hemangioblastomas in von Hippel-Lindau disease. AJNR Am J Neuroradiol 2003;24(8):1570–1574

7

Cerebellopontine Angle Lesions

Lesions in the cerebellopontine angle (CPA) are invariably neoplastic, representing 5 to 10% of intracranial tumors. They are almost all benign (>95%). Vestibular schwannomas are the most common (80 to 91%), followed by meningiomas and epidermoid cysts. Of malignant etiologies, metastatic disease, particularly melanoma, is most common, and should be considered in the setting of systemic metastases, bilateral disease, thick enhancement outside of the nodular lesion, or a rapidly progressive clinical course.

Vestibular Schwannomas

Vestibular schwannomas represent 6 to 7% of intracranial tumors and 95% of intracranial schwannomas. They arise most commonly from age 40 to 70 at the Schwann–glial junction of the eight cranial nerve, which is within the internal auditory canal (IAC), and >95% emerge into the CPA, widening the porus acusticus. On computed tomography (CT), they are isodense to hypodense to brain, widen the porus acusticus, and demonstrate intense, homogeneous enhancement. They are essentially isointense to the pons on T1-weighted magnetic resonance images (T1WI) and T2-weighted magnetic resonance images (T2WI), with intense enhancement. Larger tumors commonly develop cystic degeneration with infrequent internal hemorrhage and rare calcification (**Table 7.1**).

Meningiomas

Eight and one-half percent of meningiomas originate within the posterior fossa, most along the petrous dura/CPA, where they represent 10 to 15% of CPA tumors. On CT, they are hemispheric- shaped masses, isodense to slightly hyperdense to brain, with a broad base to the petrous bone, which may demonstrate hyperostosis or invasion. They may calcify, rarely undergo cystic degeneration, and demonstrate intense homogeneous enhancement. On magnetic resonance imaging (MRI), they are isointense to gray matter with homogeneous intense enhancement, with extension along a "dural tail" common (**Table 7.1**).

Epidermoid Cysts

Epidermoid cysts are congenital lesions of ectodermal origin and intracranially are most commonly found in the CPA cistern. They can also occur in the suprasellar and parasellar regions, the quadrigeminal plate cistern, and the temporal fossa. They often insinuate around neural and vascular structures. They contain keratin and cholesterol due to desquamated epithelium. The radiologist is usually faced with differentiating these lesions from arachnoid cysts (**Table 7.2**). Epidermoid cysts often have an imaging appearance similar to cerebrospinal fluid (CSF) on CT

Table 7.1 Differentiating Features between Vestibular Schwannomas and Meningiomas

	Vestibular Schwannomas	Meningiomas
CT	Hypodense to isodense to brain	Isodense to hyperdense to brain
Enhancement	Homogeneously intense When large, heterogeneous	Homogeneously intense
Calcification	Rare	Common
Location	Centered in IAC/ porus acusticus	Broad base with petrous bone Not centered on IAC/porus acusticus
IAC	Dilated	Not dilated
T1WI	Isointense to hypointense to pons	Isointense to pons
T2WI	Isointense to hyperintense to pons	Isointense to hypointense to pons
Cystic Degeneration	Common with large tumors	Uncommon
Involvement of Other Skull Base Foramina	Uncommon	Common

Abbreviations: CT, computed tomography; IAC, internal auditory canal; T1WI, T1-weighted magnetic resonance imaging; T2WI, T2-weighted magnetic resonance imaging.

Table 7.2 Differentiating Features between Epidermoid Cysts and Arachnoid Cysts

	Epidermoid Cysts	Arachnoid Cysts
CT	Variable Fat-fluid attenuation Cisternography sometimes needed to delineate	CSF attenuation Cisternography sometimes needed to delineate
Enhancement	None May appear enhanced peripherally due to trapped vessels	None
T1WI	Variable Most are dark, but are hyperintense relative to CSF	CSF signal intensity
T2WI	Variable Most are bright, but hypointense relative to CSF Demonstrate internal architecture on CISS sequences	CSF signal intensity
FLAIR	Same intensity as T2WI	CSF signal intensity (dark)
DWI	Restricted diffusion (bright)	No restriction (dark)
Margins	Undulating margins Encase/ infiltrate vessels and nerves • Rare calcification	Sharp margins Displace nerves and vessels
Bone Changes	None	Remodels bone

Abbreviations: CISS, constructive interference steady state; CSF, cerebrospinal fluid; CT, computed tomography; DWI, diffusion weighted images; FLAIR, fluid attenuated inversion recovery; T1WI, T1-weighted magnetic resonance imaging; T2WI, T2-weighted magnetic resonance imaging.

and MRI, although attenuation can be slightly lower than CSF due to cholesterol content. On MRI, they can be similar to slightly more hyperintense than CSF on T1WI and T2WI, and subtle heterogeneity can sometimes be seen within them. Sequences such as CISS (constructive interference in steady state) and FLAIR (fluid attenuated inversion recovery), as well as diffusion weighted sequences can often better depict these lesions.

Other Lesions

Rare and uncommon lesions in the region include arachnoid cysts, cavernous malformations, 4th ventricular tumors including choroid plexus tumors and ependymomas, cysticercosis, craniopharyngiomas, hemangioblastomas, medulloblastomas and other cerebellar neoplasms, lipomas, lymphomas, neurenteric cysts, and paragangliomas.

Additional Readings

1. Bonneville F, Sarrazin JL, Marsot-Dupuch K, et al. Unusual lesions of the cerebellopontine angle: a segmental approach. Radiographics 2001;21(2):419–438
2. Krainik A, Cyna-Gorse F, Bouccara D, et al. MRI of unusual lesions in the internal auditory canal. Neuroradiology 2001;43(1):52–57
3. Smirniotopoulos JG, Yue NC, Rushing EJ. Cerebellopontine angle masses: radiologic-pathologic correlation. Radiographics 1993;13(5):1131–1147
4. Zamani AA. Cerebellopontine angle tumors: role of magnetic resonance imaging. Top Magn Reson Imaging 2000;11(2):98–107

8

Posterior Fossa Cysts and Cerebellar Malformations

A variety of cystic lesions occur in the posterior fossa, with the most common being arachnoid cysts, Dandy–Walker complex/continuum, and mega cisterna magna (**Table 8.1**). It is often difficult to differentiate between these entities due to very subtle differences between them.

Computed tomography (CT) cisternography can aid in the differentiation in certain cases, and some of these lesions can be correctly diagnosed on fetal magnetic resonance imaging (MRI). Ultrasound can also aid in the diagnosis.

Table 8.1 Differentiating Features of Arachnoid Cysts, Mega Cisterna Magna, and Dandy–Walker Complex/Continuum

	Arachnoid Cysts	Mega Cisterna Magna[c]	Dandy–Walker Complex/Continuum[f]
Cyst Location	Retrocerebellar (most commonly), supracerebellar, intracerebellar, cerebellopontine angle	Retrocerebellar	Retrocerebellar
Cyst Communicates with 4th Ventricle	No	Yes[d]	Yes[g]
Vermis Interposed between Cyst and 4th Ventricle	Yes[a]	Yes[a]	No
Tentorial Location	Normal	Normal	High
Elevation of Torcular Herophili	No[b]	No	Yes
Normally Formed 4th Ventricle/Vermis	Yes	Yes, although may be associated inferior vermian hypoplasia and/or volume loss	Vermian hypoplasia (often also of hemispheres and cephalad rotation of vermian remnant)
Posterior Fossa Size	Normal[b]	Normal[e]	Enlarged
Inner Table of Posterior Fossa Scalloping	Yes	Yes/No[e]	Yes

(Continued on page 24)

Table 8.1 *(Continued)* Differentiating Features of Arachnoid Cysts, Mega Cisterna Magna, and Dandy–Walker Complex/Continuum

	Arachnoid Cysts	Mega Cisterna Magna[c]	Dandy–Walker Complex/Continuum[f]
Communication with Ventricles / Subarachnoid Space on Cisternography	Slow if any communication	Freely	Yes
Possible Associated Findings and Additional Findings	Hydrocephalus, mass effect	Can extend into supratentorial space; may be asymmetric	Mass effect from posterior CSF collection, hydrocephalus, callosal anomalies, interhemispheric cyst, heterotopias, craniofacial anomalies, systemic anomalies, holoprosencephaly

Abbreviations: CSF, cerebrospinal fluid; MCM, mega cisterna magna.

[a] Upward rotation of the vermis may cause the vermis not to appear to be interposed in between the cyst and 4th ventricle on axial images.

[b] These features have been described in arachnoid cysts, but are not typical.

[c] Some authors have also included a MCM in the Dandy–Walker continuum.

[d] Via the normal foramen of Magendie; enlargement of the outlet of the 4th ventricle has been used as a distinguishing feature between a MCM and an arachnoid cyst by some authors.

[e] Some authors have also stated that the posterior fossa can be enlarged with a MCM, and that there can be scalloping of the inner table of the occipital bone.

[f] Blake's pouch cyst has been included by some authors in this continuum. It is characterized by lack of regression of Blake's pouch due to lack of perforation of the foramen of Magendie. Therefore, there is a retrocerebellar cyst that communicates with an enlarged 4th ventricle, without communication of the 4th ventricle with the basal subarachnoid space through the foramen of Magendie. There are no significant additional posterior fossa anomalies, although the cyst can be associated with a high position of the posterior tentorium, scalloping of the occipital bone, and the cyst may contain choroid plexus as well.

[g] This is due to hypoplastic/absent vermis.

Arachnoid Cysts

Thirteen to 30% of intracranial arachnoid cysts involve the posterior fossa and appear on CT as low-density, noncalcified, extraaxial masses that do not enhance. The higher incidence is reported in the pediatric literature, but in a study of patients of mixed ages with adult predominance, 13% of 93 arachnoid cysts occurred in the posterior fossa.

Dandy–Walker Continuum

The spectrum of anomalies defined by varying degrees of vermis hypoplasia (with cephalad rotation of the vermian remnant), retrocerebellar cyst that communicates with the 4th ventricle, and enlarged posterior fossa with elevation of the torcular Herophili has been variously termed *Dandy–Walker malformation*, *Dandy–Walker variant*, *Dandy–Walker continuum*, *Dandy–Walker spectrum*, and *Dandy–Walker complex*. This indicates that the differentiation of these entities and their etiologies are unclear, and likely represent a spectrum of severity (within which some have included mega cisterna magna and Blake's pouch cyst). Some authors have also used the term *retrocerebellar arachnoid cyst* synonymously with Blake's pouch cyst; it has been said that this cyst both does and does not communicate with the 4th ventricle, although it usually does.

Types of Posterior Fossa Cysts and Cystic Lesions

- Arachnoid cyst
- Dandy–Walker complex/variants
- Mega cisterna magna
- Blake's pouch cyst
- Cerebellar cystic astrocytomas
- Cystic hemangioblastomas
- Hydatid cysts
- Abscesses
- Epidermoid/dermoid cysts

Types of Cerebellar Malformations

- Dandy–Walker complex/continuum: Vermian hypoplasia, posterior fossa cyst, elevation of torcular herophili, enlarged posterior fossa
- Joubert syndrome (molar tooth syndrome): Severe vermian hypoplasia and dysplasia to aplasia; deep interpeduncular fossa/thin isthmus/broad parallel superior cerebellar peduncles create a so-called "molar tooth" appearance
- Congenital muscular dystrophies: Various malformations including dysplasia, hypoplasia, subcortical cysts, and cerebellar cortical abnormalities
- Rhombencephalosynapsis: Vermian aplasia with fused cerebellar hemispheres
- Congenital cytomegalovirus infection: small cerebellum, ± calcifications, cerebellar cortical and folial abnormalities
- Cerebellar hypoplasia
- Lissencephaly and cerebellar dysplasia
- Focal cerebellar cortical dysplasia
- Idiopathic diffuse cerebellar dysplasia
- Pontocerebellar hypoplasia type 1
- Cerebellar heterotopia
- Lhermitte–Duclos syndrome (dysplastic cerebellar gangliocytoma): Nonenhancing cerebellar hemisphere mass with prolonged T1- and T2-weighted relaxation and curvilinear stripes

Additional Readings

1. Barkovich AJ, Kjos BO, Norman D, Edwards MS. Revised classification of posterior fossa cysts and cystlike malformations based on the results of multiplanar MR imaging. AJR Am J Roentgenol 1989;153(6):1289–1300
2. Calabro F, Arcuri T, Jinkins JR. Blake's pouch cyst: an entity within the Dandy–Walker continuum. Neuroradiology 2000;42(4):290–295
3. Epelman M, Daneman A, Blaser SI, et al. Differential diagnosis of intracranial cystic lesions at head US: correlation with CT and MR imaging. Radiographics 2006; 26(1):173–196
4. Erdincler P, Kaynar MY, Bozkus H, Ciplak N. Posterior fossa arachnoid cysts. Br J Neurosurg 1999;13(1):10–17
5. Nelson MD Jr, Maher K, Gilles FH. A different approach to cysts of the posterior fossa. Pediatr Radiol 2004;34(9): 720–732
6. Raybaud C, Levrier O, Brunel H, Girard N, Farnarier P. MR imaging of fetal brain malformations. Childs Nerv Syst 2003;19(7–8):455–470
7. Strand RD, Barnes PD, Poussaint TY, Estroff JA, Burrows PE. Cystic retrocerebellar malformations: unification of the Dandy–Walker complex and the Blake's pouch cyst. Pediatr Radiol 1993;23(4):258–260
8. Tan EC, Takagi T, Karasawa K. Posterior fossa cystic lesions–magnetic resonance imaging manifestations. Brain Dev 1995;17(6):418–424

9

Meningeal Enhancement

Normal Meningeal Enhancement

Enhancement of the normal meninges on T1-weighted spin-echo magnetic resonance images (MRIs) is generally in short segments or less than 50% of the total meningeal area. Patterns of meningeal enhancement that may represent an abnormality include increased length and percentage of meningeal enhancement and nodularity. However, on post-contrast spoiled three-dimensional (3D) gradient echo (GRE) T1-weighted MRIs, a much larger percentage of the meningeal area can enhance and there can also be longer segments of enhancement and larger continuous areas of enhancement. This is thought to be due to the greater spatial resolution of the 3D GRE sequences as well as decreased signal in the calvarial diploic space on these sequences.

Abnormal Meningeal Enhancement

Postcraniotomy patients can have meningeal enhancement, presumably related to postoperative inflammation, and this can be localized to the area of the craniotomy or be generalized. Meningeal enhancement involving the dura-arachnoid and the pia can occur in pathologic conditions such as neoplasm, including lymphomatous and metastatic involvement, as well as in inflammatory or infectious processes such as bacterial or viral meningitis, sarcoidosis,

chemical meningitis, subarachnoid or subdural hemorrhage, or idiopathic inflammation. In neoplastic involvement, there may be primary dural disease that seeds the subdural space, spreading to the arachnoid or the spread may be in the opposite direction. Alternatively, the neoplasm may involve the subarachnoid space hematogenously or from spread along nerves. MRI is more sensitive than computed tomography (CT) because beam hardening limits the detection of dural enhancement, particularly near the calvarium (although CT sensitivity is improved for nodular enhancement and enhancement in spaces not adjacent to the calvarium), but MRI is no more specific, and coronal or axial images are better than sagittal images.

- *Intracranial hypotension as a cause of pachymeningeal enhancement* Intracranial hypotension causes smooth pachymeningeal enhancement and may have a characteristic wavelike pattern of enhancement along the frontal and temporal base, which has been suggested to be due to the contour of the inner margin of the skull in these regions. The enhancement also improves or resolves following successful treatment. Another finding that may be seen in intracranial hypotension is "brain sagging" (low cerebellar tonsils, flattening of the pons against the clivus, and downward displacement of the optic chiasm). The meningeal enhancement does not involve the sulci, and the morphologic abnormalities resolve within 3 to 5 months after symptom resolution.

- *Hydrocephalus as a mimic of meningeal enhancement* An appearance similar to leptomeningeal enhancement has been described in obstructive hydrocephalus; however, this was thought to be due to slow flow in pial vessels. Similar enhancement has been described in vessels distal to an occlusion during an infarction and with stagnant flow in focally dilated vessels segments.

- *Dural invasion and reaction as a cause of dural enhancement* Dural enhancement can be seen adjacent to calvarial tumors, and can be either reactive or a sign of dural invasion, with either benign or malignant lesions. Nodular or discontinuous enhancement is statistically associated with dural invasion, whereas smooth linear enhancement is more likely reactive. In a study of various craniofacial and calvarial tumors the presence of a thin hypointense line representing the epidural space overlying smoothly continuously enhancing dura has also been described as a sign indicating that the dural enhancement is due to reaction rather than invasion. In cases of invasion, this line will be absent either focally or more diffusely, and the underlying dural enhancement is more likely to be discontinuous. However, it should be pointed out that in a small percentage of cases, nonenhancing dura may still be invaded.

Causes of Pachymeningeal Enhancement

- Neoplasm, reaction, or invasion
- Lymphoma/leukemia/myeloma (rare)
- Intracranial hypotension
- Postoperative, posttherapeutic
- Ventricular shunt
- Sequela of subdural hematoma
- Infection, postinfection, or inflammatory disease (meningitis, granulomatous, etc.)
- Idiopathic

Causes of Leptomeningeal Enhancement

- Carcinomatosis
- Infectious meningitis (bacterial, viral, granulomatous)
- Subarachnoid hemorrhage
- Postoperative, after intrathecal chemotherapy or radiation therapy
- Inflammatory disease (sarcoidosis, etc.)
- Lymphoma/leukemia
- Lymphomatoid granulomatosis (uncommon)

Mimics of Meningeal Enhancement

- Slow vascular flow (hydrocephalus, distal to an occlusion, in dilated segments)

Additional Readings

1. Ahmadi J, Hinton DR, Segall HD, Couldwell WT, Stanley RB. Dural invasion by craniofacial and calvarial neoplasms: MR imaging and histopathologic evaluation. Radiology 1993;188(3):747–749
2. Arana E, Marti-Bonmati L, Ricart V, Perez-Ebri M. Dural enhancement with primary calvarial lesions. Neuroradiology 2004;46(11):900–905
3. Burke JW, Podrasky AE, Bradley WG Jr. Meninges: benign postoperative enhancement on MR images. Radiology 1990;174(1):99–102
4. Farn JW, Mirowitz SA. MR imaging of the normal meninges: comparison of contrast-enhancement patterns on 3D gradient-echo and spin-echo images. AJR Am J Roentgenol 1994;162(1):131–135
5. Phillips ME, Ryals TJ, Kambhu SA, Yuh WT. Neoplastic vs inflammatory meningeal enhancement with Gd-DTPA. J Comput Assist Tomogr 1990;14(4):536–541
6. Spelle L, Boulin A, Tainturier C, Visot A, Graveleau P, Pierot L. Neuroimaging features of spontaneous intracranial hypotension. Neuroradiology 2001;43(8):622–627
7. Sze G, Soletsky S, Bronen R, Krol G. MR imaging of the cranial meninges with emphasis on contrast enhancement and meningeal carcinomatosis. AJNR Am J Neuroradiol 1989;10(5):965–975
8. Tosaka M, Sato N, Fujimaki H, Takahashi A, Saito N. Wave-like appearance of diffuse pachymeningeal enhancement associated with intracranial hypotension. Neuroradiology 2005;47(5):362–367

10

Sellar and Parasellar Lesions

The normal pituitary gland generally measures between 4 to 7 mm in height, depending on age, sex, and pregnancy status, and generally does not exceed 10 mm. The posterior lobe is hyperintense on T1-weighted magnetic resonance [MR] images (T1WI) due to vasopressin and should always be seen in normal children and infants, although the incidence of this finding decreases with age. Sellar and parasellar lesions most commonly arise from the pituitary gland or adjacent structures such as vessels, dura, or developmental remnants. Adenomas, meningiomas, craniopharyngiomas, and vascular lesions account for ~75% of sellar and parasellar lesions.

Pituitary Adenomas

These lesions comprise 10 to 15% of all intracranial neoplasms and one third to one half of sellar and parasellar masses. They are divided into macroadenomas and microadenomas based on size.

Macroadenomas are greater than 10 mm and commonly grow into the suprasellar region, but may extend into the sphenoid sinus or bone and be more invasive, and may invade the cavernous sinus. Imaging features are detailed in **Table 10.1**. Pituitary apoplexy refers to hemorrhage and necrosis of an adenoma due to tenuous blood supply from the hypophyseal

Table 10.1 Differentiating Features between Common Sellar and Parasellar Lesions

	Macroadenomas	Meningiomas	Craniopharyngiomas
T1WI	Isointense to cortex	Isointense to cortex	Cysts isointense to hyperintense; solid component isointense or heterogeneous
T2WI	Isointense to hyperintense to cortex	Isointense to cortex, but can be variable	Cysts hyperintense; solid component heterogeneous to hyperintense
CT (non-contrast)	Isodense Generally solid	Isodense to slightly hyperdense Solid	Solid and cystic components
Enhancement	Yes	Yes	Yes
Calcifications	Rare (5%)	Uncommon	Common
Cysts	Cysts or necrosis in 5–18%	Rarely, generally small	Common (70–85%)
Sellar Enlargement	Common	Generally, no	Generally, no

Table 10.1 *(Continued)* Differentiating Features between Common Sellar and Parasellar Lesions

	Macroadenomas	Meningiomas	Craniopharyngiomas
Sellar Erosion	Common	Generally, no	Rare
Lesion Epicenter	Sella	Parasellar/suprasellar	Suprasellar
Additional Features	Multilobular upper border (6%) May invade sphenoid sinus May have adjacent dural enhancement May be hemorrhagic with fluid-fluid level "Snowman" appearance due to "waisting" at diaphragm sella	Hyperostosis CSF cleft (between mass and pituitary) Sphenoid sinus blistering (upward bulging into the meningioma) Dural "tail" and obtuse dural margins	Cysts of varying signal intensity Most heterogeneous of sellar/parasellar lesions May demonstrate a significant lipid component on MRS

Abbreviations: CSF, cerebrospinal fluid; CT, computed tomography; MRS, magnetic resonance spectroscopy; T1WI, T1-weighted magnetic resonance imaging; T2WI, T2-weighted magnetic resonance imaging.

portal system. Imaging demonstrates blood products, commonly high signal on T1WI and T2WI (T2-weighted MR images). Apoplexy is differentiated from Sheehan's syndrome, which is postpartum or peripartum pituitary hemorrhage and necrosis.

Microadenomas are less than 10 mm in size. Their appearance is

- *T1WI* Hypointense to isointense with pituitary gland; enhances less than the anterior lobe on immediate post-contrast images
- *T2WI* Generally mildly more hyperintense than the anterior lobe, but can be variable depending on cell type, and can be hypointense

There may be associated sellar erosion, focal elevation of the superior margin of the pituitary, and infundibular deviation. Dynamic images may show relatively less enhancement of an adenoma with respect to a normal gland. On delayed images taken 30 to 40 minutes following injection, adenomas may have delayed enhancement with respect to a normal pituitary gland. They may have hemorrhage resulting in high signal on T1WIs.

Meningiomas

Meningiomas are the second most common sellar/parasellar lesion; in this location, they represent 5 to 11% of all meningiomas. They are more common in women. They are generally homogeneously solid tumors; however, they may occasionally contain necrosis, scarring, cystic degeneration, and calcifications. Imaging features are detailed in **Table 10.1**.

Craniopharyngiomas

Craniopharyngiomas arise within squamous epithelial remnants or remnant ectoblastic cells of Rathke's pouch and the craniopharyngeal duct and account for 3 to 5% of all intracranial masses. There is a bimodal age distribution, occurring from 5 to 14 years of age, with a second peak at 65 to 74 years of age. They tend to recur and invade local structures and adhere to surrounding structures, including vessels. They are typically suprasellar and may extend into the sella. They can have cystic and solid components. Rim or nodular calcification is present in 80 to 87%. Calcification is more common in children (90%) than in adults (50 to 70%) The imaging features are outlined in **Table 10.1**.

Rathke's Cleft Cysts

Rathke's cleft cysts (RCCs) arise from Rathke's pouch, which forms the adenohypophysis. They are usually intrasellar and rarely calcified. They arise in the pars intermedia, and therefore the stalk is displaced anteriorly. They may contain serous or mucoid material and there may be mild enhancement of the wall. Their imaging appearance (computed tomography [CT] and MR) depends on the composition of the cyst contents. Fluid characteristics are

- *Serous*   CT: hypoattenuating; MR: hypointense T1W, hyperintense T2W
- *Mucoid/proteinaceous*   CT: high attenuation; MR: hyperintense on T1W, hypointense on T2W

They may also contain concretions, which appear as low signal, small intracystic nodules on T2WI and may be hyperintense on T1WI.

Hypothalamic and Optic Gliomas

Optic gliomas are often associated with neurofibromatosis I in children where they are usually low grade; they are often more aggressive when arising in adults. They are generally hypointense or isointense on T1WI, with enlarged visual pathway structures and they may have increased signal on T2WI extending along the course of the optic pathways. Hypothalamic gliomas are more homogeneous and often enhance. Calcifications and cysts are rare (a distinction from craniopharyngiomas).

Schwannomas

Schwannomas can involve any of the cranial nerves, with the fifth nerve the most commonly involved in the parasellar region (the vestibular branches of the vestibulocochlear nerve are the nerves most commonly involved by schwannomas overall). Lesions follow the course and location of the cranial nerves and are well marginated and fusiform. On CT, they are isodense with brain with homogeneous enhancement. On MRI, they isointense to slightly hypointense to gray matter on T1WI; hyperintense to cerebrospinal fluid (CSF) on T2WI and enhance homogeneously. Occasionally, they may be heterogeneous due to cystic, necrotic, and hemorrhagic components, particularly with larger lesions.

Aneurysms

Aneurysms are the most common lesions to occur in the cavernous sinus. They may arise from the cavernous or supraclinoid internal carotid artery or the posterior communicating or ophthalmic arteries; they can present as parasellar and suprasellar masses. They can compress adjacent structures and cause cavernous sinus syndrome. When affecting the third cranial nerve, the pupil is effected first as the pupillomotor fibers are located peripherally. On CT, small aneurysms may not be evident (but should be seen on CT angiography), but larger lesions appear as hyperdense masses with curvilinear calcification and enhancement of the lumen with or without variable amounts of mural thrombus and there may be bony remodeling. On MRI, they will have a flow void if not thrombosed and there may be a misregistration artifact in the phase-encoding direction due to flow and pulsations. If mural thrombi are present, there may be peripheral crescentic lamellae of intermediate to increased signal intensity on T1WI and intermediate, increased and/or decreased signal on T2WI with an area of low-signal flow void. If the aneurysm is fully thrombosed, it will have a heterogeneous signal due to blood products and calcification.

Arachnoid Cysts

Arachnoid cysts in the sella and parasellar region are rare, and appear as well-defined fluid signal or attenuation masses on all imaging modalities. They have mass effect on adjacent structures such as the infundibulum, optic chiasm/nerves, pituitary, hypothalamus, 3rd ventricle, and possibly the foramen of Monroe.

Dermoids

On CT, dermoids may be heterogeneous with decreased attenuation due to fat, and they may have calcification; enhancement is uncommon. On MRI, they have fat signal and may have fat fluid levels. They may be heterogeneous due to additional ectodermal elements.

Germinomas

Germinomas are tumors of germ cell origin and they generally present in the first three decades of life. When occurring in this region, germinomas can be referred to as neurohypophyseal germinomas. They may arise anywhere from the posterior lobe of the pituitary to the infundibulum. They may occur as primary tumors in the parasellar region or be secondary due to spread from the pineal region. Suprasellar germinomas have no sex predominance as opposed to pineal region germinomas, which have a male predominance. They commonly invade the hypothalamus and extend into the 3rd ventricle. On CT, they appear as hyperdense suprasellar masses with enhancement. On MRI, they are well-defined homogeneous, infiltrative masses that are generally slightly hypointense to isointense to gray matter on T1WI and isointense to hyperintense on T2WIs with enhancement. They may have cysts, but do not contain calcifications. There is often

loss of the normal hyperintensity of the posterior lobe of the pituitary on T1WIs.

Types of Sellar and Parasellar Lesions

- Pituitary adenoma
- Meningioma
- Craniopharyngioma
- Rathke's cleft cyst
- Hypothalamic/optic glioma
- Schwannoma
- Aneurysm
- Arachnoid cyst
- Dermoid
- Germinoma
- Metastasis
- Leptomeningeal carcinomatosis
- Inflammatory: Pseudotumor, Tolosa–Hunt syndrome, lymphocytic adenohypophysitis (lymphocytic infundibuloneurohypophysitis)
- Granulomatous diseases such as sarcoid, tuberculosis (TB), Langerhans cell histiocytosis: Basilar subarachnoid space enhancement with involvement of hypothalamus and infundibulum (particularly histiocytosis)
- Invasion from skull base, sinonasal or pharyngeal tumors
- Perineural spread of neoplasm
- Skull base neoplasm: Chordoma, chondrosarcoma, metastases
- Hypothalamic hamartoma
- Lymphoma/Leukemia
- Choristoma (granular cell tumors, granular cell myoblastomas)
- Epidermoid
- Pituicytoma

Sellar and Parasellar Hyperintensity on T1-Weighted MRI

Normal structures and normal variations

- Posterior lobe (vasopressin)
- Anterior lobe: Pregnancy, newborn, hyperactive residual gland after treatment
- Fatty bone marrow
- Susceptibility or flow artifacts

Pathologic processes and lesions

- Hemorrhage (apoplexy, Sheehan's syndrome, hemorrhagic adenoma)
- Rathke's cleft cyst
- Craniopharyngioma
- Lipoma/dermoid
- Sphenoid sinus mucocele

Types of Infundibular Lesions

- Langerhans cell histiocytosis
- Granulomatous diseases (TB, sarcoid)
- Metastases (no blood–brain barrier)
- Lymphocytic adenohypophysitis (infundibular neurohypophysitis)
- Germinoma
- Lymphoma, leukemia
- Pituicytoma

Additional Readings

1. Bonneville F, Cattin F, Marsot-Dupuch K, Dormont D, Bonneville JF, Chiras J. T1 signal hyperintensity in the sellar region: spectrum of findings. Radiographics 2006; 26(1):93–113
2. Bonneville JF, Bonneville F, Cattin F. Magnetic resonance imaging of pituitary adenomas. Eur Radiol 2005;15(3):543–548
3. Donovan JL, Nesbit GM. Distinction of masses involving the sella and suprasellar space: specificity of imaging features. AJR Am J Roentgenol 1996;167(3):597–603
4. Johnsen DE, Woodruff WW, Allen IS, Cera PJ, Funkhouser GR, Coleman LL. MR imaging of the sellar and juxtasellar regions. Radiographics 1991;11(5):727–758
5. Kanagaki M, Miki Y, Takahashi JA, et al. MRI and CT findings of neurohypophyseal germinoma. Eur J Radiol 2004;49(3):204–211
6. Pisaneschi M, Kapoor G. Imaging the sella and parasellar region. Neuroimaging Clin N Am 2005;15(1):203–219
7. Ruscalleda J. Imaging of parasellar lesions. Eur Radiol 2005;15(3):549–559

11

Dermoid Cysts and Lipomas

Dermoid cysts are rare, nonneoplastic, congenital, ectodermal inclusion cysts. Lipomas are nonneoplastic and result from the maldifferentiation of the primitive meninx. Both lesions are extraaxial and contain fat, although the fat content of dermoid cysts is variable.

Differences in natural history, pathology, and treatment of these lesions confers significance to differentiation by imaging (**Table 11.1**). Ruptured dermoids present with a pathognomonic imaging appearance with scattered speckling of abnormal T1 shortening within the

Table 11.1 Differentiating Features between Lipomas and Dermoid Cysts

	Lipomas	Dermoid Cysts
Location	Usually midline interhemispheric fissure (~50%)	Midline
		Suprasellar
	Quadrigeminal/superior cerebellar cistern (15–25%)	Parasellar
		Posterior fossa
	Suprasellar/interpeduncular (15%)	Frontonasal
	Uncommon	Orbital region
	Cerebellopontine angle, sylvian fissure, surface of hemispheres	
CT	Homogeneous	Can be heterogeneous
	Hypoattenuating	Hypoattenuating: Typically similar to fat, but can be similar to fluid; rarely is it more dense
	Fat density −40 to −100 HU	
T1WI	Homogeneously hyperintense	Hyperintense
	Signal drops with fat saturation	Partially suppresses with fat saturation
		May see fat-fluid levels
T2WI	Homogeneously hypointense	Heterogeneous
Chemical Shift Artifact	Present, particularly in large lipomas	Less frequently present
Enhancement	None	Unruptured: Can have peripheral enhancement
		Ruptured: Intense pial enhancement

(Continued on page 34)

Table 11.1 (*Continued*) Differentiating Features between Lipomas and Dermoid Cysts

	Lipomas	**Dermoid Cysts**
Calcification	Central or peripheral May be present in interhemispheric lipomas ~50% of interpeduncular cistern/suprasellar lipomas ossify (osteolipomas) Not common in other locations	Uncommon, but may have peripheral calcification

Abbreviations: CT, computed tomography; T1WI, T1-weighted magnetic resonance imaging; T2WI, T2-weighted magnetic resonance imaging; HU, Hounsfield units.

subarachnoid space, sulci, and ventricles with characteristic fat-fluid levels. The characteristic computed tomography (CT) appearance is fat–cerebrospinal fluid (CSF) levels in the ventricles. Other presentations include fat densities within the sulci and subarachnoid spaces, and occasionally an extraaxial or combined extraaxial and intraaxial mass. The only other consideration (for the MRI imaging appearance of fat signal in the CSF space) would be prior intrathecal administration of Pantopaque, which can be confirmed by history or by correlating with hyperdense foci on unenhanced head CT.

Associated Anomalies

Lipomas, especially in the midline, can be associated with corpus callosum and septal anomalies, other brain anomalies, and rarely with vascular anomalies. The degree and type of associated anomaly is related to the location and size of the lipoma, which is concordant with the idea that lipomas are congenital malformations and not neoplasms or hamartomas. Rarely, lipomas may be located off midline in the cortical sulci, where they may be associated with cortical dysplasias or abnormal vasculature. Although not formally evaluated in the literature, tiny lipomas along the falx are not uncommonly seen and are considered incidental findings.

Dermoid cysts are associated with skeletal dysraphisms and fibrous bands or dermal sinus tracts to the skin.

Differential Diagnosis

Not many lesions are similar in appearance and location to these lesions.

- Craniopharyngiomas: Generally have enhancing components; may be hyperintense on T1WIs and have calcification, but do not contain fat
- Teratomas: Usually occur in the parenchyma (infants) or pineal region; have enhancing components
- Epidermoids: Generally occur off midline; follow CSF in density and signal intensity except they have restricted diffusion
- Lipomatous meningioma: Resembles typical meningiomas in shape; dural-based
- Rathke's cleft cyst: Usually intrasellar, less commonly purely suprasellar and anterior to the infundibulum; variable imaging appearance
- Ectopic posterior: Located between the hypothalamus and sella; hyperintense on T1WI

Additional Readings

1. Bonneville F, Cattin F, Marsot-Dupuch K, Dormont D, Bonneville JF, Chiras J. T1 signal hyperintensity in the sellar region: spectrum of findings. Radiographics 2006;26(1):93–113

2. Osborn AG, Preece MT. Intracranial cysts: radiologic-pathologic correlation and imaging approach. Radiology 2006;239(3):650–664

3. Saatci I, Aslan C, Renda Y, Besim A. Parietal lipoma associated with cortical dysplasia and abnormal vasculature: case report and review of the literature. AJNR Am J Neuroradiol 2000;21(9):1718–1721

4. Sinson G, Gennarelli TA, Wells GB. Suprasellar osteolipoma: case report. Surg Neurol 1998;50(5):457–460

5. Smirniotopoulos JG, Chiechi MV. Teratomas, dermoids, and epidermoids of the head and neck. Radiographics 1995;15(6):1437–1455

6. Smith AS, Benson JE, Blaser SI, Mizushima A, Tarr RW, Bellon EM. Diagnosis of ruptured intracranial dermoid cyst: value MR over CT. AJNR Am J Neuroradiol 1991;12(1):175–180

7. Yildiz H, Hakyemez B, Koroglu M, Yesildag A, Baykal B. Intracranial lipomas: importance of localization. Neuroradiology 2006;48(1):1–7

12

Pineal Region Lesions

When approaching masses in the pineal region, one must determine if the mass actually arises in the pineal gland or from surrounding structures. The differential diagnosis for pineal region lesions is broad and includes pineal gland lesions, tectal and thalamic astrocytomas, meningiomas, and vascular malformations. Pineal region lesions are relatively infrequent in adults, where they account for 0.4 to 1% of intracranial tumors. However, in children, pineal region tumors represent 3 to 8% of intracranial tumors.

Assuming that the lesion can be localized to the pineal gland, the differential diagnosis includes pineal cysts, tumors of pineal cell origin, germ cell tumors, and rarely metastases and astrocytomas arising from pineal stromal cells. Germ cell tumors are the most common; they are predominately germinomas followed by teratomas. Germinomas account for ~40% of pineal region tumors. The vast majority of pineal germinomas occurs in males. Pineocytomas and pineoblastomas are relatively rare, and represent less than 15% of pineal region tumors. Unfortunately, pineal region tumors have no pathognomonic imaging features. Of all the pineal region tumors, teratomas have the greatest potential for being definitively identified via imaging if they contain fat, but a fair number of intracranial teratomas do not have discernible fat on imaging. The displacement peripherally ("exploding") or "engulfing" of the native pineal calcification has also been described as a differentiating feature between germinomas and pineoblastomas and pineocytomas (**Table 12.1**).

Table 12.1 Differentiating Features between Pineal Cysts, Germinomas, Pineocytomas, and Pineoblastomas

	Pineal Cysts	Germinomas	Pineocytomas	Pineoblastomas
Age/Sex	More common in adults, M = F	10–20 years, overwhelmingly male	>20 years, M = F	<10 years, M = F
Serologic Markers	None	Placental alkaline phosphatase, occasionally HCG	None	None
Non-contrast CT	Hypodense	Hyperdense	Heterogeneous or homogeneous Isodense or hyperdense Can be hypodense*	Heterogeneous Usually hyperdense

Table 12.1 *(Continued)* Differentiating Features between Pineal Cysts, Germinomas, Pineocytomas, and Pineoblastomas

	Pineal Cysts	Germinomas	Pineocytomas	Pineoblastomas
Calcification	Displaces calcification eccentrically	"Engulfs" calcification	"Explodes" calcification May have internal calcifications	"Explodes" calcification May have internal calcifications
CT Contrast Enhancement Pattern	Thin, peripheral	Avid, homogeneous	Heterogeneous, homogeneous, or at times thin, peripheral	Heterogeneous
T1WI (Pre-contrast)	Hypointense, but variable depending on cyst content composition	Hypointense or isointense	Heterogeneous isointense to heterogeneous*	Heterogeneous, hypointense to isointense
T2WI	Hyperintense, but variable depending on cyst content composition	Isointense to mildly hyperintense	Heterogeneous, isointense to hyperintense*	Heterogeneous, predominantly isointense
T1WI (Post-contrast) Enhancement Pattern	Thin, peripheral that may be due to residual pineal gland Wall thickness generally not greater than 2 mm.	Avid, homogeneous	Heterogeneous, homogeneous, or at times thin, peripheral	Heterogeneous

Abbreviations: CT, computed tomography; F, female; HCG, human chorionic gonadotropin; M, male; T1WI, T1-weighted magnetic resonance imaging; T2WI- T2-weighted magnetic resonance imaging.

* May mimic a cyst on non-contrast CT or MRI

A major diagnostic dilemma is differentiating pineal cysts from pineocytomas. Unfortunately, there can be an overlap in the imaging features of pineal cysts and a small fraction of pineocytomas, with some reports of predominantly cystic pineocytomas, although cystic pineocytomas generally have walls thicker than 2 mm and many have nodularity of the wall or a peripheral nodule. Most series, however, have described pineocytomas with a solid or heterogeneous component comprising a significant percentage of the lesion (**Table 12.1**).

Types of Pineal Region Lesions

Germ Cell Lesions

• Germinoma
• Teratoma (highly heterogeneous with honeycomb-like pattern due to cysts, calcification, and fat)
• Mixed
• Embryonal (rare)
• Yolk sac (rare)
• Choriocarcinoma (rare)

Astrocytomas

- Tectal
- Thalamic
- Splenium of the corpus callosum
- Pineal (rare)

Pineal Parenchymal Lesions

- Pineoblastoma
- Pineocytoma
- Intermediate

Meningioma

- Tentorial
- Posterior 3rd ventricle (rare)

Vascular Malformations

- Arteriovenous malformations
- Vein of Galen malformation

Other Types of Lesions

- Epidermoid, lipoma
- Lymphoma (rare)
- Ependymoma (rare)
- Melanoma (rare)
- Metastases (rare)

Additional Readings

1. Engel U, Gottschalk S, Niehaus L, et al. Cystic lesions of the pineal region–MRI and pathology. Neuroradiology 2000;42(6):399–402
2. Korogi Y, Takahashi M, Ushio Y. MRI of pineal region tumors. J Neurooncol 2001;54(3):251–261
3. Mandera M, Marcol W, Bierzynska-Macyszyn G, Kluczewska E. Pineal cysts in childhood. Childs Nerv Syst 2003;19(10–11):750–755
4. Nakamura M, Saeki N, Iwadate Y, Sunami K, Osato K, Yamaura A. Neuroradiological characteristics of pineocytoma and pineoblastoma. Neuroradiology 2000;42(7):509–514
5. Reis F, Faria AV, Zanardi VA, Menezes JR, Cendes F, Queiroz LS. Neuroimaging in pineal tumors. J Neuroimaging 2006;16(1):52–58
6. Smirniotopoulos JG, Rushing EJ, Mena H. Pineal region masses: differential diagnosis. Radiographics 1992;12(3): 577–596

13

Arterial Infarcts versus Venous Infarcts

Infarct is the third leading cause of death in industrialized countries. Infarct may be due to arterial or venous causes; arterial causes are more common. Venous infarcts most often affect young adults and children; in adults, ~75% occur in women. The main differentiating feature between arterial and venous infarcts is that arterial infarcts conform to an arterial distribution reflecting the pathophysiology of occluded inflow. Venous infarcts, which are caused by outflow occlusion and cerebral edema, do not (**Table 13.1**). Venous thromboses

Table 13.1 Differentiating Features between Computed Tomography and Magnetic Resonance Imaging of Arterial and Venous Infarcts

	Arterial Infarct	Venous Infarct
CT **Vascular**	Dense MCA Enhancement of vessels due to slow and/or collateral flow Filling defect	Dense vein or dural sinus on non-contrast images ("cord sign" in cortical veins) Enhancement around clot ("delta sign" in superior sagittal sinus) • May see collateral medullary veins
Parenchymal	Early acute: Low density in insular ribbon, lentiform nucleus, and/or cortex conforming to all or part of a vascular distribution; sulcal effacement Late acute/subacute: Well demarcated low density conforming to all or part of a vascular distribution; swelling	Low density and/or hemorrhage not in an arterial vascular distribution May involve superficial or deep structures depending on veins involved May have bilateral relatively symmetric medial cortical or thalamic lesions; swelling
MRI	Edema/restricted diffusion in an arterial distribution Lack of flow void in arterial vessels	Edema/restricted diffusion generally not in an arterial distribution May have hemorrhage Abnormal signal in dural sinus Lesions may be relatively symmetric as on CT
CTA/MRA/ Conventional Angiography	Arterial occlusion or filling defect	Venous occlusion or filling defect

Abbreviations: CT, computed tomography; CTA, computed tomography angiography; MCA, middle cerebral artery ; MRA, magnetic resonance angiography; MRI, magnetic resonance imaging.

most commonly involve the sagittal and transverse sinuses; less commonly, the cortical veins and the deep venous system are involved. Venous infarcts are more frequently hemorrhagic and involve the white matter rather than the cortex. In venous sinus thrombosis, areas of edema may be reversible and not progress to infarction.

Causes of Venous Infarcts

- Hypercoagulable states such as hematologic disorders, coagulopathies, oral contraceptives, dehydration, pregnancy, and some paraneoplastic and inflammatory conditions
- Infection
- Trauma
- Compression by neoplasm
- Idiopathic

Causes of Arterial Infarcts

- Large vessel thromboembolic disease
- Cardioembolic disease (up to 20% of all cases have a cardiac source)
- Small vessel vasoocclusive disease (lacunar infarcts: atherosclerosis, hypertension, diabetes mellitus)
- Vasculitis (infectious and inflammatory)
- Vasospasm (fibromuscular dysplasia, secondary to subarachnoid blood, meningitis, moya moya)
- Hypercoaguable states (oral contraceptives, Protein C/S deficiencies, Antithrombin III deficiency,
- Factor V Leyden, antiphospholipid antibodies, leukemia)
- Hematologic disorders (including sickle cell and other anemias
- Drug-induced (cocaine, amphetamines, heroin; can be due to hypertension or direct)
- Proinflammatory states (elevated homocysteine, C reactive protein levels)

Additional Readings

1. Manelfe C, Cognard C, Laval C, et al. Intracranial vascular involvement of brain pathologies and venous occlusions. Eur Radiol 1998;8(7):1106–1115
2. Mullins ME, Grant PE, Wang B, et al. Parenchymal abnormalities associated with cerebral venous sinus thrombosis: assessment with diffusion-weighted MR imaging. AJNR Am J Neuroradiol 2004;25(10): 1666–1675
3. Stam J. Thrombosis of the cerebral veins and sinuses. N Engl J Med 2005;352(17):1791–1798

14

Bilateral Thalamic Lesions

Bilateral thalamic lesions are often associated with vascular causes, most commonly arterial occlusions (basilar artery, i.e., "top of the basilar syndrome") or deep venous occlusion. Top of the basilar syndrome can be associated with bilateral or unilateral lesions. Bilateral paramedian thalamic infarcts have also been described due to occlusion of an unpaired thalamic perforating artery. Cerebral venous thrombosis can involve the superficial cortical veins, the dural sinuses, and/or the deep venous system (basal vein [of Rosenthal], internal cerebral veins, and vein of Galen). Deep cerebral venous thrombosis is the least common type of cerebral venous thrombosis. It is important to consider deep venous thrombosis as the etiology of bilateral acute thalamic lesions. The lesions seen in venous thrombosis may be reversible, and not progress to infarcts. Deep venous thrombosis should especially be considered if the patient is a young woman. Imaging features can help to differentiate deep venous thrombosis from arterial causes of bilateral thalamic lesions (**Table 14.1**).

Table 14.1 Differentiating Features between Deep Venous Thrombosis and Basilar Tip Thrombosis

	Deep Venous Thrombosis	Arterial Infarct
Generalized Edema	Yes	No
Areas Affected	Bilateral symmetric thalami, basal ganglia, and corona radiata	Midbrain, thalami, occipital lobes, and posterior fossa
Hemorrhages	Yes; tends to spread from center to periphery; may be multifocal	Less common and tends to begin at margins
Vessels	Dense veins (cord sign) and/or dural sinuses on non-contrast CT Venous sinus filling defects on enhanced CT/MRI or MRA	Dense basilar artery/P1 segments Arterial occlusion on CTA/MRA, contrast enhanced studies
Multiple Infarcts in Multiple Arterial Territories	Yes	No
Diffuse Dural/Pial (Gyral, Falcine, or Tentorial) Enhancement	Yes	No

(Continued on page 42)

Table 14.1 *(Continued)* Differentiating Features between Deep Venous Thrombosis and Basilar Tip Thrombosis

	Deep Venous Thrombosis	**Arterial Infarct**
DWI	Vasogenic edema, without restricted diffusion (although may have restricted diffusion, which may be reversible)	Cytotoxic edema Restricted diffusion
Margins	Irregular	Sharp

Abbreviations: CT, computed tomography; CTA, computed tomography angiography; DWI, diffusion weighted imaging; MRA, magnetic resonance angiography; MRI, magnetic resonance imaging.

Other etiologies rarely cause relatively symmetric, diffuse bilateral thalamic lesions. Thalamic gliomas are uncommon, and bilateral thalamic gliomas are rare. Several inflammatory or postinfectious processes can occasionally cause bilateral thalamic lesions. Acute necrotizing encephalopathy is most commonly seen in Asia, with most reported cases coming from Japan. It occurs in children following a viral illness and characteristically manifests bilateral symmetric thalamic lesions. Additional lesions are also seen in the periventricular white matter, cerebellar medulla, putamen, and upper brainstem tegmentum and may have ringlike enhancement. The distribution of lesions can be similar to Leigh's syndrome, although in that process, lesions are more frequent in the basal ganglia, and can be found in the periaqueductal gray, spinal cord, inferior olivary nuclei, and substantia nigra. Variant Creutzfeldt–Jakob disease has the characteristic finding of an abnormal signal within the pulvinar of the thalamus bilaterally ("pulvinar sign"); it also may have abnormal signal in the dorsomedial nuclei ("hockey-stick sign") and periaqueductal gray. Limbic encephalitis (as seen in paraneoplastic syndromes) can also occasionally involve the thalamus bilaterally.

Causes of Bilateral Thalamic Lesions

In the majority of these pathologies, extrathalamic lesions will also be present.

- Arterial/venous infarcts
- Deep venous thrombosis
- Gliomas
- Acute demyelinating encephalomyelitis
- Encephalitis (influenza, Japanese encephalitis)
- Acute necrotizing encephalopathy
- Leigh syndrome
- Variant Creutzfeldt–Jakob disease
- Limbic encephalitis
- Benign intracranial hypertension
- Cat-scratch disease (may have associated meningeal enhancement)
- Alpers' syndrome (may have associated increased signal in the occipital lobe)
- Wernicke encephalopathy (thiamine deficiency)
- Lupus
- Fungal abscess or toxoplasmosis
- Syphilis (may be associated with HIV/AIDS).
- Carbon monoxide poisoning
- Posterior fossa arteriovenous fistula (frequently caused by occlusion of petrosal sinuses and veins, with vascular steal phenomenon and redirection of flow)

Additional Readings

1. Barkhof F, Valk J. "Top of the basilar" syndrome: a comparison of clinical and MR findings. Neuroradiology 1988;30(4):293–298
2. Bell DA, Davis WL, Osborn AG, et al. Bithalamic hyperintensity on T2-weighted MR: vascular causes and evaluation with MR angiography. AJNR Am J Neuroradiol 1994;15(5):893–899
3. Greenough GP, Mamourian A, Harbaugh RE. Venous hypertension associated with a posterior fossa dural arteriovenous fistula: another cause of bithalamic lesions on MR images. AJNR Am J Neuroradiol 1999; 20(1):145–147
4. Mihara M, Sugase S, Konaka K, et al. The "pulvinar sign" in a case of paraneoplastic limbic encephalitis associated with non-Hodgkin's lymphoma. J Neurol Neurosurg Psychiatry 2005;76(6):882–884
5. Mizuguchi M. Acute necrotizing encephalopathy of childhood: a novel form of acute encephalopathy prevalent in Japan and Taiwan. Brain Dev 1997;19(2): 81–92
6. Prakash M, Kumar S, Gupta RK. Diffusion-weighted MR imaging in Japanese encephalitis. J Comput Assist Tomogr 2004;28(6):756–761
7. Weidauer S, Nichtweiss M, Lanfermann H, et al. Wernicke encephalopathy: MR findings and clinical presentation. Eur Radiol 2003;13(5):1001–1009
8. Zeidler M, Sellar RJ, Collie DA, et al. The pulvinar sign on magnetic resonance imaging in variant Creutzfeldt-Jakob disease. Lancet 2000;355(9213): 1412–1418

15

Intracranial Hemorrhages

Intracranial hemorrhages are commonly encountered; they can have a variety of causes with differing appearances on imaging depending on the age of the hematoma. They are generally classified into five distinct stages: hyperacute (<12 hours), acute (12 hours to 2 to 3 days), early subacute (2 or 3 to 7 days), late subacute (8 days to 1 month), and chronic (>1 month to years). Characteristic imaging appearances have been described on magnetic resonance imaging (MRI) for blood in intraparenchymal hematomas at these different stages based on the presence of blood products, their oxygenation states, and breakdown products. However, these descriptions have recently been shown to only partly correspond to the actual appearance of hematomas. The characteristic intraparenchymal hematoma appearance has been detailed elsewhere, but will be summarized here for easy reference (**Table 15.1**). Computed

Table 15.1 Progression of Appearance of Blood on Magnetic Resonance Imaging

Stages	MRI Signal Characteristics
Hyperacute	T1WI: Iso or hypo, T2WI: Hyper
Acute	T1WI: Iso or hypo, T2WI: Hypo
Early subacute	T1WI: Hyper, T2WI: Hypo
Late subacute	T1WI: Hyper, T2WI: Hyper
Chronic	T1WI: Iso or hypo, T2WI: Hypo

Abbreviations: Hypo, hypointense; hyper, hyperintense; iso, isointense; MRI, magnetic resonance imaging; T1WI, T1-weighted MRI; T2WI, T2-weighted MRI.

tomography (CT) is often the modality initially used when a patient presents with acute hemorrhage.

The hematoma appearance can vary based on its age and various characteristics including hematocrit level and anticoagulation status of the patient. Hyperacute blood can appear isodense to brain, but soon becomes hyperdense, and then decreases in density in the late subacute and chronic stages passing through a stage where it is isodense to brain. Ultimately, a small low-density cavity may remain. Anemia and anticoagulation can result in the acute hematoma being intermediate in density, but active bleeding must also be considered if hypodense areas are seen.

Intracranial hemorrhages can occur in any location or combination of locations, and the distribution can suggest the etiology. It can be subarachnoid, subdural, epidural, parenchymal, or intraventricular, and it can occur supratentorially or infratentorially. One common diagnostic dilemma usually occurs when trying to determine whether a parenchymal hematoma is due to an underlying lesion such as a metastasis or vascular malformation; or if it is "primary" and due to etiologies such as hypertension, amyloid angiopathy; or systemic causes such as coagulopathy, anticoagulation, liver failure, medications (including substance abuse), pregnancy; or dural sinus thrombosis. Some authors consider hemorrhage due to coagulopathy and medications as secondary hemorrhages along with hemorrhage due to neoplasms and vascular malformations; with primary hemorrhages only those that are due specifically to pathology related to small vessels as in hypertension or amyloid angiopathy. However, for the radiologist it is most important to exclude an underlying neoplasm or vascular malformation, so we will consider these separately from the true primary or systemic causes.

Another common dilemma is determining if a subarachnoid hemorrhage (SAH) is due to an aneurysm or other cause.

Distinguishing Primary from Secondary Parenchymal Hemorrhages

Destian et al. identified features helpful in distinguishing secondary from primary hemorrhages:

- Hemorrhage secondary to neoplasms evolve more slowly than primary hemorrhages.
- Secondary hematomas tend to develop hyperintensity on T1-weighted MR images (T1WI) and T2-weighted MR images (T2WI) within the hematoma rather than at the periphery (where it will begin in primary hematomas) or to be asymmetric if peripheral.
- If a secondary hematoma develops a low-signal hemosiderin ring, it will tend to be thin.
- The chronic stages of secondary hematomas are hyperintense on T1WI and T2WI.
- Tumor-induced hemorrhages may demonstrate a mixed pattern of signal intensities due to multiple episodes of bleeding.

This same study did not find the degree of surrounding edema to be helpful when it was mild to moderate, but the authors suggest that when more extensive surrounding edema is present, the likelihood of an underlying neoplasm is higher. Generally, acute primary hematomas induce little surrounding edema compared with hemorrhages related to an associated neoplasm.

Although hemorrhages related to vascular malformations and neoplasms can occur anywhere, primary hemorrhages preferentially occur in the basal ganglia, thalami, subcortical white matter, brainstem, and cerebellum. Hemorrhagic contusions favor the anterior temporal and anteroinferior frontal lobes. Findings that suggest an underlying vascular cause such as an aneurysm or arteriovenous malformation (AVM) include SAH (more commonly with aneurysms than AVMs) particularly in the basilar cisterns, sylvian fissures, anterior interhemispheric fissure, or predominantly in the posterior fossa; hemorrhage in the temporal lobe or with intraventricular extension; abnormal intracranial calcifications; and prominent vascular structures. Follow-up MRI and/or angiography may be necessary to exclude an underlying vascular or neoplastic lesion in young patients and other patients without a known underlying clinical cause for spontaneous hemorrhage. It is known that angiograms performed at the time of hemorrhage may not demonstrate an underlying AVM, and that cavernous malformations are characteristically "occult" on angiography. These and other underlying lesions may become evident on delayed follow-up imaging and or may be diagnosed only in surgical specimens.

Distinguishing Aneurysmal from Nonaneurysmal Subarachnoid Hemorrhages

When encountering a patient with nontraumatic SAH, it is most important to exclude an aneurysm as the cause. The typical distribution for aneurysmal subarachnoid hemorrhage is mentioned in the previous paragraph. The entity known as nonaneurysmal perimesencephalic subarachnoid hemorrhage presents with SAH generally in front of the brainstem and in the interpeduncular cistern, with varying extension into the other basilar cisterns. The etiology is unclear, but is thought to be due to venous bleeding. Up to 16.6% of posterior circulation aneurysms can present with this pattern of hemorrhage, particularly if CT is not obtained until some time after the initial episode of hemorrhage, allowing for resorption and dilution of blood. An aneurysm still needs to be excluded when patients present with the characteristic CT appearance as studies have shown that up to 10% of these patients have posterior circulation aneurysms. Two normal angiograms in the absence of vasospasm are required to exclude an underlying vascular lesion, although a lesion will be found in only 2 to 24% of these patients on the second angiogram.

Distinguishing Types of Traumatic Intracranial Hemorrhages

Trauma can cause both intraaxial and extraaxial hemorrhage, depending on the mechanism of injury and severity. Epidural hematomas do not cross sutures and are lentiform (biconvex) in shape. They are generally due to arterial injury, but can originate in venous structures such as the dural sinuses, particularly in the posterior fossa. Subdural hematomas may cross sutures but not dural reflections, have a concavo-convex

configuration, and are usually due to venous causes. SAH can occur, but is generally smaller in amount and does not possess the distribution seen with aneurysmal SAH, with blood scattered in sulci or within the interpeduncular cistern. Intraventricular hemorrhage can also occur. Various parenchymal hemorrhages can arise including

- contusions, which have a predilection for the bases of the frontal lobes and the bases, tips, and lateral aspects of the temporal lobes;
- shearing injury, which generally consists of multiple small hemorrhagic foci with a predilection for the corpus callosum and septum pellucidum, as well as the gray–white matter junction including the deep periventricular white matter, basal ganglia, internal capsule, hippocampal and parahippocampal regions, brain stem, and cerebellum. These small hemorrhagic and nonhemorrhagic lesions are often better seen on MRI;
- brainstem hemorrhages, which can occur due to shearing, direct impact, and brain herniation.

Additional Readings

1. Alemany Ripoll M, Stenborg A, Sonninen P, Terent A, Raininko R. Detection and appearance of intraparenchymal haematomas of the brain at 1.5 T with spin-echo, FLAIR and GE sequences: poor relationship to the age of the haematoma. Neuroradiology 2004;46(6):435–443
2. Alen JF, Lagares A, Lobato RD, Gomez PA, Rivas JJ, Ramos A. Comparison between perimesencephalic nonaneurysmal subarachnoid hemorrhage and subarachnoid hemorrhage caused by posterior circulation aneurysms. J Neurosurg 2003;98(3):529–535
3. Besenski N. Traumatic injuries: imaging of head injuries. Eur Radiol 2002;12(6):1237–1252
4. Bradley WG Jr. MR appearance of hemorrhage in the brain. Radiology 1993;189(1):15–26
5. Destian S, Sze G, Krol G, Zimmerman RD, Deck MD. MR imaging of hemorrhagic intracranial neoplasms. AJR Am J Roentgenol 1989;152(1):137–144
6. Fewel ME, Thompson BG Jr, Hoff JT. Spontaneous intracerebral hemorrhage: a review. Neurosurg Focus 2003;15(4):E1
7. Huisman TA. Intracranial hemorrhage: ultrasound, CT and MRI findings. Eur Radiol 2005;15(3):434–440

16

Perivascular Spaces versus Lacunar Infarcts

Perivascular spaces and lacunar infarcts may appear similar and be difficult to differentiate on imaging. There are some features that can aid in this differentiation (**Table 16.1**).

Lacunar Infarcts

Lacunar infarcts are defined as small subcortical and deep infarcts (<15 mm in diameter) due to occlusion of a single deep penetrating artery and may be asymptomatic or present with specific lacunar or other neurological symptoms. They occur most frequently in the basal ganglia and internal capsule, thalamus, corona radiata, and brain stem.

Their imaging appearance varies with age. Acute lacunar infarcts are often undetectable on computed tomography (CT), but may appear as hypodensities. Magnetic resonance imaging (MRI) is much more sensitive than CT, with lacunar infarcts appearing isointense to mildly hypointense on T1-weighted MR images (T1WI) and hyperintense on T2-weighted MR images (T2WI) or fluid-attenuated inversion recovery (FLAIR) with restricted diffusion on diffusion weighted imaging (DWI) and apparent diffusion coefficient (ADC maps). A chronic lacunar infarct may be difficult to distinguish from a perivascular space. It may be cystic with CSF density and intensity on CT and MRI, respectively. It may be isointense to mildly hypointense on T1WI if not cystic. If the lacuna is

Table 16.1 Differentiating Features between Perivascular Spaces and Lacunar Infarcts

	Perivascular Space	Lacunar Infarct
Location	Basal ganglia, thalamus, white matter near vertex, subinsular, although may be seen anywhere in the brain	Basal ganglia, internal capsule, thalamus, corona radiata or pons
MRI	CSF intensity on all imaging sequences (usually)	Acute – T1WI: Isointense to mildly hypointense T2WI/FLAIR: Hyperintense Diffusion: Restricted diffusion Chronic – T1WI: Isointense to hypointense T2WI: Hyperintense FLAIR: CSF intensity to hyperintense
CT	CSF density with normal adjoining brain parenchyma	Acute – Normal to low density, possibly mild swelling Chronic – CSF density to hypodense

(Continued on page 48)

Table 16.1 (Continued) Differentiating Features between Perivascular Spaces and Lacunar Infarcts

	Perivascular Space	Lacunar Infarct
Distinguishing Features	Normal adjoining brain parenchyma without any volume loss or encephalomalacia	Acute – Appears like an infarct with restricted diffusion and may have swelling and mass effect
		Chronic – May have associated volume loss
Shape	Round, linear, oval	Wedge-shaped, oval
Age Distribution	Seen at all ages; may enlarge with advancing age	Seen typically with advanced age

Abbreviations: CSF, cerebrospinal fluid; CT, computed tomography; FLAIR, fluid-attenuated inversion recovery; MRI, magnetic resonance imaging; T1WI, T1-weighted MR images; T2WI, T2-weighted MR images.

close to the ventricular system, it may cause focal ex-vacuo dilatation of the ventricle.

Perivascular Spaces

Perivascular spaces or Virchow–Robin spaces (VRS) are pial-lined extensions of the subarachnoid space that surround blood vessels entering the brain parenchyma. However, they may not freely communicate with the remainder of the subarachnoid space and may contain interstitial fluid rather than cerebrospinal fluid (CSF). They are most commonly found and are often largest in the inferior basal ganglia at the level of the anterior commissure. They can also be seen within the white matter near the vertex. With advancing age, VRS can be seen elsewhere in the basal ganglia, the thalami, hippocampi, dentate nuclei, cerebellum, and white matter, and can become widened, particularly near the anterior commissure. The presence of enlarged perivascular spaces has also been associated with hypertension, cerebral arteriosclerosis, trauma, Parkinson's disease, cerebral autosomal dominant arteriopathy with subcortical infarcts and leukoencephalopathy (CADASIL), diabetes, and cognitive decline in older patients

On CT, perivascular spaces appear as CSF density foci. On MRI, they generally follow CSF intensity on all imaging sequences, although they may not always contain simple fluid and therefore occasionally have a signal different from CSF. They generally do not have any associated gliosis or abnormal signal in the adjoining brain parenchyma unless very large ("giant perivascular spaces") and are generally round, punctuate, or linear. Except in the brain stem and lower basal ganglia, lesions 3 × 2 mm or greater in diameter are more likely to be lacunes; although within the lower part of the basal ganglia, perivascular spaces are often larger, so they cannot be differentiated on size alone. Brain stem lesions were more commonly found to be infarcts in one study, whereas giant perivascular spaces have been found to occur most commonly in the thalami and midbrain.

Causes of and Conditions Associated with Enlarged Perivascular Spaces

- Hypertension
- Dementia
- White matter lesions
- Aging
- Encephalitis/meningitis
- Neurosarcoidosis
- Posttraumatic (high convexity)
- Cryptococcal meningitis/meningoencephalitis
- Mucopolysaccharidosis
- Parkinson's disease
- CADASIL
- Cerebral arteriosclerosis
- Diabetes
- Normal variant

Additional Readings

1. Barkhof F. Enlarged Virchow-Robin spaces: do they matter? J Neurol Neurosurg Psychiatry 2004;75(11): 1516–1517
2. Bokura H, Kobayashi S, Yamaguchi S. Distinguishing silent lacunar infarction from enlarged Virchow-Robin spaces: a magnetic resonance imaging and pathological study. J Neurol 1998;245(2):116–122
3. Braffman BH, Zimmerman RA, Trojanowski JQ, et al. Brain MR: pathologic correlation with gross and histopathology. 1. Lacunar infarction and Virchow-Robin spaces. AJR Am J Roentgenol 1988;151(3): 551–558
4. Brown JJ, Hesselink JR, Rothrock JF. MR and CT of lacunar infarcts. AJR Am J Roentgenol 1988;151(2): 367–372
5. Inglese M, Bomsztyk E, Gonen O, et al. Dilated perivascular spaces: hallmarks of mild traumatic brain injury. AJNR Am J Neuroradiol 2005;26(4): 719–724
6. Ozturk MH, Aydingoz U. Comparison of MR signal intensities of cerebral perivascular (Virchow-Robin) and subarachnoid spaces. J Comput Assist Tomogr 2002;26(6):902–904
7. Salzman KL, Osborn AG, House P, et al. Giant tumefactive perivascular spaces. AJNR Am J Neuroradiol 2005;26(2):298–305

17

Intracranial Manifestations of Human Immunodeficiency Virus

Human immunodeficiency virus (HIV) infection is associated with various neurological manifestations in 40 to 70% of acquired immune deficiency syndrome (AIDS) patients, including primary effects of HIV, opportunistic infection, neoplasia, and vascular disease. Infections can be focal or diffuse. Cerebral toxoplasmosis is the most common mass lesion, HIV encephalopathy is the most common cause of neurological disease, and cytomegalovirus encephalitis (CMV) is the most common opportunistic viral infection found in AIDS patients. Other common infections include progressive multifocal leukoencephalopathy (PML), cryptococcal meningitis, and neurosyphilis. CMV generally has an appearance similar to primary HIV on magnetic resonance imaging (MRI) (diffuse white matter hyperintensity on T2-weighted MR sequences). However, it rarely presents as a peripherally enhancing mass, or as a necrotizing meningoencephalitis with associated subependymal enhancement, a finding that can also be seen in advanced herpes zoster, and less commonly with other herpes viruses. Another common central nervous system (CNS) lesion is primary CNS lymphoma, which has been shown to be associated with Epstein–Barr virus in almost 100% of cases.

Based on MRI appearance, the lesions may be divided into

- *Diffuse white matter disease* HIV encephalopathy (HIVE) and diffuse CMV encephalitis
- *Patchy white matter disease* HIVE, PML, herpes encephalitis

- *Focal mass with enhancement* Toxoplasmosis, lymphoma, Cryptococcus, mycobacteria, CMV, neurosyphilis, bacterial and fungal abscesses (Nocardia, Bartonella, Rhodococcus)
- *Focal mass without enhancement* Cryptococcus (gelatinous pseudocysts, cryptococcomas, enlarged perivascular spaces), toxoplasmosis, and atypical primary CNS lymphoma. The lack of enhancement may be due to severely depressed cell-mediated immunity.
- *Focal enhancement without mass* Toxoplasmosis, cerebral infarct, viral encephalitis, bacterial cerebritis, PML (generally nonenhancing, but occasional faint peripheral enhancement; enhancement may be related to inflammatory reaction or may occur due to improved immune response following therapy [IRIS-immune reconstitution inflammatory syndrome] may occasionally be diffuse or speckled).
- *Focal lesion, without mass effect or enhancement* PML (no mass effect) and diffusely infiltrating primary CNS lymphoma (subtle mass effect)
- *Meningitis/meningeal disease* HIV meningoencephalitis, Cryptococcus, mycobacterial infection (basal meningitis), neurosyphilis, metastatic systemic lymphoma
- *Ventriculitis* CMV, herpes virus (especially advanced herpes zoster virus), Cryptococcus
- *Cerebrovascular disease* Tuberculosis (TB)/ cryptococcal meningitis can result in arteritis/ thrombosis and cerebral infarcts, neurosyphilis (vasculitis), CMV, Varicella zoster virus

When faced with white matter lesions in an AIDS patient, some features can help to differentiate HIV encephalitis from PML. They are listed in **Table 17.1**.

Toxoplasmosis and Lymphoma

The two most common enhancing intracranial masses in AIDS patients are lymphoma and toxoplasmosis. It can be difficult to differentiate the two with conventional computed tomography (CT) and MRI (**Table 17.2**). Fluorodeoxyglucose positron emission tomography (FDG PET) and thallium-201 single photon emission computed tomography (SPECT) are very useful in differentiating lymphoma from toxoplasmosis. Lymphoma accumulates tracer, whereas toxoplasmosis does not. The size of the lesion may play a role, with sensitivity and specificity measured at 100% and 89%, respectively, for thallium-201 SPECT for lesions ≥ 2 cm, but not meeting statistical significance for lesions <2 cm.

Table 17.1 Differentiating Features between HIV Encephalopathy and Progressive Multifocal Leukoencephalopathy

	HIVE	PML
Etiology	Direct HIV involvement	JC papovavirus. AIDS-defining disease caused by reactivation of virus when cell-mediated immunity is impaired.
		Tropism for oligodendrocytes causes demyelinating disease
Diagnosis	Neuropsychological testing	CSF polymerase chain reaction for JC papovavirus
		Definitive diagnosis is only by brain biopsy.
CT	Atrophy, white matter hypodensities	Single or multiple confluent hypodense white matter lesions predominantly in parietooccipital white matter
MRI	Diffuse confluent, bilateral symmetric white matter lesions	Asymmetric patchy white matter lesions
	T1WI: Isointense	T1WI: Hypointense – lesions become more hypointense as disease progresses
	T2WI: Hyperintense	T2WI: Hyperintense
		Central areas of necrosis can occur.
Location	Centrum semiovale /periventricular white matter	Parietal predominance
	Relative sparing of arcuate fibers and posterior fossa structures	May involve posterior fossa, basal ganglia, and thalamus
		Subcortical and/or central white matter
		Scalloped appearance due to arcuate fiber involvement
Distribution	Diffuse white matter	Multifocal and asymmetric Unifocal
	Occasionally patchy distribution of lesions	
	Uncommon: Basal ganglia and small white matter lesions	
Enhancement	No	Occasional
Mass Effect	No	No
Atrophy	Yes	No
MTR	Relatively less decrease in MTR (38–40%)	Profound decrease in MTR (22–26%) early in the disease (due to demyelination) and significantly lower than HIV white matter lesions

(Continued on page 52)

Table 17.1 *(Continued)* Differentiating Features between HIV Encephalopathy and Progressive Multifocal Leukoencephalopathy

	HIVE	PML
Proton MRS'	↑ Myoinositol ↑ Cho ↓ NAA[†]	↑ Cho Variable myoinositol Substantial ↓ in NAA Lactate peak present in 75%
Angiography	May have findings similar to primary CNS angiitis with multifocal stenoses of small and medium arteries[††]	AV shunting and parenchymal blush in some patients due to small vessel proliferation and perivascular inflammatory changes incited by presence of JC papovirus in infected oligodendrocytes May be normal

Abbreviations: AIDS, acquired immune deficiency syndrome; AV, arteriovenous; Cho, choline; CNS, central nervous system; CSF, cerebrospinal fluid; CT, computed tomography; HIV, human immunodeficiency virus; HIVE, human immunodeficiency virus encephalopathy; MRA, magnetic resonance angiography; MRI, magnetic resonance imaging; MTR, magnetization transfer ratio; MRS, magnetic resonance spectroscopy; NAA, *N*-acetyl aspartate; PML, progressive multifocal leukoencephalopathy; T1WI, T1-weighted magnetic resonance images; T2WI, T2-weighted magnetic resonance images.

* The lesions of HIV and PML may be differentiated by their appearance on the T1WI, with the PML lesions hypointense and the HIV lesions isointense.

[†] May be seen before conventional MRI findings

[††] The role of HIV in the pathogenesis is uncertain. In addition, many of the patients reported had MRA rather than conventional angiography.

Table 17.2 Differentiating Features between Toxoplasmosis and Lymphoma

	Toxoplasmosis	Lymphoma
FDG PET	Not metabolically active	Metabolically active
Thallium SPECT	Thallium index <2	Thallium index >2
CT	Isodense or hypodense; may have subtle hyperdense center	Hyperdense
MRI	T1WI: Hypointense	T1WI: Hypointense or isointense
	T2WI: Isointense or hypointense; may have hyperintense center	T2WI: Hypointense or isointense; may have hyperintense areas of necrosis
MR Spectroscopy[†]	NAA/Cr ↓ lipid ↑, Cho ↓, lactate ↑ [††]	NAA/Cr ↓ lipid ↑ Cho ↑, lactate ↓ [††]
Diffusion Weighted Imaging (compared to white matter)	Increased signal ADC ratio[†††] of 1.6 is very specific	Mildly increased to decreased signal ADC ratio[†††] not greater than 1.6 and usually lower
Enhancement	Solid or ring Wall enhancement is thin.	Solid Heterogeneous Ringlike Wall enhancement is thick and irregular May have central necrosis

Table 17.2 *(Continued)* Differentiating Features between Toxoplasmosis and Lymphoma

	Toxoplasmosis	Lymphoma
Surrounding Edema	Yes	Yes
Solitary or Multiple	More commonly multiple Solitary in 14%	Multifocal in 50%
Location	Peripheral white matter or deep nuclei (thalami, basal ganglia)	Periventricular white matter, corpus callosum, subependymal

Abbreviations: ADC, apparent diffusion coefficient; Cho, choline; Cr, creatinine; CT, computed tomography; FDG PET, fluorodeoxyglucose positron emission tomography; MRI, magnetic resonance imaging; MRS, magnetic resonance spectroscopy; ms, milliseconds; NAA, *N*-acetyl aspartate; SPECT, single photon emission computed tomography; T1WI, T1-weighted magnetic resonance images; T2WI, T2-weighted magnetic resonance images; TE, Echo Time.

* Thallium index: The ratio of counts per pixel of the lesion compared to counts per pixel of control region

† Studies comparing ratios have shown that differentiation of toxoplasmosis and lymphoma cannot be differentiated at 135 ms TE H1-MRS using commonly used metabolite ratios. Others have shown it is possible to differentiate them at short TE (30 ms) using values normalized to the contralateral normal side.

†† Compared with contralateral normal brain

††† ADC ration: Ratio of ADC of lesion to ADC of normal white matter

Additional Readings

1. Young RJ, Ghesani MV, Kagetsu NJ, et al. Lesion size determines accuracy of thallium-201 brain single-photon emission tomography in differentiating between intracranial malignancy and infection in AIDS patients. AJNR Am J Neuroradiol 2005;26(8):1973–1979
2. Hurley RA, Ernst T, Khalili K, et al. Identification of HIV-associated progressive multifocal leukoencephalopathy: magnetic resonance imaging and spectroscopy. J Neuropsychiatry Clin Neurosci 2003;15(1):1–6
3. Camacho DL, Smith JK, Castillo M. Differentiation of toxoplasmosis and lymphoma in AIDS patients by using apparent diffusion coefficients. AJNR Am J Neuroradiol 2003;24(4):633–637
4. Sibtain NA, Chinn RJS. Imaging of the central nervous system in HIV infection. Imaging 2002;14(1):48–59
5. Thurnher MM, Post MJ, Rieger A, et al. Initial and follow-up MR imaging findings in AIDS-related progressive multifocal leukoencephalopathy treated with highly active antiretroviral therapy. AJNR Am J Neuroradiol 2001;22(5):977–984
6. Berkefeld J, Enzensberger W, Lanfermann H. Cryptococcus meningoencephalitis in AIDS: parenchymal and meningeal forms. Neuroradiology 1999;41(2): 129–133

18

Hyperdense and Calcified Lesions on Computed Tomography

There are numerous causes for intracranial calcifications and for lesions to appear hyperattenuating (dense) on non-contrast computed tomography (CT) scans.

Hyperdense Lesions

There are a variety of causes for lesions to be hyperdense (hyperattenuating) on CT scanning. One of the most common causes is hemorrhage, but other etiologies include dense cellularity, mucinous or proteinaceous lesions, and partial or "psammomatous" calcification. Some metabolic and toxic processes can also result in dense lesions, although the mechanisms are not well understood.

Lesions that May Appear Hyperdense on Non-contrast CT

Neoplastic Lesions

- Highly cellular, hemorrhagic, or calcified neoplasms
- "Round blue cell tumors" (high cellularity with high nuclear to cytoplasmic ratio)
- Lymphoma
- Primitive neuroectodermal tumors (PNET)
- Medulloblastoma
- High-grade ependymoma
- Germinoma
- Choroid plexus papilloma/carcinoma
- Meningioma (mild)
- Metastases (may be due to cellularity, blood, mucin, calcification): melanoma, adenocarcinoma, choriocarcinoma, renal cell, carcinoma, osteosarcoma

Mucin or Protein-Containing Lesions

- Colloid cyst (may vary in attenuation)
- Craniopharyngioma (cystic areas)
- Rathke's cleft cyst: occasionally
- Mucinous metastases

Vascular Lesions

- Hemorrhagic tumors:
  Glioblastoma multiforme (GBM)
  Metastases (renal cell, choriocarcinoma, melanoma)
- Cavernous malformation: may be due to calcium, blood, or combination of both; may have stippled appearance
- Aneurysm with clot (or just with mildly dense blood): may have calcification of wall
- Arteriovenous malformation (AVM): may be increased density due to calcium in walls, may have associated parenchymal atrophy, low density or mass effect, and large draining veins, etc.
- Hemorrhage from any cause

Lesions Caused by Infectious/ Inflammation

- Toxoplasmosis (generally hypodense, but may have hyperdense central area)

Metabolic

- Non-ketotic hyperglycemia (with hemiballism-hemichorea): unilateral basal ganglia hyperdensity, may be contralateral putamen and/or caudate; cause unknown, possibly due to petechial hemorrhage or gemistocytes
- Methanol intoxication (due to hemorrhagic infarction of putamen)

Calcified Lesions

Calcifications can occur normally within the brain, and can be seen in characteristic locations such as the globus pallidus, pineal gland, choroid plexus, dura (where they may be actual ossifications), and habenula, as well as in blood vessels due to atherosclerosis. Many other processes can also lead to intracranial calcifications in varying distributions. Calcification can be seen in various toxic or metabolic processes, such as lead poisoning, where it has been shown to be vascular and more extensive in the cerebellum. In hyperparathyroidism, hypoparathyroidism, and pseudohypoparathyroidism, calcification generally involves the basal ganglia, dentate nuclei, and thalami, but can also involve the periventricular and peripheral white matter, occasionally causing subcortical or cortical calcifications, and can occasionally involve the dura including the tentorium. Degenerative diseases such as Fahr's disease can have calcification in a distribution similar to that of hypoparathyroidism.

Other hereditary syndromes, such as Gorlin syndrome (basal cell nevus syndrome) can have intracranial calcifications (dural, particularly falcine) as major diagnostic features. Some of the neurocutaneous syndromes have characteristic calcifications, such as Sturge–Weber (gyral calcifications) and tuberous sclerosis (calcifications of subependymal nodules and tubers). Occasionally, prior injuries such as infarcts, trauma, or hematomas can calcify. Various infections can calcify. Cysticercosis, in its inactive form, can have parenchymal or subarachnoid calcifications generally measuring between 2 and 10 mm as the sequela of previous infection. Although calcified lesions are relatively uncommon in some series of tuberculosis (TB), tuberculomas are characterized by the so-called target sign described as a central calcification with surrounding enhancement, and can demonstrate other patterns of parenchymal calcification. Calcification of the meninges can also result from tuberculous meningitis. Congenital infections commonly result in parenchymal calcifications. Various neoplasms, including metastases can also calcify, as can vascular lesions.

Lesions that May Appear Calcified on Non-contrast CT

Vascular Lesions

- Arteriosclerosis
- AVM
- Aneurysm
- Sturge–Weber
- Old hematoma
- Cavernous malformation

Congenital Lesions

- Sturge–Weber
- Tuberous sclerosis
- Cockayne syndrome

Neoplasms

- Craniopharyngioma
- Germ cell tumor
- Meningioma
- Certain gliomas
- Choroid plexus papillomas/carcinomas

- Metastases (such as osteosarcoma, gastrointestinal (GI) tract adenocarcinomas, lung, breast)

Posttherapy-/Infection-/ Inflammation-/ Injury

- Cysticercosis
- TB
- Granulomas
- Congenital infections (TORCH group – toxoplasma gondii, rubella, cytomegalovirus (CMV), herpes [including varicella zoster], and HIV)
- Treated toxoplasmosis
- Prior infarct, trauma, hematoma (all relatively uncommon)

Idiopathic/Hereditary

- Idiopathic: Globus pallidus, dura, choroid plexus, habenula
- Fahr's disease
- Gorlin syndrome (basal cell nevus syndrome)
- Mitochondrial diseases

Metabolic

- Lead poisoning (especially cerebellum)
- Hypoparathyroidism, pseudohypoparathyroidism, hyperparathyroidism
- Vitamin D intoxication (particularly in patients with hyperparathyroidism)

Iatrogenic

- Pantopaque (not calcification, but may appear similar to calcification)

Additional Readings

1. Slone HW, Blake JJ, Shah R, et al. CT and MRI findings of intracranial lymphoma. AJR Am J Roentgenol 2005;184(5):1679–1685
2. Osborn AG. Diagnostic Imaging. Salt Lake City, UT: Amirsys; 2004
3. Marshman LA, Chawda SJ, David KM. Change in CT radiodensity of a colloid cyst of the third ventricle: case report and literature review. Neuroradiology 2004;46(12):984–987
4. Kimonis VE, Mehta SG, Digiovanna JJ, et al. Radiological features in 82 patients with nevoid basal cell carcinoma (NBCC or Gorlin) syndrome. Genet Med 2004;6(6):495–502
5. Castillo M. Imaging of neurocysticercosis. Semin Roentgenol 2004;39(4):465–473
6. Grossman RI, Yousem DM. Neuroradiology: The Requisites (Requisites in Radiology). 2nd ed. Philadelphia, PA: Mosby; 2003; xvi, 908

19

Corpus Callosum Lesions

A variety of lesions may involve the corpus callosum, although callosal involvement in many of these processes is relatively uncommon. Multiple sclerosis (MS) most commonly involves the corpus callosum, with small lesions at the inferior aspect of the corpus callosum (the callosal septal interface) in up to 93% of cases. There can be associated atrophy of the corpus callosum and acute lesions can enhance. Differential diagnosis can be aided by the detection of additional lesions in a distribution characteristic for MS. Diffuse axonal injury (shearing injury) commonly involves the corpus callosum, most commonly the splenium, and callosal involvement has been associated with a worse prognosis. Lymphoma and glioblastoma multiforme are the most common neoplasms to demonstrate callosal involvement, although other high-grade glial neoplasms can cross the corpus callosum. These lesions commonly enhance and may extend bilaterally in what has been referred to as a "butterfly" pattern. A nonnecrotic bulky infiltration of the corpus callosum is suggestive of lymphoma. Ischemic lesions of the corpus callosum often occur off midline and do not extend to the superior or inferior surfaces. Hydrocephalus can result in indentation, thinning, or abnormal signal along the superior aspect of the corpus callosum due to the effect of the falx. Lipomas, while not callosal lesions per se, commonly occur in the callosal region and may be associated with callosal dysgenesis.

Marchiafava–Bignami is a rare syndrome associated with alcohol abuse. It can affect the genu and splenium in the acute form, and the callosal body in the subacute and chronic forms. It generally spares the superior and inferior margins of the corpus callosum ("sandwich sign"), and can be associated with hemorrhage and additional white matter lesions.

Differential Diagnosis of Entities that May Effect the Corpus Callosum

Common Entities

- Multiple sclerosis

Less Common Entities

- Acute disseminated encephalomyelitis (ADEM)
- Trauma/diffuse axonal injury
- Lymphoma
- Glioblastoma/high-grade glioma
- Infarct
- Hydrocephalus
- Arteriovenous malformation

Rare Entities

- Pilocytic astrocytoma
- Progressive multifocal leukoencephalopathy
- Marchiafava–Bignami

Very Rare Entities

- Toxoplasmosis
- Tuberculoma

Central Splenial Lesions

Central splenial lesions are rare; they may have diffusion abnormality and abnormal signal on T2-weighted magnetic resonance [MR] images and fluid-attenuated inversion recovery (FLAIR) images.

Causes of Central Splenial Lesions

- Seizures/antiepileptic medication induced
- Encephalitis: has been described in rotavirus, *Escherichia coli* associated hemolytic uremic syndrome and encephalopathy, *Salmonella enteritis*, measles encephalopathy, influenza A, mumps, varicella zoster, adenovirus, and it has been reported in clinically mild cases of encephalitis.
- 5-FU Encephalopathy

Additional Readings

1. Yeh IB, Tan LC, Sitoh YY. Reversible splenial lesion in clinically mild encephalitis. Singapore Med J 2005; 46(12):726–730
2. Gadda D, Carmignani L, Vannucchi L, et al. Traumatic lesions of corpus callosum: early multidetector CT findings. Neuroradiology 2004;46(10):812–816
3. Bourekas EC, Varakis K, Bruns D, et al. Lesions of the corpus callosum: MR imaging and differential considerations in adults and children. AJR Am J Roentgenol 2002; 179(1):251–257
4. Friese SA, Bitzer M, Freudenstein M, et al. Classification of acquired lesions of the corpus callosum with MRI. Neuroradiology 2000;42(11):795–802

20

Abnormal Basal Ganglia Signal on Magnetic Resonance Imaging

There are a limited number of causes of hyperintensity within the basal ganglia on T1-weighted magnetic resonance (MR) images (T1WI) without correlates on CT or T2 weighted sequences. This finding is most commonly seen in patients who have chronic liver disease or who are on parenteral nutrition. In parenteral nutrition, it is thought to be due to the deposition of trace elements such as manganese, mainly in the globi pallidi and subthalamic nuclei, and/or reaction to these elements. These findings have been shown to regress on follow-up imaging one year following cessation of manganese administration. In patients with chronic liver disease, increased signal is seen in the globus pallidus and portions of the internal capsules and cerebral peduncles. Increased signal has been described in patients with cirrhosis and portal-systemic collaterals receiving blood from an enlarged superior mesenteric vein. While the signal abnormality is essentially on T1WI, abnormalities can also be seen on the proton density images due to the contribution from T1 shortening.

Although rare, acute chorea-ballism associated with hyperglycemia also demonstrates hyperintensity on T1WI without abnormality on T2-weighted MRI (T2WI). In hemorrhage, the hyperintensity on T1WI is thought to be due to methemoglobin. In etiologies such as evolving infarct, hemorrhage, Wilson's disease, and encephalitis, there is associated abnormality on the T2WI. There is associated hyperattenuation on CT in patients with hemorrhage and calcification, and hypoattenuation is present in other etiologies such as encephalitis, Wilson's disease, neurofibromatosis, or hypoxic-ischemic encephalopathy.

Neurodegenerative diseases and inborn errors of metabolism have a predilection for involvement of the basal ganglia, and dysmyelinating disorders can also affect the basal ganglia as well as white matter tracts. These lesions generally manifest as hyperintense on T2WI. Leigh syndrome has preferential involvement of the putamen. Most other inborn errors of metabolism favor the globus pallidus.

Lymphoma commonly involves the basal ganglia with up to 33% of CNS lymphoma involving the deep gray matter structures, although the supratentorial white matter is the most common location. The lesions are most commonly hypointense on the T2WI, but may be hyperintense and may also have surrounding edema, most commonly in immuno-compromised patients, where there also may be central necrosis. Neurofibromatosis type I patients can have lesions that are hyperintense on T1WI within the basal ganglia, predominantly the globus pallidus, which extend into the internal capsule and anterior commissure. These lesions are thought to represent either hamartomas or heterotopias, and usually resolve by adulthood. These lesions can also have focal signal abnormality on T2WI, and additional T2WI-hyperintense lesions can be seen elsewhere.

Causes of Hyperintensity within the Basal Ganglia on T1-Weighted MRI

Common Causes

- Parenteral nutrition (manganese and/or astrogliotic reaction to manganese)
- Chronic liver disease
- Subacute infarct, hemorrhagic infarct, hemorrhage

Uncommon Causes

- Wilson's disease (copper deposition; more commonly hypointense)
- Japanese encephalitis (due to hemorrhage within lesions)
- Calcification (generally isointense to hypointense on T1/T2WI)
- Neurofibromatosis type I
- Hypoxic/anoxic injury (hypoxic-ischemic encephalopathy, hypoglycemia) (due to petechial hemorrhage and/or lipid laden macrophages)
- Methanol intoxication (due to hemorrhage)
- Acute chorea-ballism with hyperglycemia

Causes of Hyperintensity on T2-Weighted MRI

Common Causes

- Infarct
- Hypoxic-ischemic encephalopathy, diffuse brain injury

- Toxic-metabolic causes (carbon monoxide, cyanide, hydrogen sulfide, hypoglycemia, etc.)
- Viral encephalitis
- Neurofibromatosis

Uncommon/Rare Causes

- Lymphoma (may be hypointense due to high cellularity and increased nuclear-cytoplasmic ratio)
- Osmotic myelinolysis (central pontine/ extrapontine myelinolysis)
- Wilson's disease
- Inborn errors of metabolism
  - Leigh syndrome (basal ganglia, brainstem, thalami, with dominant involvement of the putamen)
  - Mitochondrial cytopathies
  - Lactic acidosis
  - Glutaric acidemia type 2
  - Methylmalonic academia
  - Propionic academia
  - Maple syrup urine disease
- Hallervorder–Spatz
- Dysmyelinating disorders (Canavan disease, metachromatic leukodystrophy)
- Methanol intoxication (may have lower signal if associated with hemorrhage)

For a table differentiating features of childhood basal ganglia lesions, see Ho et al.

Additional Readings

1. Blanco M, Casado R, Vazquez F, et al. CT and MR imaging findings in methanol intoxication. AJNR Am J Neuroradiol 2006;27(2):452–454
2. Ho VB, Fitz CR, Chuang SH, et al. Bilateral basal ganglia lesions: pediatric differential considerations. Radiographics 1993;13(2):269–292
3. Koeller KK, Smirniotopoulos JG, Jones RV. Primary central nervous system lymphoma: radiologic-pathologic correlation. Radiographics 1997;17(6):1497–1526
4. Lai PH, Chen C, Liang HL, et al. Hyperintense basal ganglia on T1-weighted MR imaging. AJR Am J Roentgenol 1999;172(4):1109–1115
5. Mirowitz SA, Sartor K, Gado M. High-intensity basal ganglia lesions on T1-weighted MR images in neurofibromatosis. AJR Am J Roentgenol 1990;154(2):369–373
6. Mirowitz SA, Westrich TJ. Basal ganglial signal intensity alterations: reversal after discontinuation of parenteral manganese administration. Radiology 1992;185(2): 535–536

21

Hydrocephalus

Hydrocephalus can be either noncommunicating (intraventricular obstructive hydrocephalus [IVOH]) or communicating (extraventricular obstructive hydrocephalus [EVOH]), referring to whether obstruction to cerebrospinal fluid (CSF) flow is within the ventricular system to the outflow tracts of the 4th ventricle (including the cerebral aqueduct and foramen of Monroe) – noncommunicating – or outside the ventricular system – communicating. A common diagnostic dilemma is determining whether ventricular enlargement is due to hydrocephalus or atrophy. Several findings can help differentiate the various forms of hydrocephalus from atrophy (**Table 21.1**).

Normal pressure hydrocephalus is a communicating hydrocephalus syndrome, in which hyperdynamic aqueductal CSF flow such as demonstrated by a flow void on spin-echo proton density image, or by increased aqueductal stroke volume on phase contrast magnetic resonance imaging (MRI), suggests the diagnosis

Table 21.1 Differentiating Features between Atrophy, Communicating Hydrocephalus, and Noncommunicating Hydrocephalus

	NPH/Communicating Hydrocephalus (EVOH)	Noncommunicating Hydrocephalus (IVOH)	Atrophy
Enlargement of Ventricles with Respect to Sulci	Disproportionate (ventricles and sylvian fissures larger than sulci) Sulci may be heterogeneous in size.	Disproportionate (ventricles larger than sulci)	Proportionate (ventricles and sulci enlarged to similar degree)
Perihippocampal Fissures	Compressed	Compressed	Enlarged
Aqueductal CSF Flow	Hyperdynamic	Diminished	Normal
Obstructing Lesions or Compression of Components of Ventricular System	No	Yes	No
Other Findings	3rd and lateral ventricles may be rounded, enlarged inferior recesses of 3rd ventricle, transependymal edema (if acute/exacerbated)		

Abbreviations: CSF, cerebrospinal fluid; EVOH, extraventricular obstructive hydrocephalus; IVOH, intraventricular obstructive hydrocephalus; NPH, normal pressure hydrocephalus.

as well as shunt responsiveness. In atrophy, CSF flow is generally not hyperdynamic as cerebral blood flow is decreased; therefore, there is less CSF displacement from the ventricles during systole (and less inflow during diastole).

Enlargement of the perihippocampal sulci can differentiate hydrocephalus from atrophy, particularly that related to Alzheimer's disease, for which dilatation of the perihippocampal sulci can be a predictor. In cognitively normal elderly individuals, the hippocampi remain normal from 60 to 75 years of age, but lose volume from 76 to 90 years. As the transverse fissure (and other perihippocampal sulci) does not communicate with the temporal horns, the perihippocampal sulci can be compressed in hydrocephalus rather than enlarged in Alzheimer's disease or age-related atrophy.

Additional Readings

1. Bradley WG. Normal pressure hydrocephalus: new concepts on etiology and diagnosis. AJNR Am J Neuroradiol 2000;21(9):1586–1590
2. Kim MH, Shin KM, Song JH. Cine MR CSF flow study in hydrocephalus: what are the valuable parameters? Acta Neurochir Suppl (Wien) 1998;71: 343–346
3. Holodny AI, George AE, Golomb J, et al. The perihippocampal fissures: normal anatomy and disease states. Radiographics 1998;18(3):653–665
4. Bradley WG Jr, Scalzo D, Queralt J, et al. Normal-pressure hydrocephalus: evaluation with cerebrospinal fluid flow measurements at MR imaging. Radiology 1996; 198(2):523–529

22

Restricted Diffusion

Diffusion weighted imaging (DWI) has primarily been discussed for its use in identifying acute infarcts. One of the additional main uses for DWI is in characterizing cystic lesions. The main differential considerations in this case are necrotic tumor versus abscess. Usually, brain abscesses have restricted diffusion and necrotic primary tumors or metastases do not. Magnetic resonance (MR) spectroscopy can supplement the DWI findings in equivocal cases or for a more definitive diagnosis. It has been suggested that high apparent diffusion coefficient (ADC) in abscesses may be due to a response to antibiotics. DWI is also commonly used to differentiate epidermoid cysts (restricted diffusion) from arachnoid cysts (no restricted diffusion). With increased clinical experience, many other causes of restricted diffusion and uses for DWI have been identified.

Causes of Restricted Diffusion

Common Causes

- Epidermoid
- Infarct (both arterial and venous)   Acute, sub-acute, generally up to 7 days
- Abscess   Except cysticercosis and toxoplasmosis

Less Common Causes

- 5FU toxicity: White matter, corpus callosum, can be seen early on

- Anoxic-ischemic encephalopathy: Involves both white matter (may be an early finding) and gray matter
- Carbon monoxide poisoning: May have abnormal signal and restricted diffusion in the white matter early on; white matter lesions may then resolve
- Creutzfeldt–Jacob disease: Cortex, basal ganglia
- Cyclosporin A toxicity: Corona radiata
- Demyelinating: Acute disseminated encephalo-myelitis, multiple sclerosis
- Incomplete rim: May be only mildly hyperintense on DWI
- Osmotic myelinolysis (central pontine myelinolysis): Pons; may precede findings on other sequences and CT; may involve extrapontine locations
- Seizures: Status epilepticus, generalized tonic-clonic, mesial temporal sclerosis (potentially in precipitating event)
- Venous thrombosis: May be reversible and not lead to infarction

Rare Causes

- Antiepileptic: medication-induced splenium lesions
- Encephalitis: Rotavirus (splenium), measles encephalopathy (T2-weighted MR images [T2WI], DWI, splenium), Salmonella enteritis (T2WI, DWI, splenium)
- Kearns–Sayre syndrome: Deep, gray nuclei and myelinated white matter tracts

- Methotrexate toxicity: Fronto-parietal corona radiata and splenium of corpus callosum
- Phenylketonuria: Same locations as T2WI abnormalities; mainly parietooccipital and periventricular, but can be frontal and sub-cortical when more severe
- Toxic/metabolic disorders: Maple syrup urine disease, Leigh, Wilson, and Canavan diseases

(although some of these processes also can have elevated diffusion, so this is not a helpful differentiating feature)
- Wernicke encephalopathy: Thalami, tectum, periaqueductal in the acute stage

Additional Readings

1. Bergui M, Zhong J, Bradac JB, et al. Diffusion-weighted images of intracranial cyst-like lesions. Neuroradiology 2001;43(10):824–829
2. Camacho DL, Smith JK, Castillo M. Differentiation of toxoplasmosis and lymphoma in AIDS patients by using apparent diffusion coefficients. AJNR Am J Neuroradiol 2003;24(4):633–637
3. Hakyemez B, Aksoy U, Yildiz H, et al. Intracranial epidermoid cysts: diffusion-weighted, FLAIR and conventional MR findings. Eur J Radiol 2005;54(2):214–220
4. Hartmann M, Jansen O, Heiland S, et al. Restricted diffusion within ring enhancement is not pathognomonic for brain abscess. AJNR Am J Neuroradiol 2001;22(9):1738–1742
5. Sener RN. Diffusion magnetic resonance imaging patterns in metabolic and toxic brain disorders. Acta Radiol 2004;45(5):561–570
6. Szabo K, Poepel A, Pohlmann-Eden B, et al. Diffusion-weighted and perfusion MRI demonstrates parenchymal changes in complex partial status epilepticus. Brain 2005;128(Pt 6):1369–1376
7. Thurnher MM, Castillo M. Imaging in acute stroke. Eur Radiol 2005;15(3):408–415

II Head and Neck

23

Focal Calvarial Lesions

Fibrous Dysplasia

Fibrous dysplasia is a developmental condition in which fibroosseous tissue replaces normal marrow within a portion of one (monostotic – 70 to 80%) or more bones (polyostotic). Polyostotic fibrous dysplasia (20 to 30%) involves multiple bones, and may have extensive skeletal involvement. Any bone may be involved, but the hip, proximal femur, tibia, cranial, and facial bones are most common. Although reported incidences vary, craniofacial and jaw involvement occurs in up to 50% of patients with polyostotic disease and in up to 25% of patients with monostotic disease.

Given the varied appearances of fibrous dysplasia, the differential diagnosis is extensive and includes ossifying fibroma, Paget's disease of bone, aneurysmal bone cyst, giant cell tumor, brown tumor of hyperparathyroidism, Langerhans cell histiocytosis, osteomyelitis, metastases, primary bone neoplasms, and unicameral bone cyst (**Table 23.1**).

Metastases

Metastatic neoplasms are discussed in Chapter 24 and in Chapters 141 and 142.

Table 23.1 Differentiating Features between Fibrous Dysplasia, Metastases, and Primary Bone Neoplasms*

	Fibrous Dysplasia	**Metastases**	**Primary Bone Neoplasms**
Bone Scan	Accumulates radioisotope Pathological fracture may also raise uptake.	Multiple areas of increased activity[†]	Solitary area of increased activity
MRI	T1WI: Low-to-intermediate signal intensity equal to muscle T2WI: Heterogeneous; commonly hyperintense to skeletal muscle but may be low, intermediate and/or high signal Enhancement: Patchy central, rim, homogeneous	T1WI: Low signal T2WI: Variable, may depend on degree of sclerosis; generally hyperintense; more conspicuous on FSE with fat saturation, STIR, IRFSE Enhancement: Generally, although may be variable due to degree of sclerosis	T1WI: Low-to-intermediate signal T2WI: Intermediate- to-high signal May have central areas of necrosis with blood products Enhancement: Heterogeneous (depends on cell-type and grade)

(Continued on page 68)

Table 23.1 *(Continued)* Differentiating Features between Fibrous Dysplasia, Metastases, and Primary Bone Neoplasms*

	Fibrous Dysplasia	Metastases	Primary Bone Neoplasms
CT Scan	Ground glass matrix with expansion of the bone Lytic or sclerotic May be heterogeneous with sclerotic foci Sclerotic more common in skull base and facial bones	May be lytic or sclerotic	Destructive ±periosteitis ±soft tissue mass Osteoid matrix in osteosarcoma Chondroid matrix (rings and arcs) in chondrosarcoma Destruction with relative maintenance of fat planes in chordoma
Distinguishing Features	Bone expansion May have fluid-fluid level Occasionally homogeneous on MRI Can narrow foramina and impinge neural structures	Often multiple lesions present	Depends on type Skull base involvement most common Solitary lesion

Abbreviations: CT, computed tomography; FSE, fast spin echo; IRFSE, inversion recovery fast spin echo; MRI, magnetic resonance imaging; STIR, short tau inversion recovery; T1WI, T1-weighted magnetic resonance imaging; T2WI, T2-weighted magnetic resonance imaging.

* See also Chapter 141

† Except myeloma

Primary Bone Neoplasms

The majority of primary skull lesions occur at the skull base where the most common lesions are chordoma and chondrosarcoma. Osteosarcoma, the most common primary tumor of bone, only rarely affects the head, where maxillary and mandibular lesions outnumber those of the calvarium or skull base. It may be related to prior radiation exposure or may develop secondary to Paget's disease or fibrous dysplasia. Rarely, hemangiomas can involve the skull. Although multiple myeloma commonly involves the skull, plasmacytomas are uncommon but can involve the calvarium, the skull base, or present as soft tissue masses of the head and neck.

Primary Bone Neoplasms Involving the Skull Base and Jugular Foramen

These are discussed in Chapters 25 and 26.

Additional Readings

1. Maroldi R, Ambrosi C, Farina D. Metastatic disease of the brain: extra-axial metastases (skull, dura, leptomeningeal) and tumour spread. Eur Radiol 2005;15(3):617–626
2. Murphey MD, Robbin MR, McRae GA, et al. The many faces of osteosarcoma. Radiographics 1997;17(5): 1205–1231
3. Pancholi A, Raniga S, Vohra PA, Vaidya V, Prajapati A, Mansingani S. "Imaging features of extramedullary plasmacytoma of skull base with multiple myeloma"- a rare case. Ind J Radiol Imag 2006;16(1):29–32
4. Shah ZK, Peh WC, Koh WL, et al. Magnetic resonance imaging appearances of fibrous dysplasia. Br J Radiol 2005;78(936):1104–1115
5. Singh AD, Chacko AG, Chacko G, et al. Plasma cell tumors of the skull. Surg Neurol 2005;64:434–438
6. Wenig BM, Mafee MF, Ghosh L. Fibro-osseous, osseous, and cartilaginous lesions of the orbit and paraorbital region. Correlative clinicopathologic and radiographic features, including the diagnostic role of CT and MR imaging. Radiol Clin North Am 1998;36(6): 1241–1259 xii.

24

Diffuse Calvarial Lesions

Processes that cause diffuse calvarial lesions are generally related to systemic or metabolic processes, metastases, or Paget's disease. The imaging appearance is quite variable, with some diseases causing lytic lesions, others causing sclerotic lesions, and still others giving a mixed pattern – even one that may change over the course of the disease, such as in Paget's disease. Often differentiating these lesions is not a diagnostic dilemma because of characteristic appearance (Paget's disease or diffuse metastases), or relevant clinical history.

Paget's Disease

Paget's disease of bone is a fairly common skeletal disease of uncertain etiology characterized by excessive and abnormal remodeling of bone with an imbalance between bone resorption and formation. The calvarium and skull base are commonly involved, as are the spine and pelvis. Basilar invagination can occur in the setting of skull base involvement. Although not initially a diffuse lesion, Paget's disease can progress to involve much of the calvarium.

The disease begins with a lytic phase, which appears as a destructive process affecting the inner and the outer tables of the skull. Classic teaching is that the inner table is spared, but this is not supported by the current literature. Later, there is a "mixed phase," which is characterized by coarsened trabeculae of increased volume, cortical thickening, and a heterogeneous signal

intensity on magnetic resonance imaging (MRI). The findings of cortical and trabecular thickening and preservation of areas of T1-hyperintense fatty marrow distinguishes Paget's disease from neoplastic infiltration. Areas of fibrovascular change are hypointense on T1-weighted MR images (T1WI) (with hyperintensity on T2-weighted MR images [T2WI]) giving the marrow a heterogeneous appearance, and enhance following contrast administration. In the final, blastic phase, osteoblastic activity supervenes and produces sclerotic areas, initially in a background of lysis. This patchy rounded sclerosis is described as a "cotton wool appearance" on the skull x-ray. Later in the blastic stage, there may be decreased marrow signal on all pulse sequences as the volume of the marrow cavity is decreased. Bone enlargement can occur at any stage. Computed tomography (CT) also demonstrates the plain radiographic imaging features of initial loss of trabeculae, followed by cortical and trabecular thickening with spared areas of fatty marrow, bony expansion, and eventually sclerosis. Sarcomatous degeneration, an uncommon sequela, presents on MRI and CT with cortical destruction, "mass-like" marrow replacement, and soft tissue masses.

Metastases

Diffuse calvarial metastasis may be sclerotic such as those arising from primary neoplasms of the prostate gland, breast, lung, stomach, and urinary bladder. In sclerotic metastases, there is new bone deposition in preexisting trabeculae and/or in the intratrabecular space, with trabecular thickening, marginal obscurity (the "silhouette" sign – where intratrabecular bone deposition obscures the margins of the trabeculae), and homogeneous dense sclerosis. Alternately, lytic metastases arise most commonly from lung, breast, and other adenocarcinomas due to increased osteoclastic activity. Renal and thyroid metastases are almost always lytic. Metastases can also demonstrate a mixed pattern. A technetium 99 (Tc-99m) bone scan is the most cost-effective and widely used imaging modality for evaluating for the presence of metastases, with metastasis generally demonstrating increased activity/uptake. MR is more sensitive than a bone scan for the detection of metastases, and CT and MR can better evaluate for associated soft tissue masses and cortical destruction. Metastases characteristically demonstrate low signal intensity on T1WI and variable (but generally hyperintense) signal on T2WI depending on the degree of sclerosis, with enhancement variable and best evaluated on fat suppressed T1WI (see Chapters 141 and 142).

Other Diffuse Bone Lesions

Multiple myeloma produces diffuse bone lesions that are lytic and "punched out" on plain radiographs. CT scanning is more sensitive for detecting lytic lesions, which may also demonstrate diffuse osteopenia, and rarely sclerosis. However, the true extent of disease is best demonstrated on MRI where solitary lesions are hypointense on T1WI, and diffuse disease produces diffusely decreased marrow signal on T1WI. Lesions are generally hyperintense on T2WI, and are best seen on fat-saturated sequences. Enhancement is variable and best demonstrated on fat-suppressed T1WI. Osteoporosis can also result in osteopenia.

Renal osteodystrophy may mimic malignancy because it can have a lytic or sclerotic appearance and can produce expansile masses (brown tumors). Other conditions that can cause bony sclerosis include myelofibrosis, fibrous dysplasia, fluorosis, mastocytosis, sickle cell disease, osteopetrosis, and tuberous sclerosis (see Chapters 141 and 142).

Additional Readings

1. Angtuaco EJ, Fassas AB, Walker R, et al. Multiple myeloma: clinical review and diagnostic imaging. Radiology 2004;231(1):11–23
2. Frank JA, Ling A, Patronas NJ, et al. Detection of malignant bone tumors: MR imaging vs scintigraphy. AJR Am J Roentgenol 1990;155(5):1043–1048
3. Scutellari PN, Giorgi A, De Sario V, Campanati P. Correlation of multimodality imaging in Paget's disease of bone. Radiol Med (Torino) 2005;110(5–6):603–615
4. Shah ZK, Peh WC, Koh WL, et al. Magnetic resonance imaging appearances of fibrous dysplasia. Br J Radiol 2005;78(936):1104–1115
5. Smith SE, Murphey MD, Motamedi K, et al. From the archives of the AFIP. Radiologic spectrum of Paget disease of bone and its complications with pathologic correlation. Radiographics 2002;22(5):1191–1216
6. Tigges S, Nance EP, Carpenter WA, et al. Renal osteodystrophy: imaging findings that mimic those of other diseases. AJR Am J Roentgenol 1995;165(1):143–148
7. Vanel D, Dromain C, Tardivon A. MRI of bone marrow disorders. Eur Radiol 2000;10(2):224–229

25

Skull Base Lesions

Many lesions can involve the skull base, with the majority due to extension of adjacent tumors or infection, or metastases. Primary skull base neoplasms are relatively uncommon. The most frequent primary malignancies are chordoma and chondrosarcoma and these lesions are often confused with each other. However, there are imaging features that can aid in their differentiation (**Table 25.1**).

Table 25.1 Differentiating Features between Chordomas and Chondrosarcomas

	Chordoma	Chondrosarcoma
Location	Clivus along sphenooccipital synchondrosis; less commonly petrous apex, sellar region, sphenoid sinus[a]	Generally off midline in skull base around petrooccipital fissure involving the petrous apex and clivus
CT	Expansile hyperattenuating soft tissue mass with lytic bone destruction and irregular calcifications; may have low attenuation areas[b]	Bone destruction; soft tissue mass with chondroid matrix
Enhancement	Moderate to marked; generally heterogeneous; may have "honeycomb" pattern	Heterogeneous; may be mild peripheral and septal ("pepper and salt appearance")
MRI	T1WI: Intermediate to low signal[c] T2WI: High signal with low signal septa[d, e]	T1WI: Low to intermediate[f] T2WI: High signal with low signal areas[g]
Vascular Effects	Vascular encasement and displacement are common, narrowing is rare	Vascular encasement and displacement are common, narrowing is rare
Calcifications	Irregular, either trapped bone or dystrophic; may have chondroid matrix	Chondroid matrix (linear, globular, arc-like)

Abbreviations: CT, computed tomography; MRI, magnetic resonance imaging; T1WI, T1-weighted MR images; T2WI, T2-weighted MR images.

[a] Intracranial (32% of chordomas).

[b] Thought to represent areas of myxoid and gelatinous material.

[c] May have small areas of hyperintensity related to blood or proteinaceous mucous.

[d] Low signal areas may be present due to calcification, hemorrhage, or proteinaceous mucous.

[e] Chondroid chordomas may not be as hyperintense as typical chordomas.

[f] May have punctate areas of hyperintensity on T1WI due to trapped yellow marrow.

[g] Low signal on all sequences may be due to matrix as well as fibrous or fibrocartilaginous elements.

Chordomas

Chordomas are tumors that arise from neuroectodermal remnants, and two types occur, typical or chondroid. They are generally midline tumors, and commonly occur related to the sphenooccipital synchondrosis, but can occasionally occur off midline. They are located in the skull base in 32%, spinal in 33%, and sacral in 29% of patients with the sacral lesions generally occurring in an older age group (20 to 40 years old versus 40 to 60 years old).

Chondrosarcomas

Chondrosarcomas are the third most common primary tumor of bone, although only 2% occur in the craniofacial region, with most affecting the skull base. Chondrosarcomas generally occur off midline and are often centered at synchondroses, namely the petrooccipital synchondrosis, with the majority in the petrous apex. The second most common location is the clivus (where they may be near the sphenooccipital synchondrosis. Most patients are between 30 to 44 years old. Chordomas and chondrosarcomas may appear similar; however, the appearance of a chondroid matrix and midline (chordoma) or off-midline (chondrosarcoma) location are the main differentiating imaging features, but in some cases they may be indistinguishable on imaging.

There is some overlap in the pathology, which can involve the skull base with lesions affecting the petrous apex and jugular foramen also extending into this region (see also Chapters 23, 24, 26, and 38).

Types of Lesions that Involve the Central Skull Base

Congenital/Developmental Lesions

- Cephaloceles
- Ecchordosis physaliphora

Inflammatory/Infectious/Miscellaneous Lesions

- Extension of sinus or mastoid disease
- Fungal disease
- Paget's disease
- Fibrous dysplasia
- Radiation necrosis
- Cholesterol granuloma (temporal bone region origin)
- Histiocytosis (rare)

Neoplasms

- Chordoma
- Chondrosarcoma
- Nasopharyngeal carcinoma: Extension to skull base directly and along cranial nerves
- Juvenile nasopharyngeal angiofibroma: Arises in region of sphenopalatine foramen and usually presents as nasopharyngeal or posterior nasal mass; may invade into sphenoid sinus or into temporal fossa; vascular
- Meningiomas: Associated with hyperostosis, blistering; signal similar to brain on noncontrast images; enhances
- Pituitary tumors, usually adenomas: May involve sphenoid sinus, ethmoids, nasopharynx
- Rhabdomyosarcoma: Children, skull base invasion common from nasopharyngeal muscular primary
- Metastases: More common than primary bone lesions – lytic or sclerotic depending on primary; enhance
- Perineural spread (PNS) of head and neck primary neoplasm: Squamous cell carcinoma and adenoid cystic carcinoma are the most common primary neoplasms associated with PNS
- Plasmacytoma/myeloma
- Lymphoma
- Dermoid/epidermoid
- Schwannoma
- Paraganglioma (temporal bone region origin; jugular foramen region origin)
- Endolymphatic sac tumor (temporal bone region origin, rare)
- Giant cell tumor (rare)
- Chondroblastoma, enchondroma (rare)

Additional Readings

1. Erdem E, Angtuaco EC, Van Hemert R, Park JS, Al-Mefty O. Comprehensive review of intracranial chordoma. Radiographics 2003;23(4):995–1009
2. Laine FJ, Nadel L, Braun IF. CT and MR imaging of the central skull base. Part 2. Pathologic spectrum. Radiographics 1990;10(5):797–821
3. Lowenheim H, Koerbel A, Ebner FH, Kumagami H, Ernemann U, Tatagiba M. Differentiating imaging findings in primary and secondary tumors of the jugular foramen. Neurosurg Rev 2006;29(1):1–11 discussion 12–13
4. Mehnert F, Beschorner R, Kuker W, Hahn U, Nagele T. Retroclival ecchordosis physaliphora: MR imaging and review of the literature. AJNR Am J Neuroradiol 2004; 25(10):1851–1855
5. Meyers SP, Hirsch WL Jr, Curtin HD, Barnes L, Sekhar LN, Sen C. Chondrosarcomas of the skull base: MR imaging features. Radiology 1992;184(1):103–108
6. Murphey MD, Walker EA, Wilson AJ, Kransdorf MJ, Temple HT, Gannon FH. From the archives of the AFIP: imaging of primary chondrosarcoma: radiologic-pathologic correlation. Radiographics 2003;23(5):1245–1278

26

Jugular Foramen Lesions

The most common neoplasms to be found in the jugular foramen are paragangliomas (glomus jugulotympanicum), schwannomas, or meningiomas (**Table 26.1**). A mimic of pathology in this region is heterogeneous enhancement within the jugular bulb on magnetic resonance imaging (MRI) due to mixing of blood and turbulence. A number of developmental variants also occur in this region, often better delineated on computed tomography (CT).

Table 26.1 Differentiating Features between Common Jugular Foramen Lesions

	Meningioma	Schwannoma	Glomus Jugulotympanicum
Posterior Fossa Involvement	Yes "En plaque" spread along dura	Yes Follows nerves superomedially toward lateral brainstem May be large and displace cerebellum	Uncommon Generally in larger tumors Not initial route of spread
Extracranial Involvement	Confined to nasopharyngeal carotid space	Nasopharyngeal carotid space May have a "dumbbell" appearance (intracranial and extracranial involvement)	Generally confined to nasopharyngeal carotid space
Bone Changes	"Permeative irregular" or "permeative sclerotic" appearance extending in all directions Normal bone density/architecture Hyperostosis not typical*	Expansion of jugular foramen with smooth sclerotic margins Without diploic space invasion "Scalloped" appearance	Localized skull base invasion with enlargement of jugular foramen and initially superolateral extension to hypotympanum Loss of bone density/architecture; destruction of caroticojugular spine and bony labyrinth "Permeative destructive" and "moth-eaten" appearance

Table 26.1 *(Continued)* Differentiating Features between Common Jugular Foramen Lesions

	Meningioma	Schwannoma	Glomus Jugulotympanicum
Middle Ear Involvement	Occasional	No	Common, particularly hypotympanum
CT	Dural-based, well-circumscribed mass Can have calcifications	Intracranial and extracranial components May be heterogeneous and have cystic degeneration (if large) No calcification	Soft tissue mass with intense, usually homogeneous enhancement
T1WI	Isointense to hypointense	Hypointense	Hypointense
T2WI	Intermediate	Hyperintense	Hyperintense
MRI - Contrast Enhancement	Moderate to Intense	Intense	Intense Homogeneous "Drop-out phenomena" with high-dose gadolinium and dynamic imaging[†]
MRI Flow Voids	No	Occasionally around periphery in large lesions	Yes
Other Salient Feature(s)	Dural tail	No dural tail Compress jugular vein/bulb	Invade the jugular bulb/vein and may have intraluminal growth "Salt-and-pepper" appearance (in tumors >1 cm) on short and long TR sequences Intense focal early (4 hour) uptake on indium-111 octreotide scan
Angiography	Avascular or hypovascular; may have a faint blush	Avascular or hypovascular	Hypervascular mass with enlarged feeding arteries, early draining veins, and intense blush

Abbreviations: CT, computed tomography; MRI, magnetic resonance imaging; T1WI, T1-weighted MR images; T2WI, T2-weighted MR images; TR, repetition time.

* May be present adjacent to more typical meningiomas that extend into the jugular foramen

[†] "Drop-out" phenomenon: On standard dose imaging, T1 shortening increases; hence, there is a rise in signal intensity following administration of a paramagnetic contrast agent. With high dose dynamic imaging (>0.3 mmol/kg), the magnetic susceptibility effect leads to initial predominant T2WI shortening (decreased signal intensity) and subsequently, the signal will then increase and T1WI shortening will become evident.

Schwannomas

Schwannomas of the jugular foramen usually arise from the ninth (glossopharyngeal) nerve and are rare.

Meningiomas

Primary jugular foramen meningiomas are uncommon and appear to behave differently than typical meningiomas that invade the jugular foramen secondarily. They are characterized by extensive infiltration of the skull base with involvement of neural canals and temporal bone structures.

Paragangliomas

Glomus jugulotympanicum tumors are paragangliomas that arise from either the tympanic branch of the glossopharyngeal nerve (Jacobson nerve), the auricular branch of the vagus nerve (Arnold nerve), or the jugular bulb, and occur along the dome of the jugular bulb or along the course of the two nerves, with 25% along the mucosa of the cochlear promontory (Jacobson's nerve). They are the second most common neoplasm of the temporal bone; they account for 60 to 80% of primary tumors of the jugular foramen.

Other Lesions and Anatomic Variants

Additional differential considerations in the jugular bulb region are enlarged jugular foramen, a high riding or dehiscent jugular bulb, jugular vein thrombosis, metastases, lymphoma, and primary bone lesions.

Differential Diagnosis of Jugular Foramen Lesions

Normal Variants

- Asymmetric jugular bulb
- High jugular bulb
- Dehiscent jugular bulb
- Jugular diverticulum

Neoplasms

- Paragangliomas
- Meningiomas
- Schwannomas
- Metastases

Miscellaneous Diagnoses

- Jugular vein thrombosis

Additional Readings

1. Caldemeyer KS, Mathews VP, Azzarelli B, Smith RR. The jugular foramen: a review of anatomy, masses, and imaging characteristics. Radiographics 1997;17(5): 1123–1139
2. Eldevik OP, Gabrielsen TO, Jacobsen EA. Imaging findings in schwannomas of the jugular foramen. AJNR Am J Neuroradiol 2000;21(6):1139–1144
3. Macdonald AJ, Salzman KL, Harnsberger HR, Gilbert E, Shelton C. Primary jugular foramen meningioma: imaging appearance and differentiating features. AJR Am J Roentgenol 2004;182(2):373–377
4. Rao AB, Koeller KK, Adair CF. From the archives of the AFIP. Paragangliomas of the head and neck: radiologic-pathologic correlation. Armed Forces Institute of Pathology. Radiographics 1999;19(6):1605–1632

27

Sinonasal Lesions

The majority of pathology within the sinonasal region is benign, with the overwhelming pathology being inflammatory disease. Of malignancies, squamous cell carcinoma makes up the majority. Because there is considerable overlap between nasal lesions and sinus lesions, and sinus lesions can invade the nasal cavity and vice-versa, these lesions will be discussed together as sinonasal lesions. Many of these lesions cannot be differentiated on imaging; however, some broad generalizations can be made regarding sinonasal malignancy and inflammatory processes (**Table 27.1**).

- Most malignancies have intermediate signal intensity on T2-weighted magnetic resonance images (T2WI), are heterogeneous, and have invasion of local structures. The exceptions are some salivary tumors and benign tumors such as some neuromas.

- Inflammatory tissue, including polyps, muceceles, retention cysts, and mucosal inflammation (including posttreatment inflammatory changes) generally have high-signal intensity on T2WI. However, mucoceles may have varying signal intensity based on composition and hydration status, although contrast can differentiate mucoceles from tumor by showing a peripherally enhancing rim. Another exception is mature granulation tissue, which may be intermediate in signal and indistinguishable from neoplasm.
- Lesions such as Wegener's granulomatosis can present with extensive destruction with little associated soft tissue mass.
- Polyps and inverted papilloma can cause bone expansion and remodeling without destruction.

Table 27.1 Differentiating Features between Inflammatory and Neoplastic Sinonasal Lesions

	Inflammatory Tissue*	Neoplasm	Mucocele
Signal on T1WI	Generally intermediate[†]	Generally intermediate	Generally intermediate; may be high[†]
Signal on T2WI	High[†]	Intermediate[††]	Generally high, but can be variable[†]
Enhancement	May be diffuse or peripheral	Solid or homogeneous	Peripheral
Bony Changes on CT	Remodeling, sclerosis, thinning	Erosion, destruction, invasion	Remodeling, dehiscence

Abbreviations: CT, computed tomography; T1WI, T1-weighted magnetic resonance images; T2WI, T2-weighted magnetic resonance images.

* Mature granulation tissue may appear similar to tumor.

[†] Secretions can vary based on protein composition and hydration and can be hypointense to hyperintense on T1WI and T2WI (see Chapter 28).

[††] With the exception of minor salivary tumors and some neural tumors, which can be hyperintense

- Location can play a role: inverted papillomas generally arise along the lateral nasal cavity, juvenile angiofibromas arise in the region of the sphenopalatine foramen and are very vascular, sinonasal undifferentiated carcinomas (SNUC) and esthesioneuroblastomas tend to be large when diagnosed and can both arise in the superior nasal cavity and ethmoid region

Lesions that Can Occur in the Sinonasal Region

Benign/Nonaggressive Lesions

- Osteoma, fibrous dysplasia, fibroosseous lesions, ossifying fibroma
- Wegener's granulomatosis
- Encephalocele, dermoid/epidermoid, nasal glioma
- Juvenile nasopharyngeal angiofibroma (centered in sphenopalatine foramen, vascular)
- Inflammatory (retention cysts, mucosal thickening, secretions, polyps, and mucoceles)

Malignant/Aggressive Lesions

- Squamous cell carcinoma (SCC) – most common malignancy (nonspecific mass with bony destruction 80 to 90% – maxillary sinus most common, then ethmoid)
- Neuroendocrine tumors:
    - Esthesioneuroblastoma (originates from olfactory epithelium and generally centered at the cribriform plate and may have intracranial extension)
    - SNEC (sinonasal neuroendocrine carcinoma), SNUC – commonly arise from ethmoid sinuses and superior nasal cavity
    - These tumors generally occur more anteriorly than nasopharyngeal carcinoma

- Minor salivary gland (4 to 10%) – high grade: intermediate signal on T2WI; lower grade: higher signal on T2WI
- Nonsalivary adenocarcinomas
- Inverted papilloma (has associated squamous cell carcinoma approximately in 5.5 to 27%)
- Non-Hodgkin's lymphoma
- Nasal cavity invasion from adjacent SCC, meningioma, chordoma
- Fibrous histiocytoma, sarcomas (rhabdomyosarcoma, osteosarcoma, chondrosarcoma, etc.)
- Metastases: Renal cell (most common)
- Melanoma (septum most commonly, then turbinates)

Additional Readings

1. Allbery SM, Chaljub G, Cho NL, Rassekh CH, John SD, Guinto FC. MR imaging of nasal masses. Radiographics 1995;15(6):1311–1327
2. Das S, Kirsch CF. Imaging of lumps and bumps in the nose: a review of sinonasal tumours. Cancer Imaging 2005;5:167–177
3. Kendi AT, Kara S, Altinok D, Keskil S. Sinonasal ossifying fibroma with fluid-fluid levels on MR images. AJNR Am J Neuroradiol 2003;24(8):1639–1641
4. Lanzieri CF, Shah M, Krauss D, Lavertu P. Use of gadolinium-enhanced MR imaging for differentiating mucoceles from neoplasms in the paranasal sinuses. Radiology 1991;178(2):425–428
5. Som PM, Shapiro MD, Biller HF, Sasaki C, Lawson W. Sinonasal tumors and inflammatory tissues: differentiation with MR imaging. Radiology 1988;167(3): 803–808

28

Abnormal Sinus Density and Signal

The signal and density of material related to inflammatory disease within the paranasal sinuses are generally intermediate to low on T1-weighted magnetic resonance (MR) images (T1WI), high on T2-weighted MR images (T2WI), and intermediate to lower density on computed tomography (CT), corresponding to their composition being ~95% water. However, this can be variable, depending primarily on the protein concentration of the material and the degree of hydration and viscosity. When protein concentration begins to rise, initially the signal becomes hyperintense on the T1WI and remains hyperintense on the T2WI, and then with further increase it begins to decrease on the T2WI. With further elevation in protein content however, the signal decreases on all sequence and eventually can become a signal void, without enhancement. This signifies desiccated solid or very viscous and semisolid contents. Often, these sinuses will have thin enhancing tissue, which is hyperintense on the T2WI around the periphery of the sinus or this signal will only be present in small areas within the sinus. Therefore, areas of signal void within otherwise opacified sinuses on MR imaging (MRI) do not necessarily signify air pockets as on CT scans. In addition, other substances (see the following subsection) can also mimic an aerated sinus. Because the imaging features of sinus pathology may be ambiguous on MRI, it is important always to obtain a CT scan in cases of sinus inflammatory disease.

Causes of Abnormal Sinus Signal and Density

The following signal abnormalities may involve part or all of a sinus.

Causes of Signal Void Sinus on MRI

Low or absent signal on T1WI and T2WI (signal usually lower on T2WI than T1WI). All signal void sinuses have increased density on CT except air.

- Inspissated, desiccated, concentrated, proteinaceous secretions (if sinus is either enlarged, with thickened walls, or has evidence of polyps [may be most evident only on postcontrast images], always consider an obstructed sinus with inspissated secretions.)
- Fungal sinusitis/mycetoma (probably due to above rather than paramagnetic effects)
- Calcification/bone
- Enamel (as in dentigerous cyst)
- Osteomas
- Fibrosis
- Air
- Acute hemorrhage

Causes of Hyperdense Sinus on CT

- Desiccated, proteinaceous secretions
- Fungal/mycetoma
- Polyps
- Hemorrhage
- Calcification

Additional Readings

1. Dillon WP, Som PM, Fullerton GD. Hypointense MR signal in chronically inspissated sinonasal secretions. Radiology 1990;174(1):73–78
2. Som PM, Dillon WP, Curtin HD, Fullerton GD, Lidov M. Hypointense paranasal sinus foci: differential diagnosis with MR imaging and relation to CT findings. Radiology 1990;176(3):777–781
3. Som PM, Dillon WP, Fullerton GD, Zimmerman RA, Rajagopalan B, Marom Z. Chronically obstructed sinonasal secretions: observations on T1 and T2 shortening. Radiology 1989;172(2):515–520
4. Yousem DM. Imaging of sinonasal inflammatory disease. Radiology 1993;188(2):303–314

29

Orbital Vascular Lesions

Vascular lesions represent a significant fraction of orbital masses and, as in the rest of the body, their characterization and classification are controversial, with frequent proposals for revision. Two of the more common lesions are varices and cavernous hemangiomas (**Table 29.1**).

Orbital Varix

Varices are the most common venous malformation of the orbit, and represent local dilation of one or more abnormal venous channels. They have been subcategorized as distensible and nondistensible, based on the presence of expansion with increased venous pressure or lack thereof. They are also characterized as primary or secondary based on the presence of associated intraorbital or intracranial arteriovenous shunts. Some have classified these lesions, especially the primary and nondistensible lesions, along a spectrum of orbital venous abnormalities with lymphangiomas. They are unilateral, more often left-sided, and

Table 29.1 Differentiating Features between Orbital Venous Varix and Cavernous Hemangioma

	Venous Varix	Cavernous Hemangioma
Age	Before 4th decade	Middle age (mean = 43 years old)
Gender Predilection	None	Predominantly female (70%)
Location	Mostly extraconal, superior	Mostly intraconal, lateral
Valsalva, etc.	Enlarges lesion	No effect
CT	Slightly hyperdense	Hypodense to muscle
	Appearance depends on thrombus/ hemorrhage	May have microcalcifications or phleboliths
	May have phleboliths	
T1WI	Hypointense to muscle*	Hypointense to muscle and fat
T2WI	Hypointense to muscle, flow voids*	Hyperintense to muscle with internal septations and hypointense fibrous rim
Angiography	Shows feeding and draining vessels, especially CTA	Occult MRI: No flow related enhancement
Dynamic Imaging/Enhancement	Early homogeneous enhancement, early washout	Slow progressive enhancement with delayed washout

Abbreviations: CT, computed tomography; CTA, CT angiography; MRI, magnetic resonance imaging; T1WI, T1-weighted MR images; T2WI, T2-weighted MR images.

* If thrombosed, will have signal of blood products.

more commonly related to and parallel to the superior ophthalmic vein than the inferior ophthalmic vein. The radiographic triad of an enlarged orbit with venous lakes and phleboliths is rarely seen. They are intensely enhancing, well-defined round or elongated mass lesions within or outside the muscular cone that taper toward the apex and may only be evident with provocative maneuvers such as Valsalva. Their precontrast density and intensity depends on the presence of thrombus or hemorrhage.

Cavernous Hemangioma

Cavernous hemangiomas are common lesions throughout the body, and are the most common orbital vascular lesions found in adults. They are said to be the most common primary orbital tumor in adults. Their etiology, natural history, histology, and imaging features are poorly understood, leading to controversial and conflicting classification systems. They typically present within the lateral aspect of the intraconal space, but can be found throughout the orbit. They are best characterized by dynamic multiphasic contrast-enhanced imaging, where they demonstrate slow progressive enhancement with persistence on delayed imaging.

They are well-defined, sharply marginated ovoid to round lesions, developing lobulations when large. They are homogeneously hypodense to muscle on unenhanced computed tomography (CT), isointense to muscle on T1-weighted magnetic resonance [MR] images (T1WI), and hyperintense with internal septations on T2-weighted MR images (T2WI) – a diagnostic feature when present.

Other Vascular Lesions

Lymphangiomas (more recently referred to as venous-lymphatic [venolymphatic] malformations) consist of varying degrees of venous and lymphatic components and may appear as multicystic lesions with variable associated enhancement of the venous component, as well as associated blood products. Capillary hemangiomas are vascular neoplasms that occur generally in infants. Hemangiopericytomas are vascular tumors that arise from pericytes and occur rarely in the orbit. They may behave more aggressively, but may appear similar to cavernous hemangiomas on imaging. However, they may have infiltrative margins and bony erosion and lack of hyperintensity on T2WI, which could differentiate them. Arteriovenous malformations as well as aneurysms can also occur.

Additional Readings

1. Ansari SA, Mafee MF. Orbital cavernous hemangioma: role of imaging. Neuroimaging Clin N Am 2005;15(1): 137–158
2. Ball WS, Towbin RB, Kaufman RA. Pediatric case of the day. Orbital varix. Radiographics 1987;7(6):1181–1182
3. Bilaniuk LT. Orbital vascular lesions. Role of imaging. Radiol Clin North Am 1999;37(1):169–183, xi.
4. Secil M, Soylev M, Ada E, Saatci AO. Orbital varices: imaging findings and the role of color Doppler sonography in the diagnosis. Comput Med Imaging Graph 2001;25(3):243–247
5. White JH, Fox AJ, Symons SP. Diagnosis and anatomic mapping of an orbital varix by computed tomographic angiography. Am J Ophthalmol 2005;140(5): 945–947

30

Orbital Lymphoproliferative and Inflammatory Disorders

Lymphoproliferative disorders can involve the orbit, and can be suggested by certain imaging characteristics. It can be difficult to separate benign (orbital pseudotumor, reactive lymphoid hyperplasia) from malignant (lymphoma) lymphoproliferative disorders based on imaging features, as they share many features in common (**Table 30.1**).

Orbital Pseudotumor

An orbital pseudotumor is an idiopathic nongranulomatous inflammation of the orbital contents, which is not related to an infection, neoplasm, or systemic disease. An orbital pseudotumor frequently involves the muscle cone or lacrimal gland, but can involve essentially any or all

Table 30.1 Differentiating Features between Lymphoma and Orbital Pseudotumor

	Lymphoma	Pseudotumor
Sites of Involvement	Commonly, the lacrimal gland, extraconal space (anterior and superior), extraocular muscles	Can involve any or all orbital structures Lacrimal gland most common site; extraocular muscles common
CT	Non-contrast: Isodense to slightly hyperdense to muscle/brain Mild to moderate diffuse enhancement	Soft tissue mass with no specific density values Variable, but often moderate contrast enhancement
MRI	T1WI: Isointense to mildly hyperintense to muscle T2WI: Isointense to hyperintense to muscle T1 +C Moderate to marked enhancement	T1WI: Hypointense to muscle T2WI: Isointense; may be hypointense if fibrotic T1 +C Moderate diffuse enhancement
Margins	May be well-defined mass, but may be infiltrative where lesion abuts orbital fat	Depends on site of involvement – well defined if involving lacrimal gland or muscles, or poorly defined and infiltrative
Bony Changes	Lesions tend to mold to bone and orbital structures without destruction; destruction generally only in aggressive lesions	Bony remodeling and foraminal expansion

(Continued on page 84)

Table 30.1 *(Continued)* Differentiating Features between Lymphoma and Orbital Pseudotumor

	Lymphoma	Pseudotumor
Atypical Features	Infiltrative appearance to fat May appear inflammatory	May extend through foramen, especially to cavernous sinus or temporal fossa
F18-FDG PET	Increased metabolic activity	? Not reported*

Abbreviations: CT, computed tomography; FDG PET, fluorodeoxyglucose positron emission tomography; MRI, magnetic resonance imaging; T1 +C, T1-weighted MR images with contrast; T1WI, T1-weighted MR images; T2WI, T2-weighted MR images.

*A case report has reported increased metabolic activity in pseudotumor, but no large series has been published.

orbital structures (myositis, dacryoadenitis, periscleritis, trochleitis, perineuritis and its diffuse form) and can occasionally extend through fissures into adjacent structures. Tolosa–Hunt syndrome is a variant of an orbital pseudotumor; it involves the orbital apex and cavernous sinus and is associated with a painful ophthalmoplegia. Imaging appearance varies depending on the site involved and can include lacrimal gland enlargement; scleritis; infiltration or thickening of extraocular muscles involving tendinous insertions; poorly circumscribed, infiltrative mass or well-circumscribed mass; infiltration of the intraconal fat and/or along the optic nerve sheath complex. Biopsy is usually required to differentiate benign from malignant lesions; however, clinical and radiographic findings can often provide some differentiation and a response to steroids can be highly suggestive of pseudotumor.

Lymphoma

The orbit can be involved by lymphoma either primarily or secondarily, and each has been found to occur with a near equal incidence. In addition, any structure of the orbit can be involved, with the sites of most frequent involvement being the lacrimal gland, extraconal space, and extraocular muscles, respectively. Other sites of involvement can include the eyelids, conjunctiva, and lacrimal sac, and rarely the optic nerve. When primary lymphoma involves the orbit, it is

usually a non-Hodgkin's lymphoma and often a low-grade mucosa-associated lymphoid tissue (MALT) lymphoma. Orbital involvement can uncommonly occur in leukemias and cause a focal mass (granulocytic sarcoma [chloroma]) or infiltration of the orbital fat, optic nerve, or globe (where the choroid is most frequently involved), and it may also involve the lacrimal glands and extraocular muscles.

Thyroid Eye Disease

Thyroid eye disease (TED; Graves disease, thyroid-related orbitopathy) can also provide an imaging differential diagnostic dilemma for the radiologist, and occasionally the clinician. Imaging findings generally consist of extraocular muscle involvement classically sparing the tendinous insertions, whereas pseudotumor characteristically involves the muscle belly as well as the tendinous insertions. TED typically involves the inferior rectus, then the medial and superior rectus, and is associated with eyelid edema and is uncommonly unilateral. Additional imaging findings include increased orbital fat, stretching of the optic nerve, proptosis, low signal in the muscles on computed tomography (CT), and high signal on magnetic resonance imaging (MRI). Pseudotumor may involve one or more muscles. Rarely, lymphoma can simulate these diseases and involve only the extraocular muscles. Tendinous sparing can also be a feature of malignancies.

Differential Diagnosis for Lesions with Similar Appearance to Lymphoma or Orbital Pseudotumor

- Differential can be very broad depending on sites of involvement and can include lacrimal gland tumors, as well as causes of myositis and thyroid ophthalmopathy.
- Neoplasm: Lymphoma, metastasis, histiocytosis, lipogranuloma, fibrosarcoma
- Inflammatory: Sarcoidosis, Sjögren disease, Wegener's granulomatosis, amyloidosis, fibromatosis
- Infection: Orbital cellulitis

Differential Diagnosis of Extraocular Muscle Enlargement

Common

- Thyroid ophthalmopathy
- Myositis/pseudotumor

Uncommon

- Carotid: cavernous fistula
- Neoplasm

Rare

- Autoimmune diseases: Myasthenia gravis, systemic lupus erythematosus, scleroderma, Wegener's granulomatosis
- Postviral, postvaccine
- Paraneoplastic
- Sarcoidosis
- Amyloidosis
- Cysticercosis
- Lyme disease
- Trichinosis
- Inflammatory bowel disease
- Whipple's disease

Additional Readings

1. Gufler H, Laubenberger J, Gerling J, Nesbitt E, Kommerell G, Langer M. MRI of lymphomas of the orbits and the paranasal sinuses. J Comput Assist Tomogr 1997;21(6):887–891
2. Sullivan TJ, Valenzuela AA. Imaging features of ocular adnexal lymphoproliferative disease. Eye 2006;20(10):1189–1195
3. Valvassori GE, Sabnis SS, Mafee RF, Brown MS, Putterman A. Imaging of orbital lymphoproliferative disorders. Radiol Clin North Am 1999;37(1):135–150, x–xi
4. Weber AL, Romo LV, Sabates NR. Pseudotumor of the orbit. Clinical, pathologic, and radiologic evaluation. Radiol Clin North Am 1999;37(1):151–168 xi

31

Optic Nerve-Sheath Complex Lesions

The optic nerve is unique among cranial nerves, in that it is a projection of the midbrain, myelinated by oligodendroglial cells. Its orbital and intracanalicular components are invested by a nerve sheath continuous with the intracranial meninges that delineates it from the intraconal fat. As such, the unit of the optic nerve and sheath share common pathologic processes, which can be related to intraconal or intracranial pathologies.

Meningiomas

Most meningiomas occurring in the orbit are primary optic meningiomas, which develop along the intraorbital or intracanalicular segments of the optic nerve, whereas secondary lesions originate along the intracranial dura, and spread into the orbit along the sheath. There are three patterns of growth: uniform tubular enlargement of the nerve sheath complex, fusiform spindle-shaped expansion, and excrescent outgrowth (**Table 31.1**). Although lacking specificity, the "tram track sign," where a hypointense/hypodense, and often atrophic optic nerve is demonstrated within a hyperintense/hyperdense/enhancing sheath, is the classic way to establish pathology that primarily involves the optic nerve sheath. It has been described for unenhanced computed tomography (CT), where the sheath may calcify, as well as enhanced CT and magnetic resonance imaging (MRI), where the sheath enhances preferentially.

Mild enhancement around the periphery of a non-enlarged nerve sheath complex can be normal. The most common cause of the "tram track sign" is meningioma. Very rarely, schwannomas can occur involving the optic nerve sheath complex.

Optic Gliomas

The most common optic nerve lesion is the optic glioma, representing 4% of orbital tumors, 4% of intracranial gliomas, and 2% of intracranial tumors. These are most commonly sporadic, although 10 to 38% of cases are associated with neurofibromatosis type 1. These lesions are characterized by fusiform homogeneous enlargement of the optic nerve. Buckling of the nerve and cystic changes may be present. Tumors are isointense to hypointense on T1-weighted MR images (T1WI), and isointense to hyperintense to cortex and normal nerve on T2WI. Contrast enhancement is variable on CT and MRI, from non-enhancing to intense, although it is generally less than that seen with meningioma (**Table 31.1**). Almost all of these are benign lesions, representing WHO grade 1 tumors. Malignant tumors, anaplastic astrocytomas, and glioblastoma multiforme (GBM), are exceedingly rare with 30 reported cases. They are isointense to hypointense to normal optic nerve with intense and diffuse enhancement on T1WI, and isointense to hyperintense on T2-weighted MR images (T2WI).

Table 31.1 Differentiating Features between Optic Nerve Sheath Meningioma and Optic Glioma

	Meningioma	Glioma
Clinical	Middle-aged (mean = 41 years old)	Pediatric (75% present <10 years old)
Gender Predominance	Female > male	Female > male
Non-contrast CT	Enlarged to atrophic nerve with hyperdense sheath	Homogeneously enlarged nerve, may buckle
Post-contrast CT	Peripheral enhancement with hypodense nerve	Heterogeneous to homogeneous enhancement
Calcification	20–50% – may reflect slow growth	None
T1WI	Hypointense to isointense to nerve	Hypointense to isointense to nerve
Enhancement	Marked	Variable
T2WI	Isointense to hyperintense to nerve	Hyperintense to nerve ±Cystic change
Local Reaction	Bone erosion more common than hyperostosis Pneumosinus dilatans	Enlargement of optic canal does not indicate intracranial extension

Abbreviations: CT, computed tomography; T1WI, T1-weighted magnetic resonance imaging; T2WI, T2-weighted magnetic resonance imaging.

Differential Diagnosis for Lesions Intrinsic to the Optic Nerve

- Optic neuritis
- Optic glioma
- Ganglioglioma: More rapidly progressive clinical course
- Medulloepithelioma
- Hemangioblastoma: More intense diffuse enhancement
- Choristoma: Hamartomatous lesion with fat and no enhancement

- Metastatic disease: Rare; suspect if known primary elsewhere
- Leukemia/ lymphoma: Usually involves optic nerve more prominently than sheath
- Orbital pseudotumor: Painful red eye, proptosis, impaired mobility; improves with steroids; also involves retrobulbar fat, extraocular muscles, and uveosclera
- Erdheim Chester: Rare, systemic disease
- Hemorrhage: Hyperdense, nonenhancing, MR variable based on age, sequence
- Hemangiopericytoma: Exceedingly rare

Causes of the Tram Track Sign

- Meningioma: Most common cause and classic description
- Perioptic neuritis (sarcoid, viral, syphilitic, or demyelinating)

Additional Readings

1. Belden CJ. MR imaging of the globe and optic nerve. Neuroimaging Clin N Am 2004;14(4):809–825
2. Hollander MD, FitzPatrick M, O'Connor SG, Flanders AE, Tartaglino LM. Optic gliomas. Radiol Clin North Am 1999;37(1):59–71, ix
3. Kanamalla US. The optic nerve tram-track sign. Radiology 2003;227(3):718–719
4. Mafee MF, Goodwin J, Dorodi S. Optic nerve sheath meningiomas. Role of MR imaging. Radiol Clin North Am 1999;37(1):37–58, ix

32

Lacrimal Gland Lesions

A variety of lesions can present as masses of the lacrimal gland and lacrimal fossa. Lesions are generally divided into epithelial and nonepithelial lesions. Epithelial lesions include the majority of neoplasms except lymphomas. Nonepithelial lesions are lymphoma and lymphoproliferative lesions, as well as other inflammatory processes. The neoplasms that involve the lacrimal gland are similar to lesions involving the salivary glands. Pleomorphic adenoma (benign mixed tumor,

BMT) is the most common tumor. Adenoid cystic carcinoma is the most common epithelial malignancy, and is often painful, whereas BMT is generally painless. Lymphoma is the most common nonepithelial malignancy. Inflammatory and lymphoproliferative lesions make up the majority of other lesions. It is not possible to differentiate benign and malignant processes on imaging alone, and resection or biopsy may be necessary (**Table 32.1**).

Table 32.1 Differentiating Features between Common Lacrimal Gland Neoplasms and Dermoids

	Pleomorphic Adenoma (BMT)	Adenoid Cystic Carcinoma	Dermoid
CT	Bony remodeling, fossa enlargement No bony erosion Can cause bony sclerosis Well marginated without infiltration Enhance	Bony erosion May have irregular infiltrative margins Nodularity Solid mass May contain cysts Enhance Can cause bony sclerosis	Bony remodeling/scalloping without destruction Fluid or fat tissue density well-circumcised lesion Thin wall enhancement May have surrounding inflammation/inflammatory tissue
MRI	T1WI: Hypointense to isointense T2WI: Hyperintense and may be heterogeneous T1WI + C: Moderate to marked enhancement	T1WI: Isointense T2WI: Hypointense to hyperintense depending on cellularity T1WI + C: Moderate to marked enhancement Obtain MRI skull base with fat suppression to evaluate for perineural spread	T1WI: Hypointense (most) to hyperintense depending on lipid content T2WI: Hyperintense T1WI + C and fat suppression: Hypointense Thin rim enhancement May have surrounding enhancement due to inflammation or with rupture

Table 32.1 (Continued) Differentiating Features between Common Lacrimal Gland Neoplasms and Dermoids

	Pleomorphic Adenoma (BMT)	Adenoid Cystic Carcinoma	Dermoid
Calcification	Rare	More common than in BMT and is suggestive of malignancy	May have partially calcified rim
Miscellaneous	May have malignant transformation that may manifest on imaging as rapid growth and clinically with pain	May have satellite nodules Infiltrative margins and nodularity are more common than in BMT May have perineural spread	May show fluid-fluid levels or fat-fluid level May have irregular dense areas within it on CT due to clumping of epithelial debris

Abbreviations: BMT, benign mixed tumor; CT, computed tomography; MRI, magnetic resonance imaging; T1WI, T1-weighted MR images; T2WI, T2-weighted MR images; T1WI + C, T1-weighted MR images with contrast.

Congenital lesions such as dermoid cysts are relatively common lesions presenting in the periocular region, and they commonly are located in or near the lacrimal fossa and the zygomaticofrontal suture. Depending on how they are defined, they are the most common noninflammatory space-occupying lesions of the orbit. Their appearance on imaging depends on their fat content, and unruptured cysts often have associated chronic (often asymptomatic) inflammatory changes. This can incite inflammation in and around the cyst wall as well as associated fibrosis and adhesion to adjacent structures.

Differences in signal intensity on magnetic resonance imaging (MRI) can help to differentiate various lesions. Chronic dacryoadenitis has been described to have signal intensity somewhat different from that of epithelial lesions and lymphoma, with low signal on T2-weighted MR images (T2WI), isointense signal on T1-weighted MR images (T1WI), and having moderate enhancement. Lymphoma has isointensity on the T1WI, heterogeneous isointensity to slight hyperintensity on T2WI, and moderate enhancement in their series. The nonepithelial lesions such as dacryoadenitis and lymphoma have a molded configuration conforming to the globe and bone,

whereas the epithelial tumors had rounded or oval configuration.

Differential Diagnosis of Lacrimal Gland and Lacrimal Fossa Masses

- Epithelial neoplasms
  - BMT: Most common benign neoplasm
  - Adenoid cystic carcinoma: Most common epithelial malignancy
  - Mucoepidermoid carcinoma, other salivary gland tumors
  - Squamous cell carcinoma
- Orbital pseudotumor
- Lymphoma
- Lymphoid hyperplasia
- Sarcoidosis
- Dermoid and epithelial cysts
- Sjögren's syndrome, Mikulicz syndrome
- Metastasis
- Acute or chronic dacryoadenitis
- Wegener's granulomatosis
- Amyloidosis (rare)
- Kimura's disease (rare)
- Schwannoma/neurofibroma (rare)
- Extension of paranasal sinus mucocele

Additional Readings

1. Abou-Rayyah Y, Rose GE, Konrad H, Chawla SJ, Moseley IF. Clinical, radiological and pathological examination of periocular dermoid cysts: evidence of inflammation from an early age. Eye 2002;16(5): 507–512
2. Gunduz K, Shields CL, Gunalp I, Shields JA. Magnetic resonance imaging of unilateral lacrimal gland lesions. Graefes Arch Clin Exp Ophthalmol 2003;241(11): 907–913
3. Mafee MF, Edward DP, Koeller KK, Dorodi S. Lacrimal gland tumors and simulating lesions. Clinicopathologic and MR imaging features. Radiol Clin North Am 1999;37(1):219–239, xii
4. Shields JA, Shields CL. Orbital cysts of childhood–classification, clinical features, and management. Surv Ophthalmol 2004;49(3):281–299
5. Shields JA, Shields CL, Epstein JA, Scartozzi R, Eagle RC Jr. Review: primary epithelial malignancies of the lacrimal gland: the 2003 Ramon L. Font lecture. Ophthal Plast Reconstr Surg 2004;20(1):10–21
6. Sigal R, Monnet O, de Baere T, et al. Adenoid cystic carcinoma of the head and neck: evaluation with MR imaging and clinical-pathologic correlation in 27 patients. Radiology 1992;184(1):95–101

33

Salivary Gland Lesions

The parotid gland is the most common site of salivary gland neoplasms; most (80 to 85%) are benign. Although the incidence of tumors in the submandibular and sublingual glands is lower, greater than 50% of neoplasms in these glands will be malignant (up to 80% of sublingual tumors). Fifty to 80% of minor salivary gland tumors are malignant, and malignant minor salivary gland tumors are most common in the soft palate followed by the paranasal sinuses, the nasal cavity, and the tongue. Approximately 90% of parotid tumors arise in the superficial lobe. Pleomorphic adenoma is the most common tumor in the parotid gland and the most common benign tumor in all salivary glands. It has certain characteristic imaging features (**Table 33.1**). However, imaging cannot definitively differentiate benign from malignant tumors, and various malignancies can occur related to pleomorphic adenoma. Low-grade malignancies can have imaging features similar to benign tumors. Warthin's tumors are the next most common benign tumors; they have cystic and solid components, may be bilateral in 10 to 15% of cases, and the solid components have intermediate to low signal on all sequences and can have mild enhancement. The most common malignancies are mucoepidermoid carcinoma (most common malignancy in the parotid) and adenoid cystic carcinoma (most common malignancy in other salivary glands). Lymph nodes are located in and around the parotid gland and can also be involved by pathologic processes. Non-neoplastic and inflammatory lesions can also occur.

Table 33.1 Differentiating Features between Benign and Malignant Salivary Gland Neoplasms

	Pleomorphic Adenoma[a]	Lymph Nodes[b]	Malignant Tumors[c]
MRI Signal	T1WI: Intermediate T2WI: Hyperintense with heterogeneity	Low	T1WI and T2WI[c]: Low to intermediate
Enhancement	Marked, heterogeneous May "fill-in" on delayed images	Mild	Inhomogeneous, mild to moderate
CT	All lesions have similar attenuation and the only potential differentiating features are the margins or invasion of parenchyma or adjacent structures.		
Hemorrhage	No	No	Occasionally
Calcifications	Occasionally	Rare[d]	Rare[d]

(Continued on page 92)

Table 33.1 *(Continued)* Differentiating Features between Benign and Malignant Salivary Gland Neoplasms

	Pleomorphic Adenoma[a]	Lymph Nodes[b]	Malignant Tumors[c]
Margins	May be lobulated, well defined	Well defined. May be lobulated; some metastatic nodes may have ill-defined margins	Ill defined[c]
Capsule	Yes (low signal)	Yes (can't see it)	No

Abbreviations: CT, computed tomography; MRI, magnetic resonance imaging; T1WI, T1-weighted MR images; T2WI, T2-weighted MR images.

[a] The next most common benign tumor, the Warthin's tumor has intermediate to low signal intensity on all sequences, can have cystic areas (which may be hyperintense on T1WI and may be similar to the cysts seen in mucoepidermoid carcinomas) and has mild enhancement on conventional imaging, and rapid enhancement and washout on dynamic imaging.

[b] Parotid and periparotid nodes

[c] True for all high-grade tumors. However, some low-grade tumors can be well defined and can have increased signal on T2WI mimicking pleomorphic adenomas (adenoid cystic, mucoepidermoid) or have cysts mimicking Warthin's tumor (mucoepidermoid).

[d] Calcifications may be present if: there is underlying Sjögren's syndrome or sarcoidosis; if malignancy arose in a pleomorphic adenoma; in salivary duct carcinoma; in lymph nodes and inflammatory masses mainly with granulomatous diseases

Lesions that Are Hyperintense on T2-Weighted Magnetic Resonance Imaging

Common

- Pleomorphic adenoma
- Cysts
  - ○ Retention cysts
  - ○ Abscess
  - ○ First branchial cleft cysts
  - ○ Ranula
  - ○ Sialocele
  - ○ Pseudocysts
  - ○ Benign lymphoepithelial lesions (BLELs; lymphoepithelial cysts): Cysts may not be fluid signal on T1WI due to complex contents, but will only peripherally enhance if at all.
- Warthin's tumor occasionally presents as a cystic lesion with small areas of nodularity in the wall.

Occasional

- Low-grade malignancies

Uncommon/Rare

- Hemangioma and hemangiopericytoma: Also enhance and can be considered in differential along with pleomorphic adenoma
- Basal cell adenoma can rarely present as an essentially cystic lesion.

Multiple Parotid Lesions

- Warthin's tumor
- Adenopathy (metastatic, lymphoma, inflammatory)
- Oncocytoma
- Acinic cell carcinoma
- BLELs (human immunodeficiency virus [HIV], Sjögren's syndrome)

Dynamic Imaging

- Pleomorphic adenoma: Areas that are hyperintense on T2-weighted magnetic resonance images (T2WI) have slow, but prolonged enhancement; areas that are low signal intensity on T2WI have rapid enhancement.

- Warthin's tumor: Solid components show rapid enhancement and washout.
- Basal cell adenoma: Rapid and prolonged enhancement

Types of Differential Diagnosis of Salivary Gland Lesions

- Benign neoplasms
  - Pleomorphic adenoma
  - Warthin's tumor
  - Monomorphic adenomas (basal cell adenoma and myoepithelioma)
- Malignant neoplasms
  - Mucoepidermoid carcinoma
  - Adenoid cystic carcinoma
  - Lymphoma
  - Metastases
  - Squamous cell carcinoma
  - Carcinoma ex pleomorphic adenoma (usually adenocarcinoma or salivary duct carcinoma)
  - Malignant mixed tumor (carcinosarcoma)

- Non-neoplastic lesions
  - Sialadenitis (Kuttner tumor: Focal mass-like area due to chronic sialadenitis)
  - Sialolith
  - Lipoma
  - Sarcoidosis
  - Cysts (retention cysts, first branchial cleft cysts, ranula, sialocele, pseudocysts)
  - Abscess
  - BLELs /lymphoepithelial cysts/ acquired immune deficiency syndrome (AIDS-) related parotid cysts
  - Sjögren's syndrome: Can have a "salt and pepper" appearance of hypointense and hyperintense areas on T2WI images or multiple cysts of varying sizes; BLELs
  - Granulomatous diseases
  - Sialosis: Painless enlargement due to various systemic diseases or medications
  - Kimura disease

Additional Readings

1. Licitra L, Grandi C, Prott FJ, Schornagel JH, Bruzzi P, Molinari R. Major and minor salivary glands tumours. Crit Rev Oncol Hematol 2003;45(2):215–225
2. Okahara M, Kiyosue H, Hori Y, Matsumoto A, Mori H, Yokoyama S. Parotid tumors: MR imaging with pathological correlation. Eur Radiol 2003;13(Suppl 4):L25–L33
3. Okahara M, Kiyosue H, Matsumoto S, et al. Basal cell adenoma of the parotid gland: MR imaging findings with pathologic correlation. AJNR Am J Neuroradiol 2006;27(3):700–704
4. Yousem DM, Kraut MA, Chalian AA. Major salivary gland imaging. Radiology 2000;216(1):19–29

34

Thyroid Diseases and Lesions

Thyroid nodules are commonly encountered and are seen in up to 41 to 67% of the population on ultrasound and in up to 50% of the population on autopsy. The incidence of cancer in thyroid nodules sent for fine-needle aspiration (FNA) is 9.2 to 13%, regardless of how many nodules are present in the gland. In patients with multiple nodules, the cancer is in the nondominant nodule approximately one third of the time.

Calcifications

Punctate, linear, eggshell, amorphous, and nodular calcifications can occur in benign and malignant thyroid tumors. Fine punctate calcifications are more characteristic of malignancy; when found within a solid nodule on ultrasound, they have been shown to predict a threefold increase in cancer risk. However, it has been reported that 38% of patients with microcalcifications had benign lesions. Calcifications have also been shown to become more prevalent as a patient ages and as the duration of multinodular goiter grows.

Cysts and Hemorrhage

Cysts have low T1-weighted and high T2-weighted magnetic resonance (MR) signal intensities. Cysts with high thyroglobulin concentrations are hyperintense on T1-weighted MR images (T1WI) and T2-weighted MR images (T2WI). Cysts with colloid or hemorrhage may also be hyperintense on T1WI. Hemorrhagic necrosis is prevalent in high-grade malignant tumors, especially in anaplastic carcinoma (60 to 70%), and less common in low-grade tumors. Hemorrhage may occasionally occur in a large goiter.

Cancer and Metastases

Papillary thyroid carcinoma appears isodense to muscle on CT, enhances, and has low attenuation areas and calcifications within it. On MR, it is isointense to muscle on T1WI with intermediate to high signal intensity on T2WI with heterogeneous enhancement. Cystic areas may have hemorrhage or high thyroglobulin content, causing increased signal intensity on T1WI. Lymph nodes from thyroid cancer can also have cystic areas and calcifications. Follicular carcinoma is only rarely cystic; it is usually well defined and may resemble an adenoma, but can also invade adjacent structures. Anaplastic thyroid carcinoma is usually large with areas of necrosis, hemorrhage, and invasion of neighboring structures. Medullary thyroid carcinoma is usually solid and well circumscribed, but may have coarse or psammomatous calcifications and local invasion or lymph node involvement. Thyroid lymphoma is most commonly seen in patients with Hashimoto's thyroiditis, and can appear as a solitary unencapsulated mass, multiple nodules, or a large bulky mass. It often appears hypointense on T1WI and T2WI with enhancement. Malignant lesions have been shown to have a significantly higher fluorodeoxyglucose (FDG) uptake on positron emission tomography (PET)/computed tomography (CT) and when combined with being of low density (but not cystic) on non-contrast low-dose CT scan, lesions had a higher likelihood of malignancy.

Differentiating Features of Benign and Malignant Lesions

Findings Associated with Malignant Lesions

- Irregular margins and penetration of pseudo-capsule, extraglandular extension
- Irregular thickening of the capsule may be seen in benign or malignant lesions
- Benign or malignant tumors may have well-defined margins
- Nodal involvement
- Invasion of trachea or larynx
- Calcifications, particularly fine punctate calcifications
- Distant metastases

Nondifferentiating Features

- Well-defined margins
- Irregular capsular thickening
- Size: No correlation between nodule size and the likelihood of malignancy

Findings Associated with Benign Lesions

- Purely cystic
- Eggshell calcifications: Although rarely may be malignant
- Processes involving the thyroid gland

Lesions Involving the Thyroid Gland

Common Thyroid Neoplasms

- Papillary thyroid carcinoma
- Follicular carcinoma
- Anaplastic carcinoma
- Medullary thyroid carcinoma: May be seen with multiple endocrine neoplasia type 2 (MEN2) A or B
- Hurthle cell carcinoma
- Lymphoma
- Metastases
- Squamous cell carcinoma
- Tall cell variant of papillary thyroid carcinoma

Infections/Inflammatory Diseases

- Infectious thyroiditis (acute – pyogenic, fungal, viral; granulomatous; de Quervain's thyroiditis)
- Hashimoto's disease, postpartum thyroiditis, Graves' disease (autoimmune)
- Riedel's thyroiditis: May be associated with other fibrosing conditions
- Sarcoid

Other Diseases

- Goiter (diffuse nontoxic goiter, multinodular goiter, toxic multinodular goiter)

Additional Readings

1. Choi JY, Lee KS, Kim HJ, et al. Focal thyroid lesions incidentally identified by integrated 18F-FDG PET/CT: clinical significance and improved characterization. J Nucl Med 2006;47(4):609–615
2. Frates MC, Benson CB, Charboneau JW, et al. Management of thyroid nodules detected at US: Society of Radiologists in Ultrasound consensus conference statement. Radiology 2005;237(3):794–800
3. Jhaveri K, Shroff MM, Fatterpekar GM, Som PM. CT and MR imaging findings associated with subacute thyroiditis. AJNR Am J Neuroradiol 2003;24(1):143–146
4. Weber AL, Randolph G, Aksoy FG. The thyroid and parathyroid glands. CT and MR imaging and correlation with pathology and clinical findings. Radiol Clin North Am 2000;38(5):1105–1129
5. Youserm DM, Huang T, Loevner LA, Langlotz CP. Clinical and economic impact of incidental thyroid lesions found with CT and MR. AJNR Am J Neuroradiol 1997;18(8):1423–1428

35

Carotid Space Masses

Once a mass is localized to the carotid space (also known as the poststyloid parapharyngeal space in the suprahyoid neck), the differential becomes narrow and relates to structures that occur within it. It contains mainly neural and vascular structures, including the structures within the carotid sheath, the carotid artery, the internal jugular vein (IJV), and the lower four cranial nerves. The sympathetic chain and phrenic nerve do not lie within the carotid sheath, but are considered within this "space." Lymph nodes also lie in this region. Differential considerations for pathology include paragangliomas and nerve sheath tumors arising from lower cranial nerves or from the sympathetic chain. Nodal metastasis, abscess, and venous thrombosis are also differential considerations as well as an extracranial carotid artery aneurysm. Lesions such as schwannomas or paragangliomas, which arise in the carotid sheath, will be intimately related to the vessels and may involve or separate them in characteristic patterns, whereas lymph nodes generally displace the carotid and jugular vessels together. Paragangliomas are generally hypervascular and may have shunting with early draining veins. Features such as these can aid in the differentiation of these lesions (**Table 35.1**).

Paragangliomas

The most common primary neoplasms arising from the carotid space are paragangliomas and nerve sheath tumors, with paragangliomas likely the most common. The most common paraganglioma has been suggested to be the carotid body tumor. The glomus jugulare is considered as prevalent if not more prevalent than the carotid body tumor by some authors; however, it is typically found at the skull base centered on the jugular foramen and not centered within the carotid space. The third most common paraganglioma is the glomus vagale, which arises from the nodose ganglion of the vagus nerve, but can arise from anywhere along the course of the vagus nerve. Paragangliomas may be multicentric and may manifest as unilateral or bilateral lesions. Paragangliomas can also occur as part of the multiple endocrine neoplasia (MEN) syndromes. Malignant behavior of head and neck paragangliomas is the same as in the rest of the body and occurs in 2 to 13% of those afflicted.

Nerve Sheath Tumors

Most nerve sheath tumors (schwannoma/neurofibroma) of the carotid space arise from cranial nerves 9 to 12 or the sympathetic chain. Vagal tumors tend to separate the IJV and the carotid artery. Cervical sympathetic chain tumors can displace the vessels anterolaterally and rarely can splay the internal carotid artery (ICA) and the external carotid artery (ECA) mimicking a carotid body tumor. Identification of the nerve origin is not always possible, but can be helpful to predict postoperative outcome.

Table 35.1 Differentiating Features of Carotid Space Lesions

	Location/Effect on Vessels	CT	T1WI	T2WI	MRI + Gad	Angiography
Carotid Body Tumor	Carotid bifurcation Splays ICA and ECA	Well-defined soft tissue mass Avid enhancement Rarely, enhancement may be heterogeneous due to hemorrhage or thrombi	Low signal with punctuate areas of T1 shortening due to hemorrhage or slow flow Punctate or serpentine flow voids on all sequences	"Salt and pepper"* Hyperintense	Avid enhancement If partially treated may have areas of decreased enhancement	Hypervascular mass that splays ECA and ICA Feeding artery from ascending pharyngeal and ascending cervical arteries Early draining vein
Glomus Jugulare (See Chapter 26)	Centered on the jugular foramen and prefers to extend superiorly into skull base Arises from Jacobson's nerve (CN 9) or Arnold nerve (CN 10) Can extend inferiorly	Soft tissue mass expands and erodes the jugular foramen Irregular bony margins may appear moth-eaten May extend into the middle ear	Similar to above	Similar to above	Similar to above	Hypervascular mass centered on the jugular foramen May receive blood supply from several sources including the ECA, ICA, and vertebrobasilar system
Glomus Vagale	Displaces both ICA and ECA anteromedially and IJV posterolaterally Two thirds are suprahyoid above bifurcation	Grows along the long axis of the nerve	Similar to above	Similar to above	Similar to above	Hypervascular mass displaces ECA and ICA anteromedially Usually above bifurcation Supply from ascending pharyngeal and occipital arteries

(Continued on page 98)

Table 35.1 (*Continued*) Differentiating Features of Carotid Space Lesions

	Location/Effect on Vessels	CT	T1WI	T2WI	MRI + Gad	Angiography
Schwannoma	If arising from vagus nerve, displaces the carotid vessels anteromedially and the IJV posteriorly If from sympathetic chain, all vessels are generally displaced anteriorly, but occasionally can splay the ICA and ECA	Well-defined encapsulated tumor isodense to muscle Varying degrees of enhancement 20% have cystic change Occasionally calcify	Hypointense	Hyperintense, but varies with cellularity May show variable signal change due to blood products, inflammation, and fibrosis	Enhances, may be avid May have nonenhancing areas	Hypovascular to hypervascular Characteristic puddling of contrast No arteriovenous shunting No early draining vein
Neurofibroma	Arise from vagus nerve and second from the cervical sympathetic chain (6)	Isodense to muscle Can be low attenuation May mimic cyst on NCE Variable enhancement Fusiform configuration along the course of the nerve	Hypointense	Hyperintense	Variable enhancement	Not well described

Abbreviations: CN, cranial nerve; CT, computed tomography; ECA, external carotid artery; ICA, internal carotid artery; IJV, internal jugular vein; Gad, gadolinium; MRI, magnetic resonance imaging; NCE, non-contrast enhanced; T1WI, T1-weighted MR images; T2WI, T2-weighted MR images.

* The salt is high signal representing slow flow or hemorrhage and the pepper is low signal representing flow voids. This sign is not specific. Metastatic thyroid and renal cell carcinoma may have this appearance.

Neurofibromas usually arise from the vagus nerve, then second from the cervical sympathetic chain. Differentiating between neurofibroma and schwannoma may be difficult or not possible on imaging.

Aneurysms

Extracranial carotid artery aneurysms are rare. The most common causes of extracranial carotid artery aneurysms are postcarotid endarterectomy, atherosclerotic degeneration, and trauma. Most arise from the bifurcation or proximal internal carotid artery, although post-traumatic ones may occur distally. A completely thrombosed aneurysm will not opacify with intravenous contrast. The age of thrombus may also affect the magnetic resonance imaging (MRI) appearance. Aneurysm must be considered if a round mass is found close to the vessels, especially if there are calcifications or imaging findings to suggest blood products or flow.

Differential Diagnosis of Carotid Space Lesions

- Paraganglioma
  - Carotid body tumor
  - (Glomus jugulare – inferior extension from jugular foramen)
  - Glomus vagale
- Nerve sheath tumors
  - Vagus nerve (CN 10)
  - Cranial nerves 9, 11, 12
  - Sympathetic plexus
- Adenopathy
  - Metastatic disease
  - Inflammatory/infectious
  - Reactive
- Infection/abscess
- Thrombosed jugular vein
- Extracranial carotid artery aneurysm/pseudo-aneurysm/dissection
- Congenital – branchial cleft cyst
- Pseudotumors
  - Ectatic or tortuous carotid artery
  - Asymmetric jugular vein
- Rare lesions
  - Lipoma
  - Liposarcoma

Additional Readings

1. Harnsberger HR, Osborn AG. Differential diagnosis of head and neck lesions based on their space of origin. 1. The suprahyoid part of the neck. AJR Am J Roentgenol 1991;157(1):147–154
2. Rao AB, Koeller KK, Adair CF. From the archives of the AFIP. Paragangliomas of the head and neck: radiologic-pathologic correlation. Armed Forces Institute of Pathology. Radiographics 1999;19(6):1605–1632
3. Silver AJ, Mawad ME, Hilal SK, Ascherl GF Jr, Chynn KY, Baredes S. Computed tomography of the carotid space and related cervical spaces. Part II: Neurogenic tumors. Radiology 1984;150(3):729–735
4. Smoker WR, Harnsberger HR. Differential diagnosis of head and neck lesions based on their space of origin. 2. The infrahyoid portion of the neck. AJR Am J Roentgenol 1991;157(1):155–159
5. Yousem DM. Suprahyoid spaces of the head and neck. Semin Roentgenol 2000;35(1):63–71

36

Congenital Cystic Neck Masses

The most common congenital cystic lesions of the neck are thyroglossal duct cysts (most common), branchial cleft cysts, and lymphatic malformations (**Table 36.1**).

Branchial Cleft Cysts

These lesions arise in remnants of the branchial apparatus, specifically from the cervical sinus

Table 36.1 Differentiating Features between Common Congenital Cystic Neck Masses

	Branchial Cleft Cyst	Thyroglossal Duct Cyst	Lymphatic Malformation
Location	Type II (most common) along anterior aspect of sternocleidomastoid, lateral to carotid sheath; may occur anywhere along line extending to palatine tonsil Type I – parotid, periauricular	Infrahyoid more common than at hyoid level, more common than suprahyoid at or near midline	Posterior cervical region in lower neck; less common in oral cavity, axilla, mediastinum, submandibular, sublingual, or parotid regions
MRI	T1WI: Hypointense T2WI: Hyperintense If infected can have increased signal on T1WI and thicker enhancing wall	T1WI: Hypointense to hyperintense T2WI: Hyperintense If infected can have increased signal on T1WI and thicker enhancing wall	T1WI: Hypointense to hyperintense T2WI: Hyperintense If infected can have increased signal on T1WI and thicker enhancing wall
CT	Fluid density unless hemorrhagic or infected	Fluid density, but may be more dense due to proteinaceous contents, thyroid tissue, hemorrhage, or infection	Fluid density unless infected or hemorrhagic
Distinguishing Features	Can be associated with fistula or sinus tract	Remodeling of hyoid bone	Can have fluid-fluid levels due to hemorrhage; multiloculated; ill-defined margins unless infected

Abbreviations: CT, computed tomography; MRI, magnetic resonance imaging; T1WI, T1-weighted MR images; T2WI, T2-weighted MR images.

of His or cell rests. These lesions typically appear as simple cysts on computed tomography (CT) and magnetic resonance imaging (MRI), with only a thin enhancing wall. The presence of current or prior infection, however, can result in increased density of cyst contents on CT and increased signal intensity on T1-weighted MR images (T1WI), heterogeneity, wall thickening, and irregularity. Branchial cleft anomalies may be cysts, sinuses, or fistulas. They involve the first through fourth branchial clefts, with the second branchial cleft anomalies the most common.

First Branchial Cleft Cyst

First branchial cleft (FBC) anomalies account for 8% to less than 10% of all branchial cleft defects. FBC anomalies occur along a tract extending from the floor of the external auditory canal to the submandibular region. They are classically divided into type I and type II, but probably represent a spectrum of lesions. Type I lesions present as cystic masses. They are generally in a preauricular location, or in or near the parotid gland. Type II lesions present as cysts, sinuses, fistulae, or any combination thereof. They may contain skin adnexal structures and cartilage. Generally, they are located near the angle of the mandible, posterior or inferior to it.

Second Branchial Cleft Cysts

Anomalies of the second branchial apparatus account for between 92 and 99% of branchial arch anomalies. They can occur anywhere along a line from deep to the platysma along the anterior aspect of the sternocleidomastoid muscle (type I), to the parapharyngeal space at the level of the palatine tonsil (type IV). Type II is located along the anterior aspect of the sternocleidomastoid muscle just lateral to the carotid sheath and posterior to the submandibular gland and is the most common. Type III extends between the internal and external carotid arteries. An associated sinus or fistula can occur

along this course, along the anterior aspect of the sternocleidomastoid muscle at the junction of its middle and inferior thirds, and extending from the skin to the pharynx in the region of the palatine tonsil.

Third and Fourth Branchial Cleft Cysts

Anomalies of the third branchial cleft are rare. These can be located on a course extending from the anterior margin of the sternocleidomastoid, below the level of the second arch anomalies, posterior to the common or internal carotid arteries, between the hypoglossal and glossopharyngeal nerves to the piriform sinus. They can be located in the posterior cervical region where they are the second most common congenital lesion (although rare).

Fourth branchial anomalies are usually fistulas and can occur anywhere along a path from the piriform sinuses, along the tracheoesophageal grooves into the superior mediastinum and back superiorly, along the course of the common carotid arteries to the skin along the anterior border of the sternocleidomastoid in the lower neck. Cysts generally occur anterior to the thyroid gland, generally on the left, and often present when superinfected with associated thyroiditis. They may mimic laryngoceles if adjacent to the larynx.

Lymphangioma

Lymphatic malformations are composed of a spectrum of entities, which have been classified in different ways, and some classifications include lymphangiomas and cystic hygromas, among other types. There are many theories on their pathogenesis. The majority presents in childhood, where they most commonly present in the lower posterior neck. They can also involve the oral cavity, axilla, or mediastinum. They can be seen in adults in the submandibular, sublingual, and parotid regions. On CT, they are typically of fluid density, but the density may be increased if there has been hemorrhage or infection. On MRI, they generally follow fluid, being hypointense on T1WI and hyperintense on T2WI; but if there has been hemorrhage, there may be increased signal on T1-weighted images, or fluid-fluid levels present due to layering and separation of blood products. Increased signal on T1WI may also be due to increased lipid or protein content. They are often multiloculated and poorly circumscribed; although the wall may become more evident if it becomes infected. They may be diagnosed prenatally with ultrasound or MRI.

Thyroglossal Duct Cysts

Thyroglossal duct cysts (TDCs) may occur anywhere along the course of the thyroglossal duct, from the foramen cecum in the tongue to the pyramidal lobe of the thyroid gland. They are most commonly present at or below the level of the hyoid bone. Suprahyoid cysts are generally midline, and infrahyoid off midline. The hyoid may be remodeled by the TDC, and they may have a component that extends to or into the hyoid bone. On imaging, they appear as simple cysts on CT and MRI unless they become

infected or hemorrhagic, in which case they can become more dense on CT and develop wall enhancement, and develop increased signal intensity on T1WI and a thicker, enhancing wall. Signal on T1WI can also vary due to protein content. Thyroid carcinoma occurs in less than 1% of TDCs.

Differential Diagnosis of Congenital Cystic Neck Masses

- Thyroglossal duct cyst
- Branchial cleft cyst
- Lymphangioma
- Cystic metastasis
- Dermoid
- Abscess
- Necrotic lymph node
- Laryngocele
- Ectopic thymic cyst
- Cystic schwannoma (rare)

In older people, although the congenital lesions are still possible, always consider a cystic or necrotic nodal metastasis in the differential diagnosis.

Additional Readings

1. Gadiparthi S, Lai SY, Branstetter BF 4th, Ferris RL. Radiology quiz case 2. Parapharyngeal second branchial cleft cyst. Arch Otolaryngol Head Neck Surg 2004; 130(9):1121, 1124–1125
2. Imhof H, Czerny C, Hormann M, Krestan C. Tumors and tumor-like lesions of the neck: from childhood to adult. Eur Radiol 2004;14(Suppl 4):L155–L165
3. Koeller KK, Alamo L, Adair CF, Smirniotopoulos JG. Congenital cystic masses of the neck: radiologic-

pathologic correlation. Radiographics 1999;19(1): 121–146 quiz 152–153
4. Samara C, Bechrakis I, Kavadias S, Papadopoulos A, Maniatis V, Strigaris K. Thyroglossal duct cyst carcinoma: case report and review of the literature, with emphasis on CT findings. Neuroradiology 2001;43(8): 647–649
5. Som PM, Curtin HD. Head and Neck Imaging. St. Louis, MO: Mosby; 2003: 1828–1840

37

Lymph Node Disease

Lymph Node Metastasis

Cervical metastatic lymph nodes are most commonly from squamous cell carcinoma of the head and neck. Other primary neoplasms include skin cancer, thyroid cancer, and with a lower frequency, lung, breast, and abdominal malignancies. Lymphoma also can involve the head and neck. Lymphomatous nodes are typically homogeneous, but can occasionally be necrotic, particularly after therapy and occasionally prior to therapy, especially in Hodgkin's disease and Burkitt lymphoma. Squamous cell carcinoma metastatic lymph nodes are often heterogeneous, with cystic or necrotic areas, and can have irregular margins, which are suggestive of extracapsular spread.

Imaging Criteria That Are Suggestive of Malignancy

- Short axis diameter >1 cm: Except the jugulodigastric nodes, which most authors say can be slightly larger, and the lateral retropharyngeal nodes, which are of concern when over 6 mm in the setting of known malignancy. The use of different size criteria at different levels to improve sensitivity (8, 9, 6, 7 mm for levels 1 to 4 and lower, respectively) has been suggested. Criteria may be different in N0 neck because by using these standard size criteria there is a relatively low sensitivity for metastatic disease. The use of 7 mm for level 2

and 6 mm for the remainder of the neck has been suggested.
- Rounded nodes with a ratio of the long axis to short axis <2
- Central necrosis (important to distinguish from a normal fatty hilum, which tends to be peripheral)
- Heterogeneous architecture
- Cystic neck mass in adult
- Calcification may be benign or malignant; if malignant, most commonly papillary thyroid carcinoma
- Extracapsular spread (poorly defined margins, adjacent infiltration, or fat stranding)
- Grouping of three or more 8 to 10 mm nodes in a primary drainage pathway
- Decreased iron oxide uptake (when imaging with supersmall ultraparamagnetic iron oxide contrast media)
- Increased metabolic activity on F18-fluorodeoxyglucose positron emission tomography (FDG PET)

Causes of Nonmalignant Adenopathy

Some rare conditions are mentioned, as it is important to consider them as they can mimic malignancy. Biopsy is generally required for diagnosis.

- Reactive adenopathy: Follicular hyperplasia related to infections, inflammation (current or prior)

- Viral infections: Nodes are generally diffuse, numerous, and normal to mildly enlarged; etiologies include mononucleosis, varicella, measles. Many occur mainly in immunocompromised hosts such as herpes simplex virus, cytomegalovirus, and HIV.
- Bacterial adenitis most commonly due to streptococcus and may be suppurative; etiologies also include syphilis, Lyme disease, and cat scratch disease.
- Mycobacteria, fungal and protozoal: Mostly in immunocompromised patients, and includes histoplasmosis, coccidioidomycosis, Cryptococcus, *pneumocystis carinii*, and toxoplasmosis.
- Sarcoidosis
- Kimura's disease: Generally involves parotid and submandibular regions and local lymph nodes; male predominance; predominantly in Asia; associated with eosinophilia and high-plasma immunoglobulin E (IgE)
- Rosai–Dorfman disease (sinus histiocytosis with massive lymphadenopathy): Very large nodes
- Castleman's disease (angiofollicular hyperplasia): Rare benign lymphoid tissue hyperplasia; most common in the mediastinum; 14% occur in the head and neck; can be multifocal; mainly occurs in cervical nodes, then the parotid and submandibular regions and occasionally Waldeyer's ring or mucosal surfaces
- Kawasaki's syndrome
- Kikuchi–Fujimoto disease (histiocytic necrotizing adenitis): Tender cervical adenopathy; predominantly posterior triangle; generally unilateral; may be necrotic; may have low-grade fever, skin lesions
- Systemic lupus erythematosus (SLE): Can have adenopathy with necrosis
- Posttransplantation lymphoproliferative disorder (PTLD): 1 to 10% of transplants, but relatively uncommon in neck; can have a mass with necrosis of Waldeyer's ring, large nodal masses, or groups of normal to borderline large nodes
- Leukemia, lymphoma
- Reactive to foreign bodies or substances
- Langerhans cell histiocytosis
- Anti-epileptic hypersensitivity syndrome: Rare; associated with generalized adenopathy, with necrotic nodes, mucocutaneous rash, fever, and hepatitis

Causes of Calcified Cervical Nodes

Cervical nodal calcification is uncommon. Conditions that more commonly calcify in the chest, such as tuberculosis (TB) or other granulomatous diseases calcify less frequently in the neck. Nodal calcification cannot be used to distinguish between malignant and benign disease. Also central and peripheral calcifications occur with relatively equal frequency in benign and malignant diseases. Either treated or untreated neoplastic causes must be considered as the etiology for calcified nodes.

- Metastases
  - Thyroid (most common; mainly papillary thyroid carcinoma, but reported with medullary and follicular carcinomas)
  - Lung and breast mucinous adenocarcinoma
  - Rarely colon adenocarcinoma
  - Rarely squamous cell carcinoma (oral cavity or pharynx)
- Treated Hodgkin's disease/lymphoma
- TB
- Sarcoid
- Amyloidosis
- Treated sinus histiocytosis with massive lymphadenopathy (Rosai–Dorfman disease)

Additional Readings

1. Castelijns JA, van den Brekel MW. Imaging of lymphadenopathy in the neck. Eur Radiol 2002;12(4): 727–738

2. Eida S, Sumi M, Yonetsu K, Kimura Y, Nakamura T. Combination of helical CT and Doppler sonography in the follow-up of patients with clinical N0 stage neck

disease and oral cancer. AJNR Am J Neuroradiol 2003;
24(3):312–318

3. Eisenkraft BL, Som PM. The spectrum of benign and
   malignant etiologies of cervical node calcification. AJR
   Am J Roentgenol 1999;172(5):1433–1437

4. Gor DM, Langer JE, Loevner LA. Imaging of cervical
   lymph nodes in head and neck cancer: the basics.
   Radiol Clin North Am 2006;44(1):101–110 viii

5. Gormly K, Glastonbury CM. Calcified nodal metastasis
   from squamous cell carcinoma of the head and neck.
   Australas Radiol 2004;48(2):240–242

6. Loevner LA, Karpati RL, Kumar P, Yousem DM, Hsu W,
   Montone KT. Posttransplantation lymphoproliferative
   disorder of the head and neck: imaging features in
   seven adults. Radiology 2000;216(2):363–369

7. Som PM, Brandwein MS. Lymph nodes. In Som PM,
   Curtin HD, eds. Head and Neck Imaging. St. Louis, MO:
   Mosby; 2003:1865–1934

8. Weber AL, Rahemtullah A, Ferry JA. Hodgkin and non-
   Hodgkin lymphoma of the head and neck: clinical,
   pathologic, and imaging evaluation. Neuroimaging
   Clin N Am 2003;13(3):371–392

38

Ear and Temporal Bone Lesions

Many pathologic entities can effect the ear and temporal bone, with the most common etiologies being inflammatory. Imaging can help differentiate between the various entities and help to determine the presence of residual/recurrent disease in the postoperative setting. One of the more common diagnostic imaging dilemmas, differentiating cholesteatoma from inflammatory tissue, particularly in the postoperative ear, will be addressed in detail here. Skull base lesions and jugular foramen lesions that can affect this region are addressed in Chapters 7, 25, and 26.

Cholesteatoma versus Chronic Otitis Media

Inflammatory processes, namely otitis media, either acute or chronic, most often affect the middle ear. The imaging characteristics of acute otitis media (AOM) include opacification of the middle ear and mastoids (otomastoiditis) without bony destruction. Complications of AOM included coalescent mastoiditis, subperiosteal, epidural or subdural abscess/empyema, petrous apicitis, dural sinus thrombosis, or associated soft tissue (Bezold's) abscess.

Chronic otomastoiditis (CO) may present with a variety of manifestations including effusion, granulation tissue, or cholesteatoma. A common diagnostic dilemma is to differentiate cholesteatoma from chronic inflammatory tissue (**Table 38.1**). Cholesteatomas are associated with bony erosion, most commonly of the scutum or ossicular chain, where the long process of the incus is most often affected. They may also erode intracranially. However, on postoperative studies, the finding of bony erosion is no longer reliable. On magnetic resonance imaging (MRI), they are moderately hyperintense to brain on T2-weighted magnetic resonance [MR] images (T2WI) and isointense on T1-weighted magnetic resonance [MR] images (T1WI) with or without moderate peripheral enhancement.

After surgery, if the middle ear and mastoidectomy defect are well aerated, the likelihood of recurrent cholesteatoma is low, and if a rounded tissue mass is present, it is high. If the mastoidectomy defect and middle ear are opacified, it can be difficult to distinguish cholesteatoma from postoperative tissue. The use of delayed post-contrast MR scanning with a 30 to 45 minute delay has been shown to have a high sensitivity and specificity for residual cholesteatoma 3 mm in size or greater. A postoperative scar will enhance on these delayed images, whereas cholesteatoma will not.

Diffusion weighted imaging (DWI) has shown promising results detecting cholesteatomas at initial presentation, but only mixed results in detecting residual cholesteatomas, where it may be hampered by artifact, and it is insensitive to small lesions. Cholesteatoma should be hyperintense on DWI. Cholesterol granuloma can have a similar appearance on DWI, but is generally hyperintense on T1WI facilitating differentiation.

Table 38.1 Differentiating Features of Cholesteatoma in Both Preoperative and Postoperative Patients from Granulation/Inflammatory Tissue

	Cholesteatoma, Preoperative	Cholesteatoma, Postoperative	Granulation/Inflammatory Tissue
T2WI	Hyperintense to brain	Hyperintense to brain	Hyperintense to brain
T1WI	Hypointense to Isointense to brain	Hypointense to Isointense to brain	Hypointense to isointense to brain
Contrast	±Peripheral enhancement	±Peripheral enhancement	+Enhancement
CT Bony Changes	Bony erosion: Characteristically of scutum, ossicles, tegmen tympani, sigmoid plate, bony labyrinth	Bony erosion less reliable	Generally no bony erosion of these areas in uncomplicated cases; however, bony erosion can occur in complicated otomastoiditis.
CT Soft Tissue	Soft tissue mass located in the middle ear, which may extend into mastoids	Rounded soft tissue mass highly predictive	Tissue within middle ear and/or mastoids
DWI	Hyperintense	Hyperintense	Hypointense

Abbreviations: CT, computed tomography; DWI, diffusion weighted imaging; T1WI, T1-weighted magnetic resonance images; T2WI, T2-weighted magnetic resonance images.

Lesions of the Ear and Temporal Bone

Many neoplasms can also involve the ear and temporal bones, and there is some overlap with lesions of the skull base and cerebellopontine angle, which often extend into this region (see Chapters 7, 25, and 26).

External Ear

Inflammatory Lesions

- Keratosis obturans
- External auditory canal cholesteatoma
- Postinflammatory medial canal fibrosis
- Malignant otitis externa

Neoplastic Lesions

- Basal and squamous cell carcinomas
- Melanoma
- Invasion from adjacent parotid tumors or squamous cell carcinoma
- Merkel cell carcinoma (rare)

- Angiosarcoma (rare)
- Tumors of glandular origin (e.g., ceruminous adenocarcinoma, adenoid cystic carcinoma [rare])
- Lymphoma (rare)

Middle/Inner Ear

Inflammatory Lesions

- Otitis media, otomastoiditis
- Cholesteatoma

Neoplastic Lesions

- Glomus tympanicum
- Metastases
- Invasion from adjacent parotid tumors or squamous cell carcinoma
- Hematopoietic malignancies
- Endolymphatic sac tumors (rare)
- Primary squamous cell carcinoma (rare)
- Giant cell tumor (rare)
- Adenocarcinoma (rare)

Mastoid/Petrous Apex

Inflammatory Lesions

- Otomastoiditis
- Cholesterol granuloma
- Petrous apicitis

Neoplastic Lesions

- Metastases
- Invasion from adjacent tumors (e.g., squamous cell carcinoma, chordoma, schwannoma, paraganglioma, meningioma, endolymphatic sac tumors)
- Chondrosarcoma

Additional Readings

1. Ayache D, Williams MT, Lejeune D, Corre A. Usefulness of delayed postcontrast magnetic resonance imaging in the detection of residual cholesteatoma after canal wall-up tympanoplasty. Laryngoscope 2005;115(4): 607–610
2. Devaney KO, Boschman CR, Willard SC, Ferlito A, Rinaldo A. Tumours of the external ear and temporal bone. Lancet Oncol 2005;6(6):411–420
3. Dubrulle F, Souillard R, Chechin D, Vaneecloo FM, Desaulty A, Vincent C. Diffusion-weighted MR imaging sequence in the detection of postoperative recurrent cholesteatoma. Radiology 2006;238(2):604–610
4. Maroldi R, Farina D, Palvarini L, et al. Computed tomography and magnetic resonance imaging of pathologic conditions of the middle ear. Eur J Radiol 2001; 40(2):78–93

39

Vocal Cord Lesions and Paralysis

Vocal Cord Paralysis

Vocal cord paralysis is usually diagnosed clinically. However, it can be an incidental finding on neck computed tomography (CT) as 35% of patients with unilateral vocal cord paralysis may be asymptomatic and may have a normal voice. Imaging is often performed to find the cause of the paralysis; however, a radiographic cause is not demonstrated in at least half of all patients. The finding of atrophy/paralysis of the pharyngeal constrictor muscles with resultant dilatation of the ipsilateral pharyngeal wall has been described to differentiate a central vagal paralysis from a peripheral paralysis. In addition, the cricothyroid muscle is innervated by the superior laryngeal nerve, which arises from the proximal vagus nerve. If atrophy of this muscle is identified, then a proximal or central vagal lesion/neuropathy is present. It is important to recognize the findings of vocal cord paralysis and not to confuse any of the findings, such as thickening of the aryepiglottic fold or fullness of the paralyzed vocal fold, with other causes such as neoplasm.

Laryngeal Neoplasm

Over 90% of laryngeal and hypopharyngeal tumors are squamous cell carcinoma. Squamous cell carcinoma can involve any or all portions of the larynx (i.e., subglottic, glottic, supraglottic).

CT and magnetic resonance imaging (MRI) are insensitive to superficial mucosal tumors without a significant exophytic component or submucosal extension. Two to five percent of laryngeal tumors will be non-squamous cell in etiology and several inflammatory and granulomatous processes can also involve the larynx.

Findings Suggestive of Vocal Cord Paralysis

- Thickening and medial positioning of the ipsilateral aryepiglottic fold*
- Dilatation of the ipsilateral piriform sinus*[††]
- Dilatation of the ipsilateral laryngeal ventricle*[††]
- Anterior and medial positioning of the ipsilateral arytenoid cartilage[†]
- Fullness of the ipsilateral true vocal cord[†]
- Paramedian cord position[††]
- Thyroarytenoid muscle atrophy (may be subtle)
- Ipsilateral subglottic fullness
- Dilatation of the ipsilateral vallecula
- Flattening of the ipsilateral subglottic arch
- Posterior cricoarytenoid atrophy

---

*Seen in greater than 75% of patients in a series by Chin et al.

[†]Seen in greater than 45% of patients in a series by Chin et al.

[††]Seen in 100% of cases (paramedian cord, piriform sinus dilation), 95% of cases (thyroarytenoid atrophy) and 90% of cases (enlarged laryngeal ventricle) in a series by Romo and Curtin.

Relatively Common Non-neoplastic Laryngeal Lesions

Except for laryngoceles, many non-neoplastic lesions are often not imaged.

- Laryngocele (saccular cyst)
- Sequela of gastroesophageal reflux (inflammation, [Reinke] edema, subglottic stenosis, vocal cord nodules, ulcers, granulomas)
- Vocal cord nodules/polyps, cysts
- Pharyngitis/supraglottitis

Uncommon/Rare Laryngeal Lesions

Although most tumors will be squamous cell tumors, many of the following neoplasms can be considered when a mass is present with intact mucosa, or if there are specific imaging features suggestive of these lesions. The inflammatory processes will often involve the mucosa.

- Vascular: Hemangioma/venous malformations (may have phleboliths); paraganglioma
- Kaposi's sarcoma
- Bone/chondroid: Chondroma, chondrosarcoma (stippled calcification, hyperintense on T2-weighted MR images [T2WI]); osteosarcoma
- Lymphoma, plasmacytoma
- Minor salivary gland tumors
- Lipomas, liposarcoma
- Laryngeal cyst
- Papilloma
- Hematoma
- Metastases (may have features in common with metastases in general from the same primary such as being hyperintense on T1-weighted MR images (T1WI) in melanoma, vascular in renal cell carcinoma, etc.)
- Inflammatory/granulomatous: Sarcoid, Wegener's granulomatosis, tuberculosis (TB), Teflon granuloma, rheumatoid arthritis, systemic lupus erythematosus (SLE), relapsing polychondritis, amyloid, reflux-related

Additional Readings

1. Becker M. Larynx and hypopharynx. Radiol Clin North Am 1998;36(5):891–920, vi
2. Becker M, Moulin G, Kurt AM, et al. Non-squamous cell neoplasms of the larynx: radiologic-pathologic correlation. Radiographics 1998;18(5):1189–1209
3. Chin SC, Edelstein S, Chen CY, Som PM. Using CT to localize side and level of vocal cord paralysis. AJR Am J Roentgenol 2003;180(4):1165–1170
4. Romo LV, Curtin HD. Atrophy of the posterior cricoarytenoid muscle as an indicator of recurrent laryngeal nerve palsy. AJNR Am J Neuroradiol 1999;20(3): 467–471

40

Head and Neck Cancer

Head and neck cancer is a collective term to describe malignant tumors of the aerodigestive tract, from the cervical esophagus through the nasal cavity, paranasal sinus and nasopharynx. Squamous cell carcinoma is the most common primary neoplasm in the head and neck, accounting for 90% of cancers arising in this region. The majority occur in the oral cavity, followed by the pharynx and larynx. Lymphoma is the second most common tumor of the head and neck: with nodal involvement most common and due to Hodgkin's disease, and extranodal involvement less frequent and due to non-Hodgkin's lymphoma. Aggressive appearing lesions within the aerodigestive tract should be assumed to be squamous cell carcinoma (or a subtype) with biopsy necessary for definitive diagnosis.

Site-Specific Differential Diagnosis of Head and Neck Cancer

Tonsil/Oropharynx

- Squamous cell carcinoma
- Lymphoma
- Adenocarcinoma
- Salivary gland tumors
- Melanoma
- Hodgkin's disease
- Sarcoma and metastatic tumors
- Lymphoepithelioma
- Plasmacytoma

- Lymphoid hyperplasia
- Thyroglossal duct cysts
- Lingual thyroid

Nasopharynx

Nasopharyngeal carcinoma occurs most commonly in the fossa of Rosenmüller and 60 to 72% of patients present with nodal metastases. It can invade locally as well as into the parapharyngeal space, carotid space, and skull base; it can also extend intracranially.

- Squamous cell carcinoma
- Lymphoma
- Minor salivary gland origin
- Benign tumors such as juvenile angiofibromas (arises in region of sphenopalatine foramen and may grow into nasopharynx)
- Thornwald cysts
- Retention cysts
- Hemangiomas
- Invasion downward from skull base tumors, meningiomas, or metastases

Oral Cavity

The palate is the most common site in the oral cavity for minor salivary gland tumors; malignant minor salivary gland tumors are most common in the soft palate.
- Squamous cell carcinoma (95% of malignancies)
- Minor salivary gland origin (adenoid cystic, pleomorphic adenoma, etc.)

- Lymphoma
- Melanoma
- Lipoma
- Dermoid/epidermoid
- Vascular (infantile hemangioma, venous or lymphatic malformations, arteriovenous malformations)
- Lingual thyroid
- Thyroglossal duct cysts
- Ranula
- Cellulitis/abscess

- Schwannoma
- Amyloidoma
- Osteomas
- Tori
- Fibrous dysplasia
- Fibroosseous lesions
- Odontogenic lesions

Larynx

See Chapter 39: Vocal Cord Lesions and Paralysis

Additional Readings

1. Chin SC, Fatterpekar G, Chen CY, Som PM. MR imaging of diverse manifestations of nasopharyngeal carcinomas. AJR Am J Roentgenol 2003;180(6):1715–1722
2. Chong VF, Fan YF. Radiology of the nasopharynx: pictorial essay. Australas Radiol 2000;44(1):5–13
3. Flis CM, Connor SE. Imaging of head and neck venous malformations. Eur Radiol 2005;15(10):2185–2193
4. Sigal R, Zagdanski AM, Schwaab G, et al. CT and MR imaging of squamous cell carcinoma of the tongue and floor of the mouth. Radiographics 1996;16(4): 787–810
5. Yousem DM, Chalian AA. Oral cavity and pharynx. Radiol Clin North Am 1998;36(5):967–981, vii

41

Lymphoma

Although squamous cell carcinoma (SCC) is the most commonly encountered neoplasm in the head and neck, lymphomas can arise in both nodal and extranodal sites in the head and neck and can be similar in appearance to squamous cell carcinomas (**Table 41.1**). The majority of head and neck lymphomas (and lymphomas in general) are non-Hodgkin's lymphomas (NHL).

Table 41.1 Differentiating Features between Lymphoma and Squamous Cell Carcinoma

	Lymphoma	SCC
Typical Appearance	Large bulky mass; occasionally infiltrative	May be mucosal lesion not evident on imaging to infiltrative enhancing lesion to bulky mass[a,b]
Associated Enlarged Lymph Nodes	Frequent	Depends on tumor site, size[c]
Ulceration and Irregular Margins	Rare	Common
CT	Homogeneous, isodense to muscle	Soft tissue density
MRI	T1WI: Intermediate	T1WI: Intermediate to mildly hypointense
	T2WI: Mildly hyperintense	T2WI: Low intermediate to high intermediate[b]
Contrast Enhancement	Yes, generally homogeneous	Yes, may be heterogeneous
Bony and Soft Tissue Invasion	Uncommon	Common
Most Common Sites	Waldeyer's ring; also, the orbit, sinonasal and salivary glands,[d,e] oral cavity, larynx, thyroid,[f] mandible, maxilla	Floor of the mouth, the tongue, soft palate, anterior tonsillar pillar, the retromolar trigone, and lip
Necrotic Nodes	Uncommon prior to treatment	Common

Abbreviations: CT, computed tomography; MRI, magnetic resonance imaging; SCC, squamous cell carcinoma; T1WI, T1-weighted MR images; T2WI, T2-weighted MR images.

[a] Appearance often depends on location. Small lesions involve the tongue, tonsil, vocal cords, and nasopharynx. Bulky lesions are more common in hypopharynx and supraglottic larynx, but may occur with advanced disease at other sites.

[b] A smaller, relatively hypointense on T2WI appearance to the tonsil has been described as a rare appearance of malignancy.

[c] Except nasopharyngeal cancer, where tumor size is unrelated to the presence of nodal metastases

[d] Parotid in up to 70 to 80%

[e] Associated with Sjögren syndrome in 20%

[f] Most commonly associated with Hashimoto's thyroiditis

Nodal involvement occurs with Hodgkin's disease in the head and neck in 24% and with NHL in 33%. The head and neck is also the second most frequent site of extranodal involvement by NHL (11 to 33%). NHL of the neck arises in lymph nodes in 65% of cases and in extranodal sites in 25 to 30% of cases. Waldeyer's ring is the most common extranodal location in the head and neck. Waldeyer's ring is the primary site of lymphoma in 5 to 10% of patients, and this area accounts for at least one third of extranodal sites of involvement. The tonsil is the most commonly involved site, followed by the nasopharynx. Including Waldeyer's ring, lymphoma can involve many of the sites that SCC involves, such as the sinonasal region and larynx, where it is usually supraglottic. Head and neck involvement by lymphoma is seen in the majority of patients with lymphoma associated with Sjögren syndrome. There may be additional findings associated with Sjögren syndrome such as lymphoepithelial lesions in the parotid glands.

Whereas lymphomas can commonly present as bulky masses, squamous cell carcinomas can present as small mucosal lesions that may not be evident on imaging with CT or MRI. Squamous cell carcinomas can also present as infiltrative lesions, or large bulky masses, with presentation often varying depending on the site of involvement. In the majority of cases, differentiation between squamous cell carcinoma, lymphoma, and other less common tumors such as minor salivary gland tumors, melanoma, or rare lesions can only be made by biopsy.

Additional Readings

1. King AD, Lei KI, Ahuja AT. MRI of primary non-Hodgkin's lymphoma of the palatine tonsil. Br J Radiol 2001;74(879):226–229
2. King AD, Yuen EH, Lei KI, Ahuja AT, Van Hasselt A. Non-Hodgkin lymphoma of the larynx: CT and MR imaging findings. AJNR Am J Neuroradiol 2004;25(1):12–15
3. Tonami H, Matoba M, Kuginuki Y, et al. Clinical and imaging findings of lymphoma in patients with Sjögren syndrome. J Comput Assist Tomogr 2003;27(4):517–524
4. Weber AL, Romo L, Hashmi S. Malignant tumors of the oral cavity and oropharynx: clinical, pathologic, and radiologic evaluation. Neuroimaging Clin N Am 2003; 13(3):443–464
5. Yasumoto M, Shibuya H, Takeda M, Korenaga T. Squamous cell carcinoma of the oral cavity: MR findings and value of T1-versus T2-weighted fast spin-echo images. AJR Am J Roentgenol 1995;164(4):981–987

42

Radiation Changes

Radiation-related changes can mimic recurrent or residual tumor, and can be difficult to differentiate from it. These changes are due to lymphatic and vascular obstruction, altered vascular permeability, and later on, fibrosis. Radiation-related changes have a characteristic pattern on both magnetic resonance imaging (MRI) and computed tomography (CT) that can help differentiate them from recurrent tumor. Radiation-related changes can affect the majority of the tissues of the head and neck. They can begin during therapy and many are present in virtually all patients from within 2 weeks following the end of therapy through 6 months following therapy. In many cases many of these changes begin to diminish after 6 months, but in some patients they can persist for much longer periods of time. The majority of patients will have laryngeal, pharyngeal, subcutaneous and epiglottic edema initially. Edema can persist, but in many patients these tissues will become fibrotic with time.

Findings Related to Radiation Changes

- Subcutaneous and deep fat edema
- Thickening of
  - Epiglottis
  - Aryepiglottic folds
  - Anterior and posterior commissures
  - Subglottic larynx
  - Posterior pharyngeal wall
  - Platysma

- Retropharyngeal and parapharyngeal edema
- Lymph node enhancement/atrophy
- Salivary gland inflammation/atrophy
- Muscle atrophy (after 8 months)
- Mastoid air cell opacification
- Paranasal sinus inflammatory changes
- Fatty replacement of marrow
- Osteoradionecrosis, chondronecrosis

Radiation-Related Changes versus Neoplasm Recurrence

The presence of a focal mass suggests neoplasm, but this finding is not specific for neoplasm, especially during radiation therapy and within the first 6 months after radiation therapy. Within the first 6 months, MRI cannot accurately differentiate tumor from radiation changes, as they can have a similar appearance (hyperintense on T2-weighted MR images (T2WI), intermediate on T1-weighted MR images (T1WI) with enhancement). After this time, due to fibrosis, tumor may be more accurately differentiated, as fibrosis will have a reduced signal on the T2WI, with low contrast enhancement. However, edema may also persist and a hypervascular scar may be present – these processes will not be accurately differentiated from neoplasm. Other findings indicative of persistent tumor following radiation have been described for laryngeal or hypopharyngeal tumors; they include a less than 50% reduction in size of the original tumor or a 1 cm or greater focal mass. A focal mass of less than 1 cm should be followed closely and correlated clinically. Serial imaging is helpful because if a mass increases in size it may be a neoplasm. Additional studies such as positron emission tomography (PET) imaging also can help differentiate tumor from treatment-related changes.

Additional Readings

1. Hermans R, Pameijer FA, Mancuso AA, Parsons JT, Mendenhall WM. Laryngeal or hypopharyngeal squamous cell carcinoma: can follow-up CT after definitive radiation therapy be used to detect local failure earlier than clinical examination alone? Radiology 2000; 214(3):683–687
2. Mukherji SK, Mancuso AA, Kotzur IM, et al. Radiologic appearance of the irradiated larynx. Part I. Expected changes. Radiology 1994;193(1):141–148
3. Nomayr A, Lell M, Sweeney R, Bautz W, Lukas P. MRI appearance of radiation-induced changes of normal cervical tissues. Eur Radiol 2001;11(9):1807–1817
4. Rabin BM, Meyer JR, Berlin JW, Marymount MH, Palka PS, Russell EJ. Radiation-induced changes in the central nervous system and head and neck. Radiographics 1996;16(5):1055–1072

III Chest

43

The Mosaic Pattern of Lung Attenuation

A mosaic pattern of attenuation, with patchy areas of increased and decreased attenuation, is nonspecific and may be seen on thin-section computed tomography (CT) of lungs when various infiltrative lung, airway, or vascular diseases are present (**Table 43.1**). When this pattern is caused by regional differences in perfusion due to vascular diseases, it is also known as *mosaic perfusion* or *mosaic oligemia.*

Differential Diagnosis of Mosaic

- Hypersensitivity pneumonitis
- Desquamative interstitial pneumonitis
- Nonspecific interstitial pneumonitis (NSIP)
- Sarcoidosis
- Pulmonary edema
- Atypical interstitial pneumonia
- Bronchiolitis obliterans

Table 43.1 Differentiating Features between the Various Diseases that May Cause CT Mosaic Lung Attenuation Pattern

Type of Disease	CT Findings		
	Attenuation	**Vessels**	**Air Trapping**
Infiltrative Lung	Ground glass	Normal size and number throughout lung	Not seen
Airway	Reduced (hypoxic vasoconstriction) Increased (regional hyperperfusion)	Decreased in size and number in areas of reduced attenuation	Seen at expiratory CT
Vascular	Reduced (obstructed flood flow) Increased (regional hyperperfusion)	Decreased in size and number in areas of reduced attenuation Increased in size and number in areas of increased attenuation	Not seen

Abbreviations: CT, computed tomography.

- Asthma
- Chronic pulmonary thromboembolism
- Pulmonary veno-occlusive disease

- Pulmonary arterial hypertension
- Polyarteritis nodosa

Additional Readings

1. Grenier P, Valeyre D, Cluzel P, et al. Chronic diffuse inter-stitial lung disease: diagnostic value of chest radiography and high-resolution CT. Radiology 1991;179: 123–128
2. Hansell DM, Wells AU, Padley SPG, Muller NL. Hypersensitivity pneumonitis: correlation of individual CT patterns with functional abnormalities. Radiology 1996;199:123–128
3. Muller NL, Miller RR. Diseases of the bronchioles: CT and histopathologic findings. Radiology 1995;196:3–12
4. Primack SL, Muller NL, Mayo JR, Remy-Jardin M, Remy J. Pulmonary parenchymal abnormalities of vascular origin: high-resolution CT findings. Radiographics 1994; 14:739–746
5. Stern EJ, Muller NL, Sewnson SJ, Hartman TE. CT mosaic pattern of lung attenuation: etiologies and terminology. J Thorac Imaging 1995;10:294–297
6. Stern EJ, Swenson SJ, Hartman TE, Frank MS. CT mosaic pattern of lung attenuation: distinguishing different causes. AJR Am J Roentgenol 1995;165:813–816
7. Worthy SA, Muller NL, Hartman TE, Swenson SJ, Padley SG, Hansell DM. Mosaic attenuation pattern on thin-section CT scans of the lung: differentiation among infiltrative lung, airway and vascular diseases as a cause. Radiology 1997;205:465–470

44

The Tree-in-Bud Pattern

One characteristic feature of bronchiolar disease is a tree-in-bud pattern on computed tomography (CT); the other is centrilobular nodules. The tree-in-bud pattern was first used as a descriptor by Im et al. to describe the appearance of the endobronchial spread of mycobacterial tuberculosis. This pattern is manifested by luminal filling of contiguous branching segments of bronchioles seen in bronchiolar disease. Bronchiolitis and bronchiolectasis are nonspecific inflammatory processes (sometimes associated with fibrotic bronchiolitis) of the small airways caused by many different conditions. Imaging of bronchiolar disease is best performed by thin-section CT.

Bronchiolar Anatomy

Bronchioles, small airways with an internal diameter of <2 mm, do not contain cartilage in their walls, consist of membranous or terminal bronchioles that are purely air conducting, and respiratory bronchioles containing alveoli in their walls, distal to the 7th or 8th generation of the tracheobronchial tree. The secondary pulmonary lobule, measures 10 to 25 mm in diameter, is the smallest portion of the lung that is surrounded by connective tissue septa. Each lobule is supplied by a lobular bronchiole (≤1 mm in diameter) and a pulmonary artery branch, both of which are located in the center of the secondary lobule. Because visibility on CT is typically limited to bronchi >2 mm in

diameter, normal lobular bronchioles cannot be seen on CT scans. However, diseased bronchioles (bronchiolar wall thickening, bronchiolar dilatation, and luminal impaction) can be visualized as a tree-in-bud pattern. This pattern is analogous to the large airway "finger-in-glove" appearance of bronchial impaction, but on a much smaller scale. Indirect signs of bronchiolar disease on CT include mosaic attenuation, air trapping, and subsegmental atelectasis especially on expiratory CT scanning.

Differential Diagnosis Based on a Tree-in-Bud Pattern

- Infections: The tree-in-bud pattern is most commonly seen with infectious causes of bronchiolitis (e.g., viral, mycoplasma, mycobacterial).
- Hypersensitivity pneumonitis due to organic or inorganic inhaled agents and respiratory bronchiolitis, due to cigarette smoking, could have similar imaging findings of poorly defined centrilobular nodules, mosaic attenuation, and ground-glass opacities.
- Immunologic disorders: Allergic bronchopulmonary aspergillosis (ABPA). The fungus proliferates in the proximal bronchi resulting in central bronchiectasis with upper lobe predominance (finger-in-glove appearance on chest radiographs). In some cases, extension of mucoid impaction to the bronchioles can have a tree-in-bud pattern on CT.

- Congenital disorders: Cystic fibrosis. It is a hereditary disease of the exocrine glands, transmitted as an autosomal recessive trait. Abnormal secretions are produced by the salivary and sweat glands, pancreas, large bowel, and tracheobronchial tree. The CT findings include bronchial wall thickening, bronchiectasis, bronchiolectasis, and mucus plugs. A large amount of bronchiolar secretions can produce a tree-in-bud pattern. Dyskinetic cilia syndromes are inherited abnormalities of ciliary structure and function. One of these syndromes, Kartagener's syndrome, is characterized by the clinical triad of situs inversus, sinusitis, and bronchiectasis. Abnormal ciliary motion in the respiratory tract results in recurrent bronchial infections that lead to bronchiectasis. Airway damage can extend to the smaller airways and this can lead to bronchiolectasis and centrilobular opacities (tree-in-bud pattern on CT).
- Neoplasms: Juvenile laryngotracheobronchial papillomatosis. Aspiration: The tree-in-bud pattern can be an uncommon presentation of commonly seen aspiration.
- Idiopathic causes: Diffuse panbronchiolitis is a chronic obstructive lung disease of obscure cause, reported almost exclusively in Asians, primarily in Japanese.[6] Most affected individuals are nonsmokers, and almost all have chronic sinusitis. The histologic features are centered around the respiratory bronchiole and consist of a transmural infiltrate composed of lymphocytes and plasma cells. Mucus and neutrophils fill the lumina of infected bronchioles.
- Obliterative bronchiolitis results from a variety of lung conditions including infection, collagen vascular disorders, inhalation of toxic fumes, and transplantation (lung and bone marrow); it is frequently idiopathic.[7] Obliterative bronchiolitis is characterized by fibrotic material in the bronchi and concentric narrowing of the bronchioles associated with submucosal and peribronchiolar fibrosis, leading to chronic airway obstruction. Findings on CT vary and include normal to thickened bronchiolar walls, bronchiolar dilatation, bronchiectasis, and air trapping (seen especially on expiratory CT scans). Centrilobular opacities from luminal impaction may also be seen. These findings could mimic those seen in asthma, panlobular emphysema, and neuroendocrine hyperplasia.
- CT findings of bronchiolar disease are seen in 10 to 40% of CT scans of patients with asthma.

Pitfalls in Diagnosing Bronchiolar Disease

Granulomatous processes that can create a false pattern of bronchiolar disease include sarcoidosis, silicosis, and Langerhans cell granulomatosis (eosinophilic granulomas). The main features that differentiate sarcoidosis from bronchiolitis are pronounced involvement of the proximal airways, perivenule perilymphatic nodularity, and lymphadenopathy. Silicosis and Langerhans cell granulomatosis involve the upper lobes predominantly and may have other characteristic findings (massive pulmonary fibrosis in silicosis and cysts in Langerhans). Follicular bronchiolitis is a form of lymphoid hyperplasia (seen in Sjögren's syndrome, rheumatoid arthritis, immunodeficiency), characterized by coalescent germinal centers distributed along airways (unlike luminal filling of contiguous branching segments of bronchioles seen in bronchiolar disease resulting in a tree-in-bud pattern). Lymphangitic carcinomatosis, from both lymphatic and hematogenous spread, can have reticulonodular pattern. This generally is not confused with a tree-in-bud pattern because the nodular and linear opacities are not contiguous.

Classification of Bronchiolar Disorders

Primary Bronchiolar Disorders

- Constrictive bronchiolitis (obliterative bronchiolitis or bronchiolitis obliterans)
- Acute bronchiolitis
- Diffuse panbronchiolitis
- Respiratory bronchiolitis (smoker's bronchiolitis)

- Mineral dust airway disease
- Follicular and lymphocytic bronchiolitis
- Other primary bronchiolar disorders (diffuse aspiration bronchiolitis, lymphocytic bronchiolitis)

Interstitial Lung Diseases with a Prominent Bronchiolar Involvement

- Hypersensitivity pneumonitis (HSP)
- Respiratory bronchiolitis-associated interstitial lung disease (ILD)/desquamative interstitial pneumonia (DIP)

- Cryptogenic organizing pneumonia (bronchiolitis obliterans organizing pneumonia [BOOP] or proliferative bronchiolitis)
- Other ILD (pulmonary Langerhans' cell histiocytosis, sarcoidosis, bronchiolocentric interstitial pneumonia)

Bronchiolar Involvement in Large Airway Diseases

- Chronic bronchitis
- Bronchiectasis
- Asthma

Additional Readings

1. Akira M, Kitatani F, Lee Y-S, et al. Diffuse panbronchiolitis: evaluation with high-resolution CT. Radiology 1988;168:433–438
2. Aquino SL, Gamsu G, Webb WR, Kee ST. Tree-in-bud pattern: frequency and significance on thin section CT. J Comput Assist Tomogr 1996;20:594–599
3. Collins J, Blankenbaker D, Stern EJ. CT patterns of bronchiolar disease: what is "tree-in-bud"? AJR Am J Roentgenol 1998;171:365–370
4. Garg K, Lynch DA, Newell JD, King TE. Proliferative and constrictive bronchiolitis: classification and radiographic features. AJR Am J Roentgenol 1994;162:803–808
5. Hartman TE, Primack SL, Lee KS, Swenson SJ, Muller NL. CT on bronchial and bronchiolar diseases. Radiographics 1994;14:991–1003
6. Im JG, Itoh H, Shim YS, et al. Pulmonary tuberculosis: CT findings – early active disease and sequential change with antituberculous therapy. Radiology 1993;186: 653–660
7. Muller NL, Miller RR. Diseases of the bronchioles: CT and histopathologic findings. Radiology 1995;196:3–12

45

Ground-Glass Opacity

Ground-glass opacity (GGO) describes a finding on high-resolution computed tomography (HRCT) of the lungs in which there is hazy increased attenuation of the lung, with preservation of bronchial and vascular margins. This should not be confused with consolidation in which bronchovascular margins are obscured. The GGO is caused by partial filling of air space, interstitial thickening, partial collapse of alveoli, normal expiration, or increased capillary blood volume. Because GGO can represent either interstitial or alveolar processes, beyond the resolution of HRCT technique, the complete differential diagnosis is long.

Differential Diagnosis of Ground-Glass Opacity

- Alveolar proteinosis: Pulmonary alveolar proteinosis is a disease of the lung that results in filling in of the alveoli by a periodic acid-Schiff-positive proteinaceous material rich in lipid. The underlying cause is speculated to be dust (particularly silica) exposure or an immunologic disturbance (caused by acquired immune deficiency syndrome [AIDS] or other immunodeficiency, hematologic or lymphangitic malignancy, or chemotherapy). Superinfections occur, most notably with nocardiosis.
- Acute chest syndrome or sickle cell disease: The opacities seen on chest CT represent pneumonia or infarction due to microvascular occlusion.

- Acute lung transplant rejection: New lung opacities in the immediate period after lung transplantation can be due to infection, rejections, reperfusion edema, or fluid overload.
- Adult respiratory distress syndrome (ARDS): It is characterized by refractory hypoxemia and respiratory distress caused by nonhydrostatic pulmonary edema. Leaky capillary membranes lead to extravasation of protein-rich fluid into the interstitial and alveolar spaces of the lung, leading to a decrease in normal inflated lung volumes and a decrease in lung compliance.
- Pulmonary hemorrhage: This can be diffuse, patchy, or focal depending on the underlying cause. Pulmonary renal syndromes that cause pulmonary hemorrhage including Goodpasture's syndrome, Wegener's granulomatosis, systemic lupus erythematosus, Henoch–Schonlein purpura, mixed connective tissue disease, and other vasculitides.
- Cryptogenic organizing pneumonia (COP; also called idiopathic bronchiolitis obliterans organizing pneumonia [BOOP]): This is a disease characterized histologically by the presence of granulation tissue plugs, which occupy and often occlude respiratory bronchioles and alveolar ducts. The CT findings of COP include GGO, nodules, or areas of consolidation with a predominant peripheral bilateral and nonsegmental distribution.

Without a history of recent trauma, a peripheral distribution of GGO on CT suggests a diagnosis of eosinophilic pneumonia, COP, sarcoidosis, or drug toxicity.

Additional Causes of Ground-Glass Opacity

- Bronchoalveolar lavage
- Bronchiolitis-associated interstitial lung disease
- Cytomegalovirus and other pneumonias (*pneumocystis carinii*)
- Cancer and lymphoproliferative disorders
- Collagen vascular disease
- Contusion
- Drug toxicity
- Desquamative interstitial pneumonitis
- Extrinsic allergic alveolitis
- Eosinophilic pneumonia
- Edema
- Fibrosis
- Granulomatous disease (e.g., sarcoidosis)

Additional Readings

1. Austin JHM, Muller NL, Friedman PJ, et al. Glossary of terms for CT of the lungs: recommendations of the Nomenclature Committee of the Fleischer Society. Radiology 1996;200:327–331
2. Bessis L, Callard P, Gotheil C, Biaggi A, Grenier P. High-resolution CT of parenchymal lung disease: precise correlation with histologic findings. Radiographics 1992;12:45–58
3. Engeler CE, Tashjian JH, Trenkner SW, Walsh JW. Ground-glass opacity of the lung parenchyma: a guide to analysis with high-resolution CT. AJR Am J Roentgenol 1993;160:249–251
4. Klein J, Gamsu G. High-resolution computer tomography of diffuse lung disease. Invest Radiol 1989;24:805–812
5. Remy-Jardin M, Remy J, Giraud F, Wattinne L, Gosselin B. Computed tomography assessment of ground-glass opacity: semiology and significance. J Thorac Imaging 1993;8:249–264
6. Swensen SJ, Aughenbaugh GL, Douglas WW, Myers JL. High-resolution CT of the lungs: findings in various pulmonary diseases. AJR Am J Roentgenol 1992;158:971–979
7. Webb WR, Muller NL, Naidick DP. High-resolution CT of the lung. 2nd ed. Philadelphia: Lippincott-Raven; 1996

46

The Halo Sign

The halo sign refers to a zone of ground-glass opacity surrounding a pulmonary nodule or mass on computed tomography (CT).

In severely neutropenic patients, the CT halo sign is highly suggestive of infection by an angioinvasive fungus, most commonly *aspergillus*. Most common risk factors for mucormycosis are uncontrolled diabetes mellitus, hematologic malignancies, treatment with corticosteroids, renal transplantation, and acquired immune deficiency syndrome (AIDS). The presence of a halo of ground-glass attenuation is usually associated with hemorrhagic nodules. Pulmonary Kaposi's sarcoma typically manifests on chest CT images as ill-defined, flame-shaped nodules, predominantly seen in a peribronchovascular distribution.

Rarely, the halo sign can be seen in post-transplantation lymphoproliferative disorders and lung cancer, especially with lipidic growth seen in bronchioalveolar carcinoma.

Not withstanding this wide spectrum of associated diseases, the CT halo sign is a useful diagnostic clue in the appropriate clinical setting and may be the first evidence of pulmonary fungal infection.

Differential Diagnosis of Diseases that Cause the Halo Sign on Computed Tomography

Infectious Diseases

- Common: *Aspergillus*
- Less common: mucormycosis, pulmonary candidiasis, coccidioidomycosis, and *Nocardia*
- Uncommon: Tuberculosis, mycobacterium avium complex, *Coxiella burnetii*, cytomegalovirus, herpes simplex virus, and myxovirus

Neoplastic Diseases

- Lung metastasis from hypervascular tumors such as angiosarcoma, choriocarcinoma, osteosarcoma, Kaposi sarcoma
- Primary lung cancer: Bronchioalveolar carcinoma (BAC)

Miscellaneous Diseases or Conditions

- Wegener's granulomatosis
- Necrotizing vasculitis
- Posttransbronchial biopsy
- Eosinophilic pneumonia
- Cryptogenic organizing pneumonia

Additional Readings

1. Carignan S, Staples CA, Muller NL. Intrathoracic lymphoproliferative disorders in the immunocompromised patient: CT findings. Radiology 1995;197: 53–58

2. Gaeta M, Caruso R, Barone M, Volta S, Casablanca G, LaSpada F. Ground-glass attenuation in nodular bronchioalveolar carcinoma: CT patterns and prognostic value. J Comput Assist Tomogr 1998;22:215–219

3. Kazerooni EA, Cascade PN, Gross BH. Transplanted lungs: nodules following transbronchial biopsy. Radiology 1995;194:209–212
4. Kuhlman JE, Fishman EK, Siegelman SS. Invasive pulmonary aspergillosis in acute leukemia: characteristic findings on CT, the CT halo sign, and the role of CT in early diagnosis. Radiology 1985;157:611–614
5. Primack SL, Hartman TE, Lee KS, Muller NL. Pulmonary nodules and the CT halo sign. Radiology 1994;190: 513–515
6. Pinto PS. The CT halo sign. Radiology 2004;230:109–110
7. Webb WR, Muller NL, Naidich DP. Diseases characterized primarily by nodular and reticulonodular opacities. In High Resolution CT of the Lung. Philadelphia, PA: Lippincott Williams and Wilkins; 2001:259–353

47

The Crazy-Paving Pattern

The crazy-paving pattern is a common finding at thin-section computed tomography (CT) of the lungs. It consists of scattered or diffuse ground-glass attenuation with superimposed interlobular septal thickening and intralobular lines; this finding has a variety of causes. **Table 47.1** details the features of some of the more common conditions associated with the crazy-paving pattern.

Differential Diagnoses Related to Crazy-Paving Pattern on CT

Infectious Disease

- *Pneumocystis carinii* pneumonia (PCP)
- Bacterial pneumonia
- Tuberculosis
- Mycoplasma pneumonia
- Chronic eosinophilic pneumonia

Neoplastic Disease

- Mucinous bronchioloalveolar carcinoma (BAC)

Idiopathic Disease

- Pulmonary alveolar proteinosis (PAP)
- Sarcoidosis
- Nonspecific interstitial pneumonia (NSIP)
- Organizing pneumonia

Disease Caused by Inhalation

- Lipoid pneumonia
- Acute respiratory distress syndrome
- Drug-induced pneumonitis
- Acute interstitial pneumonia

Table 47.1 Differentiating Features between Common Etiologies of Crazy-Paving Patterns

Condition	Salient Features
Pneumocystis carinii **Pneumonia**	History of HIV or AIDS
Pulmonary Alveolar Proteinosis	Bilateral perihilar and hilar distribution resembles pulmonary edema. The diagnosis is established by bronchioalveolar lavage.
Sarcoidosis	Associated nodules in bronchovascular distribution, lymphadenopathy
Nonspecific Interstitial Pneumonia	Diagnosis of exclusion; cellular NSIP has better prognosis than other interstitial pneumonias

Abbreviations: AIDS, acquired immune deficiency syndrome; HIV, human immunodeficiency virus; NSIP, nonspecific interstitial pneumonia.

Disease Associated with Hemorrhage

• Pulmonary hemorrhage syndromes

• Diffuse alveolar damage superimposed on usual interstitial pneumonia

Additional Readings

1. Gruden JF, Huang L, Turner J, et al. High-resolution CT in the evaluation of clinically suspected pneumocystis carinii pneumonia in AIDS patients with normal, equivocal, or nonspecific radiographic findings. AJR Am J Roentgenol 1997;169:967–975
2. Kuhlman JE. Pneumocystic infections: the radiologist's perspective. Radiology 1996;198:623–635
3. Lee KS, Kim Y, Han J, Ko EJ, Park CK, Primack SL. Bronchioloalveolar carcinoma: clinical, histopathologic, and radiologic findings. Radiographics 1997;17: 1345–1357
4. Rossi SE, Erasmus JJ, Volpacchio M, et al. "Crazy-paving" pattern at thin-section CT of the lungs: radiologic-pathologic overview. Radiographics 2003;23:1509–1519

48

The Angiogram Sign

This sign describes the visualization of normal pulmonary vascular architecture within parenchymal consolidations. Causes are

- Bronchioalveolar cell carcinoma
- Infectious or noninfectious pneumonia and pneumonitis
- Primary pulmonary lymphoma
- Passive atelectasis
- Lipoid pneumonia
- Pulmonary hemorrhage

Additional Readings

1. Im JG, Han MC, Yu EJ, et al. Lobar bronchioalveolar carcinoma: angiogram sign on CT. Radiology 1990;176: 749–753

2. Shah RM, Friedman AC. CT angiogram sign. Incidence and significance in lobar consolidation evaluated by contrast enhanced CT. AJR Am J Roentgenol 1998;170: 719–721

49

The Feeding Vessel Sign

The feeding vessel sign seen on computed tomography (CT) consists of a distinct vessel leading directly into the center of a nodule. This sign has been considered highly suggestive of septic embolism. The feeding vessel sign also occurs in pulmonary metastasis, hemorrhagic nodules, or consolidation seen in vasculitis. Septic emboli are seen most commonly in patients with infective endocarditis, patients with infective venous catheters or pacemaker leads, and in patients with periodontal disease. The characteristic CT manifestations of septic emboli include ill-defined, spherical nodules or wedge-shaped subpleural opacities, and the feeding vessel sign. Sometimes on multiplanar reconstructions, the apparent feeding vessel is shown to pass around the opacity or nodules instead of entering it. The feeding vessel, in some cases, represents a pulmonary vein, which can be traced to the left atrium.

The feeding vessel sign is a nonspecific finding; however, in combination with pleural-based wedge-shaped opacity, it may represent vasculitis. In combination with peripheral multiple ill-defined nodules in patients with indwelling venous catheters and history of fever, it may support a diagnosis of septic emboli.

Arteriovenous malformation (AVM) is a distinct entity seen with a feeding artery and a draining vein. Up to 60% of patients with pulmonary AVM will have hereditary hemorrhagic telangiectasia (HHT) or Osler–Weber–Rendu syndrome. Conversely, ~29% of patients with HHT will have pulmonary AVMs.

Additional Readings

1. Dodd JD, Souza CA, Muller NL. High-resolution MDCT of pulmonary septic embolism: evaluation of the feeding vessel sign. AJR Am J Roentgenol 2006;187:623–629
2. Hoen B, Alla F, Selton-Suty C, et al. Changing profile of infective endocarditis: results of a 1-year survey in France. JAMA 2002;288:75–81
3. Huang RM, Naidich DP, Lubat E, Schinella R, Garay SM, McCauley DI. Septic pulmonary emboli: CT-radiographic correlation. AJR Am J Roentgenol 1989;153:41–45
4. Kuhlman JE, Fishman EK, Teigen C. Pulmonary septic emboli: diagnostic with CT. Radiology 1990;174: 211–213
5. Murata K, Takahashi M, Mori M, et al. Pulmonary metastatic nodules: CT-pathologic correlation. Radiology 1992;182:331–335
6. Shiota Y, Arikita H, Horita N, et al. Septic pulmonary embolism associated with periodontal disease: reports of two cases and review of the literature. Chest 2002;121:652–654
7. Sonnet S, Buitrago-Tellez CH, Tamm M, Christen S, Steinbrich W. Direct detection of angioinvasive pulmonary aspergillosis in immunosuppressed patients: preliminary results with high-resolution 16-MDCT angiography. AJR Am J Roentgenol 2005;184: 746–751

50

Bronchiectasis

The radiological types of bronchiectasis include cylindrical, cystic, varicoid, or a combination of types. *Traction bronchiectasis* is the term used when there is bronchiolar dilatation due to pulmonary fibrosis.

Bronchiectasis can also be divided into proximal and distal types. There are fewer causes for proximal bronchiectasis; they include cystic fibrosis, allergic bronchopulmonary aspergillosis (ABPA), and tuberculosis.

Causes of Bronchiectasis

Postinfectious

- Bacterial
- Mycobacterial
- Fungal
- Viral

Congenital

- Primary ciliary dyskinesia
- α1 antitrypsin
- Cystic fibrosis
- Tracheobronchomegaly (Mounier–Kuhn)
- Cartilage deficiency (Williams–Campbell)
- Pulmonary sequestration
- Marfan syndrome

Immunodeficiency

- Primary: hypogammaglobulinemia
- Secondary: chronic lymphocytic leukemia; immunosuppression

Trapped Lung

- Right middle lung syndrome

Collagen Vascular Diseases

- Rheumatoid arthritis
- Systemic lupus erythematosus
- Sjögren's syndrome
- Relapsing polychondritis

Collagen vascular diseases more commonly result in traction bronchiectasis due to fibrosis.

Other

- Inflammatory bowel disease (ulcerative colitis and Crohn's disease)
- Young's syndrome (secondary ciliary dyskinesia)
- Yellow nail syndrome
- Foreign bodies
- Radiation fibrosis

Toxic Inhalation Leading to Bronchiectasis

- Chlorine
- Ritalin
- Heroin, cocaine, other narcotics

Most patients are expected to survive and recover with little or no residual dysfunction regardless of the severity of the initial event. However, in some cases disabling long-term sequelae, e.g., bronchiectasis, chronic airflow obstruction, bronchial hyperreactivity, asthma-like disease (reactive airways dysfunction syndrome), bronchiolitis obliterans, or residual psychophysiologic dyspnea, can occur.

Williams–Campbell Syndrome

For Williams–Campbell syndrome, there is some debate whether this disorder is congenital or acquired. The symmetric presentation and familial occurrence favors a congenital etiology. Williams–Campbell syndrome is characterized by the absence or markedly decreased amount of cartilage in the bronchi beyond the central airways. Bronchial dilatation distal to third division is seen on computed tomography (CT). There is expiratory collapse of bronchiectatic cysts. The trachea and main bronchi have normal caliber in contrast to Mounier-Kuhn syndrome, which is characterized by marked dilatation of the entire tracheobronchial tree.

Mounier–Kuhn Syndrome

Mounier–Kuhn syndrome (Tracheobronchomegaly) is divided into three subtypes. Type 1 has diffuse symmetric enlargement of the trachea and major bronchi. Type 2 has more exaggerated enlargement of the airways with occasional diverticular formation. This type is associated with frequent airway infections and severe bronchiectasis. Type 3 is characterized by large, bizarre diverticular formations, severe infections, and can lead to eventual scarring, fibrosis, and death from respiratory insufficiency. Normal tracheal diameter is 20.2 ± 3.4 mm, right main stem 16.0 ± 2.6 and the left main stem 14.5 ± 2.8. Patients with Mounier–Kuhn syndrome have greater than 3 standard deviations above the mean dimension when corrected for height.

Additional Readings

1. Hansell D. Bronchiectasis. Radiol Clin North Am 1998; 36:107–128
2. Schwartz M, Rossoff L. Tracheobronchomegaly. Chest 1994;106:1589–1590
3. Smith DL, Witherts N, Holloway B, Collins JV. Tracheobronchomegaly: an unusual presentation of a rare condition. Thorax 1994;49:840–841
4. Stern EJ. Normal trachea during forced expiration: dynamic CT measurements. Radiology 1993;187:27–31
5. Williams H, Campbell P. Generalized bronchiectasis associated with deficiency of cartilage in the bronchial tree. Arch Dis Child 1960;35:182–191

51

Tracheobronchomalacia

Tracheobronchomalacia refers to a weakness of the trachea, usually due to reduction and/or atrophy of the longitudinal elastic fibers or due to impaired cartilage integrity. Normally, the intrathoracic trachea dilates somewhat during inspiration and narrows with expiration. Tracheobronchomalacia allows an exaggeration of this normal physiologic process that may result in dynamic and ultimately even a static airway obstruction. This tracheal abnormality may be diffuse or focal.

Causes of Tracheobronchomalacia

Congenital Causes

- Seen in neonatal population, especially in premature children
- Associated with polychondritis, Mounier–Kuhn

Acquired Causes

- Posttraumatic (prolonged intubation, tracheostomy, external chest trauma, lung transplantation)
- Emphysema
- Chronic bronchitis
- Chronic inflammation (relapsing polychondritis)
- Chronic external compression of the trachea (malignancy, benign tumors, abscess, aortic aneurysm)
- Vascular rings previously undiagnosed in childhood

Additional Readings

1. Calhoun PS, Kuszyk BS, Heath DG, et al. Three-dimensional volume rendering of spiral CT data: theory and method. Radiographics 1999;19(3):745–764
2. Gilkeson RC, Ciancibello LM, Hejal RB, et al. Tracheobronchomalacia: dynamic airway evaluation with multidetector CT. AJR Am J Roentgenol 2001; 176(1): 205–210
3. Remy-Jardin M, Remy J, Artaud D, et al. Volume rendering of the tracheobronchial tree: clinical evaluation of bronchographic images. Radiology 1998;208(3): 761–770
4. Stern EJ. Normal trachea during forced expiration: dynamic CT measurements. Radiology 1993;187: 27–31

52

Asthma and Associated Conditions

Findings on High-Resolution Computed Tomography

Bronchial Abnormalities

Most of the bronchi in patients with asthma have normal or decreased internal diameters. Bronchial wall thickening is common (44 to 92%). However, in ~30 to 40% of adult patients with uncomplicated asthma, one or more bronchi are dilated. The bronchiectasis in patients with uncomplicated asthma typically is cylindrical, and the bronchoarterial diameter ratio is less than 1.5.

Bronchiolar Abnormalities

Bronchiolar abnormalities include areas of decreased attenuation and vascularity, air trapping, and small centrilobular opacities. One study reported air trapping equivalent to one pulmonary segment or more was seen in 50% of asthmatic patients compared with 14% of healthy subjects. Prominent centrilobular opacities have been reported in 10 to 20% of patients with asthma. These presumably reflect the presence of mucus stasis in bronchioles or peribronchiolar inflammation.

Parenchymal Abnormalities

These are rare and include hyperinflation, emphysema, and very rarely cysts.

Associated Conditions

- Allergic bronchopulmonary aspergillosis
- Chronic eosinophilic pneumonia: The characteristic radiologic manifestations consist of bilateral areas of consolidation, mainly affecting the peripheral regions of the middle and upper lung zones.
- Churg–Strauss syndrome: The most common high-resolution CT finding consists of patchy, nonsegmental, bilateral areas of consolidation or ground-glass opacities that have a predominantly peripheral distribution characteristic of chronic eosinophilic pneumonia. Less common manifestations include multiple solid or cavitated 1 to 3 cm pulmonary nodules, small centrilobular nodules, and intralobular septal thickening. Churg–Strauss syndrome is a multisystem disorder characterized by a combination of allergy, peripheral blood eosinophilia, and systemic vasculitis. Almost all patients with this syndrome are asthmatic and present with peripheral neuropathy, typically mononeuritis multiplex.

Additional Readings

1. Park CS, Muller NL, Worthy SA, et al. Airway obstruction in asthmatic and healthy individuals: inspiratory and expiratory thin section CT findings. Radiology 1997;203:361–367

2. Silva CIS, Colby TV, Muller NL. Asthma and associated conditions: high resolution CT and pathological findings. AJR Am J Roentgenol 2004;183: 817–824

53

Emphysema

Types of Emphysema and Associated Features

- Centrilobular emphysema
  - Predominantly affects the respiratory bronchioles in the central portion of the acinus (the central portion of secondary lobules)
  - Cigarette smoking
  - Upper lung predominance
- Panlobular emphysema
  - Involves all the components of the acinus (involves entire secondary lobules)
  - Associated with alpha-1 protease inhibitor deficiency or cigarette smoking
  - May also be seen without protease deficiency in smokers, in elderly persons, and with elicit drug abuse
  - Lower lobe predominance
- Paraseptal emphysema
  - Predominantly involves the alveolar ducts and sacs in the lung periphery with areas of destruction often marginated by interlobular septae
  - Can be isolated finding in young adults, often associated with spontaneous pneumothorax
  - Can be seen in older patients with centrilobular emphysema
  - Bullae most commonly seen with paraseptal or centrilobular emphysema
- Cicatricial or irregular emphysema
  - Occurs in patients with pulmonary fibrosis
  - Found adjacent to localized parenchymal scars or diffuse pulmonary fibrosis and in the pneumoconiosis, especially with progressive massive fibrosis
- Bullous emphysema
  - Cigarette smoking or idiopathic
  - Also called *vanishing lung syndrome*
  - Often upper lobe
  - Often asymmetric

Additional Readings

1. Thurlback WM, Muller NL. Emphysema: definition, imaging, and quantification. AJR Am J Roentgenol 1994;163:1017–1025
2. Webb WR. Emphysema and chronic obstructive pulmonary disease. In: Webb RW, Higgins CB, eds. Thoracic Imaging. Pulmonary and Cardiovascular Radiology. Philadelphia: Lippincott, Williams & Wilkins; 2005:553–574

54

Differential Diagnosis of Mediastinal Masses Based on Common Sites of Origin

Anterior Mediastinum

- Lymph node masses
- Thymic masses
- Germ cell tumors
- Thyroid masses
- Parathyroid masses
- Aneurysms
- Lipoma
- Lymphangioma and hemangioma

Anterior Mediastinum (Cardiophrenic Angle)

- Lymph node masses (particularly lymphoma and metastases)
- Pericardial cyst
- Morgagni hernia
- Thymic masses
- Germ cell tumors

Middle Mediastinum

- Lymph node masses
- Lung carcinoma
- Sarcoidosis
- Lymphoma
- Metastases
- Infections
- Foregut cyst
- Tracheal tumor
- Lipoma

- Thyroid masses
- Aneurysms
- Lymphangioma and hemangioma
- Chemodectoma
- Dilated azygos vein
- Esophageal varices
- Hernia

Posterior Mediastinum

- Neurogenic tumor
- Foregut cyst
- Meningocele
- Extramedullary hematopoiesis
- Pseudocyst
- Spine abnormalities
- Hernia
- Esophageal masses
- Varices
- Lipoma
- Lymph node masses
- Dilated azygos or hemiazygos vein
- Hernia
- Lymphangioma and hemangioma

Lymph Node Masses

Calcified Lymph Nodes

- Common:
  - Prior granulomatous diseases
  - Tuberculosis
  - Fungal infections (histoplasmosis)
  - Sarcoidosis

○ Silicosis
○ Hodgkin's disease (usually following treatment)
• Rare:
  ○ *Pneumocystis jirovecii* (*P. carinii*) pneumonia
  ○ Metastases (mucinous adenocarcinoma)
  ○ Amyloidosis
  ○ Scleroderma
  ○ Castleman's disease

Low Density/Necrotic Lymph Nodes

• Common:
  ○ Infectious granulomatous diseases
  ○ Tuberculosis
  ○ Fungal infections (histoplasmosis)
  ○ Metastases
  ○ Lung cancer
  ○ Extrathoracic malignancy

○ Lymphoma
• Rare:
  ○ Sarcoidosis

Enhancing Lymph Nodes

• Common:
  ○ Metastases (vascular tumors)
  ○ Tuberculosis
• Rare:
  ○ Castleman's disease
  ○ Sarcoidosis
  ○ Angioimmunoblastic lymphadenopathy

Thymic Masses

The features and computed tomography (CT) findings for thymic masses, germ cell tumors, and mediastinal masses, respectively, are presented in **Tables 54.1, 54.2,** and **54.3.**

Table 54.1 Features and Computed Tomography Findings of Thymic Masses

Type	Feature	CT Findings
Thymoma	Most common thymic tumor	Focal or lobulated mass
	Myasthenia gravis in 30 to 50% 10 to 30% of patients with myasthenia have thymoma. 70% noninvasive	Homogeneous or cystic, may calcify Invasion difficult to diagnose with certainty
Thymic Carcinoma	Myasthenia rare Commonly invasive	Indistinguishable from thymoma unless metastases visible (distant metastasis in 50 to 65%)
Carcinoid Tumor	Usually malignant Cushing's syndrome in 25 to 40% multiple endocrine neoplasia in 20%	Mimics thymoma Dense enhancement with contrast
Thymolipoma	Benign Often young patients Usually asymptomatic	Large, gravity dependent mediastinal mass containing fat and strands of tissue
Thymic Cysts	Uncommon Congenital or acquired	Thin-walled nonenhancing fluid Density mass close to that of water
Lymphoma and Metastases	Hodgkin's lymphoma more commonly involves thymus than non–Hodgkin's lymphoma	Homogeneous thymic enlargement is seen in lymphoma. Calcification uncommonly occurs in the absence of radiation or chemotherapy. CT findings of thymic metastases are nonspecific.

Abbreviations: CT, computed tomography.

Table 54.2 Features and Computed Tomography Findings of Germ Cell Tumors

Type	Feature	CT Findings
Teratoma	Mature teratoma is benign	Well defined, smooth, cystic
	Constitutes 60 to 70% mediastinal germ cell tumors	Teeth and bone rare
		Fluid in 90%; fat in 75%, calcification in 50%
	Occurs in children and young adults	Presents as nodular mass
	Also called dermoid cyst	Fat seen in 40%
	Immature or malignant teratoma	Invasion of mediastinal structures
		Enhancing capsule
Seminoma	30% of germ cell tumors	Large, lobulated, anterior mediastinal mass
	Mean age of 29 years	Homogeneous in attenuation
Nonseminomatous Germ Cell Tumors	Poor prognosis	Inhomogeneous in attenuation

Abbreviations: CT, computed tomography.

Enlargement of anterior mediastinal nodal group suggests lymphoma. Enlarged bilateral hilar and right paratracheal lymph nodes suggest sarcoidosis. Enlarged right paratracheal lymph nodes can be seen in tuberculosis.

Amorphous soft tissue mediastinal mass with calcifications with encasement of mediastinal structures, including superior vena cava, pulmonary arteries, and bronchi, suggest findings of fibrosing mediastinitis, which can be seen in histoplasmosis, tuberculosis, sarcoidosis, autoimmune disease, retroperitoneal fibrosis, result from drugs, or could be idiopathic.

Fat-containing masses include lipomatosis, lipoma, liposarcoma, thymolipoma, teratoma, hernias containing fat, and extramedullary hematopoiesis. Congenital or acquired cysts including bronchogenic, esophageal, neuroenteric, pericardial, and thymic cysts present as cystic low attenuation, fluid-filled masses on CT.

Table 54.3 Features and Computed Tomography Findings of Mediastinal Masses

Type	Feature	CT Findings
Thyroid Mass	10% of mediastinal masses	High in attenuation and enhanced profusely with contrast
	Almost always connected to cervical thyroid	May have cystic areas or punctuate calcifications
Parathyroid Mass	10% of parathyroid glands are ectopic	Usually small soft tissue nodule
	60% in anterior mediastinum	
	10% in posterior-superior mediastinum	
Peripheral Nerve Sheath Tumors	Present as posterior mediastinal masses	Round, elliptical, or lobulated paravertebral mass
	Common in adults	Usually lower attenuation than muscle
	One third of patients with neurofibromas have neurofibromatosis	

Abbreviations: CT, computed tomography.

Additional Readings

1. Brown LR, Aughenbaugh GL. Masses of the anterior mediastinum: CT and MR imaging. AJR Am J Roentgenol 1991;157:1171–1180
2. Do YS, Im JG, Lee BH, et al. CT findings in malignant tumors of thymic epithelium. J Comput Assist Tomogr 1995;19:192–197
3. Hoffman OA, Gillespie DJ, Aughenbaugh GL, et al. Primary mediastinal neoplasms (other than thymoma). Mayo Clin Proc 1993;68:880–891
4. Kawashima A, Fishman EK, Kuhlman JE, et al. CT of posterior mediastinal masses. Radiographics 1991;11:1045–1067
5. Lee KS, Im JG, Han CH, et al. Malignant primary germ cell tumors of the mediastinum: CT features. AJR Am J Roentgenol 1989;153:947–951
6. Patil SN, Levin DL. Distribution of thoracic lymphadenopathy in sarcoidosis using computed tomography. J Thorac Imaging 1999;14:114–117
7. Rosado de Christenson ML, Templeton PA, Moran CA. Mediastinal germ-cell tumors: radiologic and pathologic correlation. Radiographics 1992;12:1013–1030
8. Webb WR. The mediastinum: mediastinal masses. In: Thoracic Imaging. Pulmonary and Cardiovascular Radiology. In: Webb RW, Higgins CB, eds. Philadelphia: Lippincott, Williams & Wilkins; 2005: 212–270

55

High-Resolution Computed Tomography of Chronic Diffuse Infiltrative Lung Disease

The differential diagnosis in the setting of chronic diffuse interstitial lung disease relies upon recognition of specific high-resolution computed tomography (HRCT) signs. These include interlobular septal thickening, reticular densities, cystic air spaces, nodules, ground-glass attenuation, and consolidation.

Septal Thickening

In normal individuals, a few thin interlobular septa may be visualized on HRCT in the sub-pleural regions. When multiple contiguous septa become thickened, a characteristic appearance of polygonal arcades can be seen. Septal thickening may be due to fluid, cellular infiltration, fibrosis, or a combination of these. Smooth septal thickening favors pulmonary edema over lymphangitic carcinomatosis. Nodularity or beading of the septa favors the diagnosis of lymphangitic carcinomatosis. Irregular septal thickening implies the presence of underlying fibrosis and may be seen in sarcoidosis, asbestosis, and idiopathic pulmonary fibrosis.

Reticular Densities

Irregular linear areas of increased attenuation are indicative of underlying parenchymal fibrosis. In idiopathic pulmonary fibrosis, collagen vascular disease, and asbestosis, the reticulation predominantly involves the subpleural lung regions and the lower lung zones. The diagnosis of asbestosis is based on an appropriate history of exposure, presence of pleural plaques, and diffuse pleural thickening and evidence of pulmonary fibrosis. The parenchymal abnormalities in asbestosis include intralobular linear opacities, irregular thickening interlobular septa, curvilinear subpleural lines, and parenchymal bands. The reticular densities in chronic hypersensitivity pneumonitis (extrinsic allergic alveolitis) and sarcoidosis are more prominent in upper- and mid-lung zones or randomly distributed throughout all lung zones.

Cystic Airspaces

Cysts are defined as circumscribed air-containing lesions with well-defined walls.

Ancillary Findings in Interstitial Lung Disease

- Esophageal dilatation: Scleroderma or mixed connective tissue disorder
- Shoulder joint erosions/arthropathy: Rhematoid arthritis
- Calcified pleural plaques: Asbestosis
- Lymphadenopathy: Lymphangitic carcinomatosis, lymphoma, sarcoidosis

High-Resolution CT Findings in Chronic Diffuse Infiltrative Lung Disease

Septal Thickening

- Pulmonary edema
- Lymphangitic carcinomatosis

Reticular Densities

- Idiopathic pulmonary fibrosis
- Collagen vascular disease
- Asbestosis
- Chronic hypersensitivity pneumonitis
- Sarcoidosis

Cystic Airspaces

- Lymphangioleiomyomatosis
- Pulmonary Langerhans-cell granulomatosis
- End-stage (honeycomb) lung

Nodules

- Sarcoidosis
- Silicosis
- Coal worker's pneumoconiosis
- Acute hypersensitivity pneumonitis (Acute HP)

Ground-Glass Attenuation

- Acute or subacute HP
- Desquamative interstitial pneumonia (DIP)
- Idiopathic pulmonary fibrosis
- Sarcoidosis
- Pulmonary alveolar proteinosis

Consolidation

- Chronic eosinophilic pneumonia
- Cryptogenic organizing pneumonia (COP)
- Bronchioloalveolar carcinoma
- Lymphoma

Additional Readings

1. Grenier P, Valeyre D, Cluzel P, et al. Chronic diffuse infiltrative lung disease: diagnostic value of chest radiography and high-resolution CT. Radiology 1991;179:123–132
2. Leung AN, Miller RR, Muller NL. Parenchymal opacification in chronic infiltrative lung diseases: CT-pathologic correlation. Radiology 1993;188:209–214
3. McLoud TC, Carrington CB, Gaensler EA. Diffuse infiltrative lung disease: a new scheme for description. Radiology 1983;149:353–363
4. Padley SPG, Hansell DM, Flower CDR, et al. Comparative accuracy of high-resolution computed tomography and chest radiography in the diagnosis of chronic diffuse infiltrative lung disease. Clin Radiol 1991;44:222–226
5. Webb WR, Muller NL, Naidich DA. Standardized terms for high-resolution computed tomography of the lung: a proposed glossary. J Thorac Imaging 1993;8: 167–175
6. Webb WR. High-resolution computed tomography of obstructive lung disease. Radiol Clin North Am 1994; 32:745–757

56

Idiopathic Interstitial Pneumonia

The term idiopathic interstitial pneumonia (IIP) is applied to a group of disorders with distinct histologic and radiologic appearances and without a known cause. These disorders are tabulated in **Table 56.1**.

The histologic temporal and spatial heterogeneity of usual interstitial pneumonia (UIP) results in characteristic constellation of basal-predominant, peripheral-predominant reticular abnormality and honeycombing. Nonspecific interstitial pneumonia (NSIP), desquamative interstitial pneumonia (DIP), acute interstitial pneumonia (AIP), and lymphoid interstitial pneumonia (LIP) are microscopically homogeneous and are characterized by homogeneous attenuation at thin-section computed tomography (CT).

Exposure to cigarette smoke results in respiratory bronchiolitis (RB) and DIP. RB has been

Table 56.1 Findings and Differential Diagnosis of Idiopathic Interstitial Pneumonia

Morphologic Pattern	Associated Clinical Syndrome	Imaging Features	Differential Diagnosis
Usual interstitial pneumonia (UIP)	Idiopathic pulmonary fibrosis (IPF)	Reticular abnormality Honeycombing Basal, peripheral predominance often patchy	Collagen vascular diseases Asbestosis Chronic hypersensitivity pneumonitis
Nonspecific interstitial pneumonia (NSIP)	NSIP	Ground glass attenuation Reticular abnormality Basal, peripheral predominance (Fibrotic NSIP could mimic UIP; however, greater extent of honeycombing is seen in UIP.)	Collagen vascular diseases Chronic hypersensitivity pneumonitis DIP
Desquamative interstitial pneumonia (DIP)	DIP	Ground glass attenuation Cysts and/or basal and peripheral predominance	Hypersensitivity pneumonitis, NSIP

(Continued on page 144)

Table 56.1 *(Continued)* Findings and Differential Diagnosis of Idiopathic Interstitial Pneumonia

Morphologic Pattern	Associated Clinical Syndrome	Imaging Features	Differential Diagnosis
Respiratory bronchiolitis (RB)	Respiratory bronchiolitis-interstitial lung disease (RB-ILD)	Ill-defined centrilobular nodules Ground glass attenuation Upper lobe predominance	Hypersensitivity pneumonitis
Organizing pneumonia (previously called BOOP)	Cryptogenic organizing pneumonia (COP)	Basal, peripheral predominance	Infection, vasculitis, sarcoidosis, lymphoma, and Bronchioloalveolar carcinoma
Lymphoid interstitial pneumonia (LIP)	LIP	Ground glass attenuation Perivascular cysts Ill-defined centrilobular nodules Thickening of bronchovascular bundles	DIP, Hypersensitivity pneumonitis
Diffuse alveolar damage (DAD)	Acute interstitial pneumonia (AIP)	Consolidations Ground glass attenuation	Pneumonia Pulmonary hemorrhage Hydrostatic edema

Source: Adapted from Lynch DA, Travis WD, Muller NL, et al. Idiopathic interstitial pneumonias: CT features. Radiology 2005;236:10–21.

rarely reported in nonsmokers with other inhalational exposures, especially asbestos and nonasbestos dusts, as well as various fumes. For the majority of patients with respiratory bronchiolitis-interstitial lung disease (RB-ILD) and DIP, the onset of symptoms is usually in the fourth or fifth decades of life. It is considerably earlier than that noted in patients with idiopathic pulmonary fibrosis (IPF)/UIP. There is a slight male predominance, and these patients have experienced an average of over 30 years of cigarette smoking. Patients with RB-ILD and DIP commonly present with gradual onset of cough and dyspnea. Most patients with RB-ILD have relatively mild symptoms compared with those with DIP who commonly have significant dyspnea and hypoxemia.

Hypersensitivity pneumonitis is an immunologically induced inflammatory disease involving the lung parenchyma and terminal airways secondary to repeated inhalation of a variety of organic dusts and other agents in a sensitized host.

IPF is recognized as a progressive disease with a relatively poor prognosis. Complications of IPF include accelerated progression in 10 to 20% of patients (ground-glass opacities mimicking AIP with diffuse alveolar damage [DAD]), increased risk for lung cancer (estimated at 10 to 17%), and secondary infections. NSIP has a better prognosis. AIP is the idiopathic form of adult respiratory syndrome. LIP and DIP are less common, both are characterized by ground-glass opacites and are sometimes associated with cysts.

The American Thoracic Society has set major and minor criteria for the diagnosis of IPF in the absence of a surgical biopsy. One of the major criterias is the presence of typical UIP findings on thin-section CT. The cases without typical features of UIP or other interstitial pneumonia may require biopsy for accurate diagnosis and morphologic characterization.

The diagnosis of idiopathic interstitial pneumonia requires integration of the morphologic patterns identified on high-resolution CT and pathology with complete clinical evaluation.

Additional Readings

1. American Thoracic Society, European Respiratory Society. American Thoracic Society/European Respiratory Society International Multidisciplinary Consensus Classification of the Idiopathic Interstitial Pneumonias. Am J Respir Crit Care Med 2002;165: 277–304
2. Grenier P, Valeyre D, Cluzel P, et al. Chronic diffuse infiltrative lung disease: diagnostic value of chest radiography and high-resolution CT. Radiology 1991;179: 123–132
3. Leung AN, Miller RR, Muller NL. Parenchymal opacification in chronic infiltrative lung diseases: CT-pathologic correlation. Radiology 1993;188: 209–214
4. Lynch DA, Travis WD, Muller NL, et al. Idiopathic interstitial pneumonias: CT features. Radiology 2005;236: 10–21
5. Muller NL, Colby TV. Idiopathic interstitial pneumonias: high-resolution CT and histologic findings. Radiographics 1997;17:1016–1022
6. Padley SPG, Hansell DM, Flower CDR, et al. Comparative accuracy of high-resolution computed tomography and chest radiography in the diagnosis of chronic diffuse infiltrative lung disease. Clin Radiol 1991;44: 222–226
7. Ryu JH. Jeffrey, Myers JL, Swensen SJ. Bronchiolar disorders: state of the art. Am J Respir Crit Care Med 2003; 168:1277–1292
8. Webb WR, Muller NL, Naidich DA. Standardized terms for high-resolution computed tomography of the lung: a proposed glossary. J Thorac Imaging 1993;8: 167–175
9. Webb WR. High-resolution computed tomography of obstructive lung disease. Radiol Clin North Am 1994;32:745–757

57

Cystic Lung Disease

Causes for upper lobe predominant fibrocystic changes include:

- Tuberculosis
- Sarcoidosis
- Ankylosing spondylitis
- Chronic hypersensitivity pneumonitis
- Chronic Langerhans cell granulomatosis (eosinophilic granuloma)
- Drug toxicity

Causes of Focal or Multifocal Cystic Lung Disease

- Congenital

  ○ Bronchogenic cysts
  ○ Pulmonary sequestration
  ○ Congenital cystic adenomatoid malformation

- Infectious

  ○ Pulmonary tuberculosis
  ○ Coccidioidomycosis
  ○ *Pneumocystic carinii*
  ○ *Echinococcus granulosus* or *multilocularis*

- LAM
- Lymphocytic interstitial pneumonia
- Desquamative interstitial pneumonia

Pulmonary lymphangioleiomyomatosis is a rare, idiopathic cystic interstitial lung disease that affects primarily women of childbearing age. It has, however, been reported in post-menopausal women. The sporadic form presents only in women, whereas rare cases associated with tuberous sclerosis have been reported among men. It is characterized pathologically by interstitial smooth muscle proliferation. Compression of the conducting airways results in obstruction of airflow and in alveolar disruption, which leads to the development of cystic changes. Chest computed tomography (CT) shows numerous uniformly thin-walled cysts scattered in an even distribution with normal intervening lung parenchyma. The most common clinical presentation is spontaneous pneumothorax. Many patients present with chylous effusions. In an appropriate clinical setting, high-resolution CT findings can be pathognomonic. However, pathologic examination of a lung tissue specimen is recommended for confirmation of the diagnosis of lymphangioleiomyomatosis (LAM), one of the conditions that can recur after transplantation. Extrapulmonary manifestations include lymphadenopathy, abdominal (especially renal angiomyolipomas), and pelvic masses.

Additional Readings

1. Kalassian KG, Doyle R, Kao P, et al. Lymphangio-leiomyomatosis: new insights. Am J Respir Crit Care Med 1997;155:1183–1186

2. Mueller NL, et al. Disease of the Lung. Radiologic and Pathologic Correlations. Philadelphia, PA: Lippincott Williams and Wilkins; 2003

58

Pneumoconiosis

Pneumoconiosis is caused by the accumulation of inhaled particulates. Pneumoconiosis may be classified as fibrotic (involving focal nodular or diffuse fibrosis) or nonfibrotic (involving particle laden macrophages, with minimal or no fibrosis).

Types of Pneumoconiosis

- Fibrotic pneumoconiosis
  - Silicosis
  - Coal worker pneumoconiosis
  - Asbestosis
  - Berylliosis
  - Talcosis
- Nonfibrotic pneumoconiosis
  - Siderosis (from iron oxide)
  - Stannosis (from tin oxide)
  - Barytosis (from barium sulfate)

Silicosis, coal worker pneumoconiosis, and asbestosis are the three most common types of pneumoconiosis, whereas berylliosis, siderosis, stannosis, and barytosis are relatively uncommon.

Silicosis

Silicosis is caused by the inhalation of fine particles of crystalline silicon dioxide (silica). Quartz is the most common form of crystalline silica. The disease occurs in two clinical forms: acute silicosis, which manifests as alveolar silicoproteinosis, and classic silicosis, which manifests as chronic interstitial reticular nodular disease.

On computed tomography (CT), two main patterns are recognized: simple and complicated.

The simple form is characterized by multiple nodules, which are well defined and uniform in shape, and attenuation is distributed throughout both lungs. However, the nodules tend to be predominantly located in the upper lobes and posterior portions of the lungs. The nodules in simple silicosis tend to be more sharply defined than those in coal worker's pneumoconiosis are, but are otherwise indistinguishable from the latter on thin-section CT. The nodules are distributed in centrilobular, periseptal, and subpleural regions and have a perilymphatic distribution. Hilar and mediastinal lymph node enlargement may precede the appearance of parenchymal nodular lesions. The so-called eggshell calcification pattern is highly suggestive of silicosis.

Complicated silicosis or progressive massive fibrosis is characterized by large conglomerate opacities. Carcinoma and tuberculosis are potential serious complications of silicosis.

Coal Worker's Pneumoconiosis

Coal worker's pneumoconiosis is caused by exposure to washed coal, which is nearly free of silica. Its histologic basis is very different from that of silica. Tissue specimens from patients with coal worker's pneumoconiosis demonstrate two characteristic morphologic features: coal macules and progressive massive fibrosis. The coal macules range in size from 1 to 5 mm and are characterized by solid anthracotic pigmentation without intervening fibrotic tissue. The macules contain pigment-laden macrophages that surround the bronchioles in the lobular core; thus, the distribution of the macules is primarily centrilobular. The small nodules are slightly ill defined and smaller than those of silicosis. Otherwise, the CT features are similar to those of silicosis.

Asbestosis

Asbestosis is diffuse interstitial pulmonary fibrosis that occurs secondary to the inhalation of asbestos fibers. Thin-section CT can demonstrate thickened intralobular and interlobular lines, subpleural curvilinear lines, pleural-based irregular small nodules, hazy patches of increased attenuation, and small cystic spaces with lower lobe predominance. Honeycombing is a common finding in advanced stage disease, predominantly in the lung periphery and the posterior regions. Thin-section CT findings in patients with asbestosis are similar to those in patients with idiopathic pulmonary fibrosis (IPF). The fibrotic changes, however, are more often basal and subpleural in IPF than that in the asbestosis group. The presence of parietal pleural thickening (pleural plaques) in association with lung fibrosis is the most important feature distinguishing asbestosis-induced pulmonary fibrosis from IPF. The two most important complications of asbestosis are pulmonary fibrosis and malignancy, which includes malignant pleural or peritoneal mesothelioma.

Berylliosis

Berylliosis is a chronic granulomatous disease caused by exposure to beryllium dust or fumes, characterized by accumulation of CD4+ T cells and macrophages in the lower respiratory tract. Exposure to beryllium may occur in the manufacture of ceramics, nuclear weapon production, and the aerospace industry. Granulomas in berylliosis are histopathologically indistinguishable from those in other granulomatous diseases such as sarcoidosis. However, the granulomatous reaction derives from an immunopathologic process due to beryllium-specific CD4+ T lymphocytes in lung tissue. Thin-section CT findings of berylliosis are similar to those of granulomatous lung disease such as sarcoidosis.

Hard Metal Pneumoconiosis

Hard metal pneumoconiosis, or hard metal lung disease, is caused by exposure to dust produced in the hard metal industry (e.g., during the processing of tungsten carbine and cobalt, sometimes with the admixture of other metals). The histopathologic manifestations of hard metal disease range from bronchitis to subacute fibrosing alveolitis to interstitial fibrosis. Obliterative bronchiolitis is reported to be the earliest manifestation of hard metal disease. Thin-section CT findings consist of bilateral ground glass opacities or consolidation, extensive reticular opacities, and traction bronchiectasis. In advanced cases, parenchymal distortion and honeycombing may be seen. Because these patterns are similar to those of other idiopathic interstitial pneumonias, including idiopathic pulmonary fibrosis and nonspecific interstitial pneumonia, a diagnosis of hard metal lung disease should be based on combined occupational, clinical, radiologic, and pathological findings.

In general, a diagnosis of pneumoconiosis should be made by taking a history of occupational exposure to inorganic dust or fumes with the pathologic and radiologic findings.

Additional Readings

1. Chong S, Lee KS, Chung MJ, Han J, Kwon OJ, Kim TS. Pneumoconiosis: comparison of imaging and pathologic findings. Radiographics 2006;26:59–77
2. Fraser R. Muller NL, Colman N. Inhalation of inorganic dust (pneumoconiosis). In: Fraser R, Muller N, Colman N, eds. Diagnosis of Diseases of the Chest. 4th ed. Philadelphia, PA: Saunders; 1999: 2386–2484
3. International Labour Organization (ILO). Guidelines for the Use of ILO International Classification of Radiographs of Pneumoconioses. Geneva, Switzerland: ILO; 1980
4. McLoud TC. Occupational lung disease. Radiol Clin North Am 1991;29:931–941
5. Weil I, Jones R, Parkes W. Silicosis and related diseases. In: Parkes W, ed. Occupational Lung Disorders. 3rd ed. London, UK: Buttersworth; 1994: 285–339

59

Radiation and Drug-Induced Lung Disease

Radiation-Induced Lung Disease

Radiologic manifestations are usually confined to the lung tissue within the radiation port and are dependent on the interval after completion of treatment. The radiological changes are expected 8 weeks after 4000 rad, and 1 week earlier for each 1000 rad increments above 4000. In the acute phase (2 to 6 weeks), radiation injury typically manifests as ground-glass opacity or as consolidation; in the late phase, it typically manifests as traction bronchiectasis, volume loss, and scarring. However, the use of oblique beam angles and newer irradiation techniques such as three-dimensional conformal radiation therapy or hypofractionated stereotactic radiotherapy can result in an unusual distribution of these findings. Awareness of the typical and atypical manifestations of radiation-induced lung disease can be useful in differentiating from infection, recurrent malignancy, lymphangitic carcinomatosis, and radiation-induced tumors. Findings such as the late appearance or enlargement of a pleural effusion, development of consolidation, opacification of a previously demonstrated air bronchogram, a mass, or cavitation suggest recurrence of malignancy and/or infection. Because radiation pneumonitis can have increased fluorodeoxyglucose (FDG) uptake that mimics recurrent disease, fluorodeoxyglucose positron emission tomography (FDG PET) is best performed at least 3 months after completion of radiation therapy or before lung radiation-induced lung injury. FDG PET has, however,

high negative predictive value, and focal opacities with low FDG uptake can be followed radiographically.

Approximately 10% of patients receiving lung radiation will develop clinical disease usually 2 to 6 months after the initiation of therapy. Radiographic changes following radiation therapy can be seen in up to 42% of patients. Drug toxicity can be synergistic and may occur even if the drugs and radiotherapy are separated in time, as many as 10% of patients receiving chemotherapeutic agents will develop an adverse drug reaction in their lungs. The most common drugs resulting in lung toxicity are bleomycin, methotrexate, carmustine, busulfan, and cyclophosphamide.

Drug-Induced Lung Disease

The high-resolution computed tomography (CT) findings of drug-induced lung disease reflect the histologic findings (**Table 59.1**).

- Diffuse alveolar damage (DAD): Chest radiographs show bilateral heterogeneous or homogeneous opacities, often in a mid- or lower lung distribution, mimicking pulmonary edema. Progression to diffuse opacification is common. High-resolution CT in early DAD typically shows scattered or diffuse areas of ground-glass opacity. Fibrosis typically develops within 1 week and progressive fibrosis may be manifested

Table 59.1 Principal Histopathologic Manifestations of Pulmonary Drug Toxicity

Mechanism of Injury	Drugs
Diffuse alveolar damage	Bleomycin, busulfan, carmustine, cyclophosphamide, mitomycin, melphalan, gold salts
Nonspecific interstitial pneumonitis	Amiodarone, methotrexate, carmustine, chlorambucil
Cryptogenic organizing pneumonia	Bleomycin, gold salts, methotrexate, amiodarone, nitrofurantoin, penicillamine, sulfasalazine, cyclophosphamide
Eosinophilic pneumonia	Penicillamine, sulfasalazine, nitrofurantoin, nonsteroidal anti-inflammatory drugs, para-aminosalicylic acid
Pulmonary hemorrhage	Anticoagulants, amphotericin B, cytarabine (ara-C), penicillamine, cyclophosphamide
Hypersensitivity pneumonitis	Methotrexate

by marked architectural distortion and honeycombing.

- Nonspecific interstitial pneumonia: In the early stages of nonspecific interstitial pneumonia (cellular NSIP), scattered or diffuse areas of ground-glass opacity may be seen. Later (fibrotic NSIP), findings of fibrosis (traction bronchiectasis, honeycombing) predominate in a basal distribution.
- Cryptogenic organizing pneumonia (COP): Previously called bronchiolitis obliterans organizing pneumonia (BOOP), CT often shows patchy areas of subpleural and peribronchial consolidations, ground-glass opacities, linear opacities, centrilobular nodules and branching linear opacities (tree-in-bud opacities), and bronchial dilatation. COP caused by pulmonary drug toxicity typically responds well to cessation of drug therapy, but treatment with corticosteroids may be required.
- Eosinophilic pneumonia: CT can be useful for demonstrating the peripheral nature of the pulmonary opacities.
- Pulmonary hemorrhage: CT usually shows bilateral, scattered, or diffuse areas of ground-glass opacities. Crazy-paving pattern may be seen.

- Hypersensitivity pneumonitis: High-resolution CT may show poorly defined centrilobular nodules and areas of ground-glass attenuation.

Differential diagnosis for drug-induced lung disease includes pulmonary edema, pneumonia, interstitial pneumonitis, and opportunistic infection. Open lung biopsy may be required to confirm the diagnosis. In some cases, drug-induced lung injury may have unique features due to the implicated drug. For example, high-attenuation consolidated areas may be seen with amiodarone pulmonary toxicity due to high iodine concentration. Associated high attenuation of the liver and spleen may also be seen.

Because drug-related pulmonary toxicity can be progressive and fatal, early recognition is important. The high-resolution CT manifestations of drug-induced disease imitate other entities such as infection, pulmonary fibrosis, and disease recurrence.

Drug-induced pulmonary toxicity can be difficult to diagnose; therefore, knowledge of the drugs most frequently involved, together with an understanding of the typical histopathologic and radiologic manifestations of toxicity by those drugs, is necessary for the institution of appropriate treatment.

Additional Readings

1. Choi YW, Munden RF, Erasmus JJ, et al. Effects of radiation therapy on the lung: radiologic appearances and differential diagnosis. Radiographics 2004;24:985–998

2. Copper JA Jr. Drug-induced lung disease. Adv Intern Med 1997;42:231–268

3. Ellis SJ, Cleverley JR, Muller NL. Drug-induced lung disease: high-resolution CT findings. AJR Am J Roentgenol 2000;175:1019–1024

4. Kuhlman JE, Teigen C, Ren H, Hurban RH, Mutchins GM, Fishman EK. Amiodarone pulmonary toxicity: CT findings in symptomatic patients. Radiology 1990;177: 121–125

5. McAdams HP, Rosado-de-Christenson ML, Wehunt WD, Fishback NF. The alphabet soup revisited: the chronic interstitial pneumonias in the 1990s. Radiographics 1996;16:1009–1033

6. Rossi SE, Erasmus JJ, McAdams HP, Sporn TA, Goodman PC. Pulmonary drug toxicity: radiologic and pathologic manifestations. Radiographics 2000;20:1245–1259

60

The Solitary Pulmonary Nodule

A solitary pulmonary nodule can be defined as a well- or poorly defined, roughly circumscribed, round or oval lesion measuring less than 3 cm in diameter. The only specific and reliable sign of the benign nature of a solitary lesion includes the identification of certain benign types of calcifications and the absolute absence of growth over a 2-year period. A solitary pulmonary nodule in a patient under the age of 35 years with no history of an extrathoracic malignancy is generally considered benign. Benign nodules generally have a doubling time (double in volume) of less than 1 month or more than 16 months. There is a significant overlap of growth rates among rapidly growing nodules (**Table 60.1**).

Typically, malignant nodules enhance on contrast-enhanced chest computed tomography (CT). Active granulomas and other infectious lesions, however, can also show enhancement. Similarly, positron emission tomography (PET) imaging with glucose analog F18-fluorodeoxyglucose (FDG) shows increased glucose metabolism in metabolically active processes such as malignant nodules; however, inflammatory or infectious processes can also have increased FDG activity leading to a false-positive result (**Table 60.2**).

Table 60.1 Recommendations for Follow-up and Management of Nodules Smaller than 8 mm Detected Incidentally at Nonscreening CT[a]

Nodule Size (mm)[b]	Low-Risk Patient[c]	High-Risk Patient[d]
≤4	No follow-up needed[e]	Follow-up CT at 12 mon if unchanged, no further follow-up[f]
>4 to 6	Follow-up CT at 12 mon if unchanged, no further follow-up[f]	Initial follow-up CT at 6 to 12 mon then at 18 to 24 mon if no change[f]
>6 to 8	Initial follow-up CT at 6 to 12 mon then at 18 to 24 mon if no change	Initial follow-up CT 3 to 6 mon, then at 9 to 12 and 24 mon if no change
>8	Follow-up CT at around 3, 9, and 24 mon dynamic contrast-enhanced CT, PET, and/or biopsy	Same as low-risk patient

Abbreviations: CT, computed tomography; PET, positron emission tomography.

[a] Newly detected indeterminate nodule in persons 35 years of age or older

[b] Average of length and width

[c] Minimal or absent history of smoking and of other known risk factors

[d] History of smoking or of other known risk factors.

[e] The risk of malignancy in this category (<1%) is substantially less than that in a baseline CT scan of an asymptomatic smoker.

[f] Nonsolid (ground glass) or partly solid nodules may require longer follow-up to exclude indolent adenocarcinoma.

Table 60.2 Distinguishing Characteristics of Benign versus Malignant Pulmonary Nodules

	Benign	Malignant
Margins	Smooth	Stellate, spiculated pleural tail
Size[a]	Smaller	Larger
Change in Size[b]	No change over 2 years	
Calcifications[c]	Present	Absent
CT Density	>150 HU	<100 HU
Enhancement Pattern	None or gradual enhancements <15 HU	Rapid enhancement >15 HU
Cavitation	Concentric, thin wall	Eccentric (squamous cell carcinoma), thick wall
Associated Findings	Satellite lesions	Lymphadenopathy
PET[d]	Negative	Positive

Abbreviations: CT, computed tomography; HU, Hounsfield unit; PET, positron emission tomography.

[a] Size is a relative criteria. In a given case, by itself it may not be of much significance but in general benign nodules are smaller (< 5mm).

[b] Nonsolid nodules (ground-glass attenuation) representing bronchioloalveolar cell carcinoma may have longer doubling times.

[c] Rarely minimal irregular, eccentric calcification may be seen with a malignant nodule. Benign calcification is usually diffuse and homogeneous or central and smooth. 30% of hamartomas may show "popcorn" calcification.

[d] Some malignancies, such as small bronchioloalveolar cell carcinomas or well differentiated adenocarcinomas and carcinoid tumors may not be PET avid, resulting in false-negative results.

Differential Diagnosis of Pulmonary Nodules

Granulomas

- Tuberculosis
- Histoplasmosis
- Sarcoidosis

Benign Neoplasms

- Hamartoma
- Chondroma
- Pulmonary pseudotumor

Malignant Neoplasms

- Primary lung cancer (adenocarcinoma, squamous cell and other cell types
- Metastases

- Carcinoid
- Kaposi sarcoma
- Lymphoma

Other

- Septic emboli
- Intrapulmonary lymph node
- Arteriovenous malformation
- Round atelectasis
- Round pneumonia (including cryptogenic organizing pneumonia)

The uptake of FDG with PET in nonneoplastic thoracic diseases may limit the evaluation of patients with a pulmonary nodule. Knowledge of the conditions with positive FDG uptake will provide accurate diagnosis and avoid unnecessary treatments. The fusion of the established technologies of PET and CT into a single PET/CT system promises more accurate diagnosis and staging of malignant nodules.

Additional Readings

1. MacMahon H, Austin JH, Gamsu G, et al. Guidelines for management of small pulmonary nodules detected on CT scans: A statement from the Fleishner Society. Radiology 2005;237:395–400
2. Shaefer-Prokop C, Prokop M. Lungs and tracheobronchial system. In: Prokop M, Galanski M, eds. Spiral and Multislice Computed Tomography of the Body. Stuttgart, Germany: Thieme Medical Publishing; 2003
3. Technology Forum AJR. Issues, controversies & utility of PET/CT imaging. AJR Am J Roentgenol 2005;194: S135–S155
4. Travis WD, Garg K, Franklin W, et al. Evolving concepts in the pathology and CT imaging of lung adenocarcinoma and bronchioloalveolar carcinoma. J Clin Oncol 2005; 23:3279–3287
5. Winer-Muram HT. Solitary pulmonary nodule. Radiology 2006;293:34–49

61

Lung Transplantation

Indications

Single Lung Transplantations

- Emphysema
- Idiopathic pulmonary fibrosis
- Alpha-1 antitrypsin deficiency
- Sarcoidosis
- Langerhans cell histiocytosis
- Chronic hypersensitivity pneumonitis
- Lymphangioleiomyomatosis
- Drug-induced pulmonary fibrosis

The only absolute contraindications to single lung transplantations are chronic pulmonary sepsis and uncorrectable cardiac defects.

Bilateral Lung Transplantations

- "Septic" lung diseases such as cystic fibrosis and bronchiectasis
- Primary pulmonary hypertension

Heart–Lung Transplantations

- Uncorrectable congenital heart disease

Complications

Table 61.1 provides an overview of the complications associated with lung transplantation.

Lymphoproliferative Disorders

The spectrum of expression ranges from a mild, benign polyclonal proliferation of lymphatic tissue with few if any signs and symptoms to non-Hodgkin's lymphoma. The incidence of post-transplant lymphoproliferative disorders (PTLD) after lung transplantation ranges from 6.2 to 9.4% and is twofold higher than what is seen after transplantation of other organs. Almost all cases of this disorder result from a combination of Epstein–Barr virus (EBV), stimulation of B-lymphocyte proliferation associated with a cyclosporin-inhibited regulatory mechanism of T-lymphocyte proliferation. A higher incidence of PTLD in children as compared with adults has been attributed to a greater susceptibility to EBV infection. A unique feature of this entity is that lymphoid masses may regress or disappear when immunosuppressive therapy is stopped or reduced.

Intrathoracic PTLD is most commonly characterized by the presence of discrete nodules, more often multiple than solitary. The nodules are frequently distributed in peribronchovascular and subpleural locations involving the lower and middle lung zones. The intrathoracic computed tomography (CT) findings of PTLD are similar in immunocompromised patients with or without AIDS and are usually extranodal. Less frequently, mediastinal or hilar lymph node enlargement can be a manifestation of PTLD. Thymic, pericardial, and pleural involvement has also been reported.

Table 61.1 Complications Associated with Lung Transplantation

Complication	Description	Time of Appearance
Primary Graft Failure	Mimics findings of pulmonary edema	First 24 hours
Reperfusion Edema	Mimics findings of pulmonary edema	Within 1st week
Acute Rejection	Reticular areas of increased opacity, indistinct 2–3 mm diameter nodules, ground-glass opacity and consolidation COP can often be associated with acute rejection, more often with BLT (13%) than with SLT (5%).	First week, but may occur as early as 24 hours after transplantation Most recipients experience 2 or 3 significant rejection episodes in the first 3 months. After 6 months, acute rejection becomes less common.
Infection	Bacterial or fungal CMV, PCP, bacteria, or fungi, *Aspergillus*, *Candida*	First month after transplantation After 1 month
Airway Complications	Bronchial anastomotic dehiscence, necrosis, malacia, and stenosis	Early or late
Pleural Space & Diaphragmatic Abnormalities	Pleural effusion, pneumothorax Phrenic nerve injury	Early or late
Lymphoproliferative Disorders*	Single or multiple nodules, lymphadenopathy	From 1 month to several years, peaks around 6 months after transplantation

Abbreviations: BLT, bilateral lung transplantations; CMV, cytomegalovirus; COP, cryptogenic organizing pneumonia; PCP, *Pneumocystis carinii;* SLT, single lung transplantations.

Bronchiolitis Obliterans Syndrome

The major long-term complication of lung and heart–lung transplantation is the development of bronchiolitis obliterans syndrome (BOS), which is thought to be a manifestation of chronic rejection. This complication develops in approximately one-third of patients who survive longer than 6 months and the mortality rate is 29 to 50%. BOS has been associated with multiple episodes of acute rejection and chronic cytomegalovirus infection. The clinical manifestation of BOS includes cough and progressive dyspnea. CT commonly shows bronchial dilatation and decrease in lung attenuation with narrowing of vessels, which is assumed to be due to air trapping and oligemia. Bronchial dilatation on CT can precede clinical manifestation of BOS.

Miscellaneous Complications

Other complications include herniation of native hyperinflated lung across the midline resulting in graft compression, herniation at the operative site, development of ill-defined nodular opacities, which may be associated with a linear opacity representing needle tract and cavitation after transbronchial biopsy, and lung torsion. Finally, disease recurrence in the donor lung, although rare, has been reported to occur in patients who received a transplant for sarcoidosis, panbronchiolitis, and lymphangioleiomyomatosis.

Additional Readings

1. Collins J, Muller NL, Leung AN, et al. Epstein-Barr-virus-associated lymphoproliferative disease of the Lung: CT and histologic findings. Radiology 1998;208:749–759

2. Cooper JD. Lung transplantation. In: Sabiston D & Spencer F, eds. Surgery of the Chest. 5th ed. Vol 2. Philadelphia, PA: Saunders; 1990:1950–1964

3. Garg K, Zamora MR, Tuder R, Armstrong JD, Lynch DA. Lung transplantation: indications, donor and recipient selection, and imaging of complications. Radiographics 1996;16:355–367

4. McAdams HP, Palmer SM, Erasmus JJ, et al. Bronchial anastomotic complications in lung transplant recipients: virtual bronchoscopy for noninvasive assessment. Radiology 1998;209:689–695

5. Shreeniwas R, Schulman LL, Berkmen YM, McGregor CC, Austin JHM. Opportunistic bronchopulmonary infections after lung transplantation: clinical and radiographic findings. Radiology 1996;200:349–356

6. Worthy SA, Park CS, Kim JS, Muller NL. Bronchiolitis obliterans after lung transplantation: high-resolution CT findings in 15 patients. AJR Am J Roentgenol 1997; 169:673–677

62

Pleural Effusions

Exudative versus Transudative Effusion on Computed Tomography

The most common cause of transudative effusion is congestive heart failure. The most common cause of exudative effusion is infection or pneumonia. In older patients, exudative effusions secondary to malignancy should be considered (**Table 62.1**). Thick enhancing pleural rind suggests exudative effusion. Pleural-based soft tissue nodules may be seen in malignant effusions on computed tomography (CT). Lung cancer and breast lymphomas are the cause of 75% of malignant effusions. A hematocrit effect (layering of blood products) should be looked for on the narrow mediastinal window to assess for hemothorax.

Mechanisms by which Malignancy Leads to Pleural Effusion

- Direct
  - Pleural metastasis
  - Obstruction of pleural lymphatic vessels
  - Mediastinal lymph node involvement with decreased pleural lymphatic drainage
  - Chylothorax (thoracic duct obstruction)
  - Bronchial obstruction (decreased pleural pressures)
  - Pericardial involvement
- Indirect
  - Hypoproteinemia
  - Postobstructive pneumonitis
  - Pulmonary embolism
  - Postradiation therapy

Table 62.1 The Appearance of Transudative versus Exudative Effusion on Computed Tomography

	Transudative Effusion	Exudative Effusion
Glucose	–	↑
Protein	–	↑
Blood	–	↑
LDH	–	↑
pH	–	↓
Appearance	Thin, clear	Cloudy, bloody

Chylous Effusion

Chylous effusion is due to thoracic duct obstruction or disruption. Common causes are lymphoma, trauma, lymphangioleiomyomatosis (LAM), and malignancy.

Pseudochylous Effusion/Chyliform Pleural Effusion

The pseudochylous effusion, also called cholesterol effusion, is a high-lipid effusion that is turbid or milky, but not chylous, as it does not result from the disruption of the thoracic duct. The chyliform pleural effusion is formed on the basis of a chronic pleural effusion surrounded by thickened and fibrotic and sometimes calcified pleura. The two most common causes of chyliform effusions are tuberculosis and rheumatoid arthritis. Other causes include paragonimiasis, syphilis, diabetes, Behçet's syndrome, alcoholism, or neoplastic disease. The mean duration for the effusion is 5 years before it turns chyliform. Many patients are asymptomatic. Chyliform effusions are usually unilateral.

Hepatic Hydrothorax

Hepatic hydrothorax is defined as a pleural effusion in a cirrhotic patient in the absence of significant pulmonary or cardiac disease. The predominant mechanism leading to a pleural effusion in a cirrhotic patient with ascites appears to be the movement of the ascitic fluid from the peritoneal cavity to the pleural space through the diaphragm.

Pancreatic Pleural Effusion

Pleural effusions are associated with both acute and chronic pancreatitis. Pancreatic pleural effusion typically shows a high amylase to serum ratio, pH of 7.3 to 7.35, glucose pleural fluid is equal to serum and polymorphonuclear predominant white cell count.

Additional Readings

1. Alberts WM, Salem AJ, Solomon DA, et al. Hepatic hydrothorax: cause and management. Arch Intern Med 1991;151:2383–2388
2. Dewan NA, Kinney WW, O'Donahue WJ Jr. Chronic massive pancreatic pleural effusion. Chest 1984;85: 497–501
3. Light RW. Chylothorax and pseudochylothorax. In: Light RW, ed. Pleural Diseases. 4th ed. Baltimore, MD: Williams and Wilkins, 327–343
4. Light RW. Pleural diseases. 3rd ed. Baltimore, MD: Williams and Wilkins; 1995
5. Song JW, Im JG, Goo JM, Kim HY, Song CS, Lee JS. Pseudochylous pleural effusion with fat-fluid levels: report of six cases. Radiology 2000;216:478–480

63

Pericardial Effusion

It can be difficult to differentiate benign from malignant pericardial effusion by CT or MRI. Thick enhancing pericardium and loculations suggest exudative effusion. Pericardial-based soft tissue nodules and complexity of effusion may be seen in malignant pericardial effusion.

Causes of Pericardial Effusion

- Idiopathic pericarditis
- Uremia
- Infections (bacterial, viral, fungal)
- Connective tissue disorders
- Postprocedure (iatrogenic)
- Trauma
- Postmyocardial infarction
- Radiation therapy
- Malignancy

64

Pulmonary Embolism

With the introduction of multidetector row computed tomography (MDCT), CT has been firmly established as the de facto first-line test for imaging patients with suspected pulmonary embolism (PE). Magnetic resonance imaging (MRI) for PE is indicated only in select cases, mostly with contraindication to iodinated contrast agents. Even in those cases, CT could be attempted using gadolinium DTPA (diethyl-enetriamine penta-acetic acid) as the contrast agent. CT, unlike conventional pulmonary angiography or a lung scan, can provide alternative diagnoses for patients' signs and symptoms and reveal additional findings. The newer faster, multidetector CT with improved temporal resolution not only allows diagnosis of common noncardiac causes of acute pain such as acute or chronic PE (**Table 64.1**) or aortic dissection, but the same scan can be used to evaluate the heart and coronary arteries.

Limitations of Computed Tomography

The most common reasons for nondiagnostic CT studies are poor contrast opacification of pulmonary vessels, patient motion, and increased

Table 64.1 Computed Tomography Findings in Acute versus Chronic Pulmonary Embolism (PE)

CT Finding	Acute PE	Chronic PE
Filling defect	Central	Eccentric, mural
Lumen	Occluded	Nonoccluded
Embolus attenuation	Hypodense[a]	Hyperdense
Calcification	Absent	Present
Bronchial artery collaterals	Absent	Present[b]
Caliber of involved artery	Larger	Smaller, poorly enhancing
Central pulmonary arteries	Normal[c]	Larger
Webs, recanalization	Absent	Present
Pulmonary parenchyma	Infarct[d]	Mosaic attenuation

[a] Rarely, acute embolus may be dense on unenhanced multidetector row computed tomography (MDCT).

[b] The presence of collaterals favors chronic thromboembolism over primary pulmonary hypertension as the cause of pulmonary arterial hypertension.

[c] May be larger in cases of massive PE (≥50% arterial bed involvement) resulting in acute cor pulmonale

[d] Corresponding radiographic sign is Hampton's hump. Similarly, computed tomography shows direct findings corresponding to other radiographic signs: the Knuckle and Westermark signs.

image noise due to morbid obesity. In many instances, these limitations could be resolved with improved intravenous access, a higher contrast media injection rate, the use of automated bolus triggering techniques, adaptation of tube output to patient's body type, the use of electrocardiogram (ECG) synchronized scan acquisition, etc.

Additional Readings

1. Garg K, Kemp JL, Wojcik D, et al. Thromboembolic disease: comparison of combined CT pulmonary angiography and venography with bilateral leg sonography in 70 patients. AJR Am J Roentgenol 2000;175:997–1001
2. Garg K, Sieler H, Welsh CH, et al. Clinical validity of helical CT being interpreted as negative for pulmonary embolism: implications for patient treatment. AJR Am J Roentgenol 1999;172:1627–1631
3. Kanne JP, Gotway MB, Thhoongsuwan N, Stern EJ. Six cases of acute central PE revealed on MDCT of the chest. AJR Am J Roentgenol 2003;180:1661–1664
4. Patel S, Kazerooni EA. Helical CT for the evaluation of acute pulmonary embolism. AJR Am J Roentgenol 2005; 185:135–149
5. Qanadli SD, Hajjam ME, Mesurolle B, et al. Pulmonary embolism detection: prospective evaluation of dual-section helical CT versus selective pulmonary arteriography in 157 patients. Radiology 2000;217: 447–455
6. Schoepf UJ, Costello P. Spiral computed tomography is the first-line chest imaging test for acute pulmonary embolism: yes. J Thromb Haemost 2005;3:7–10
7. Schoepf UJ, Holzknect N, Helmberger TK, et al. Subsegmental pulmonary emboli: improved detection with thin-collimation multi-detector row spiral CT. Radiology 2002;222:483–490

65

Aortic Dissection

Stanford Classification

- Stanford A: Dissection involves ascending aorta
- Stanford B: Dissection involves descending aorta (beyond left subclavian artery)

DeBakey Classification

- Type 1: Dissection involves both ascending and descending thoracic aorta
- Type 2: Dissection involves only ascending aorta
- Type 3: Dissection involves only descending aorta

Aortic Dissection versus Motion Artifact

Aortic wall motion can produce curvilinear artifacts in the proximal ascending aorta near the aortic root, which mimic a dissection. These artifacts are typically at the left anterior (12 to 1 o'clock) and right posterior (6 to 7 o'clock) locations.[1]

True versus False Lumen

The true and false lumens are usually easily distinguished. However, the distinction can occasionally be difficult. The false lumen typically has a larger cross-sectional area. The presence of an acute angle between the flap and the outer wall (the "beak" sign) is seen only in the false lumen. Slender lines of low attenuation can be seen in the false lumen (the "cobweb" sign), which represent residual strands of the media. If one lumen wraps around another in the aortic arch, the inner lumen is the true lumen. Outer wall calcification always indicates the true lumen in an acute dissection. However, the outer wall of the false lumen can calcify in a chronic dissection if the false lumen lining endothelializes.[2,3]

Features of the False Lumen in an Aortic Dissection

- Larger cross-sectional area
- Beak sign
- Cobweb sign
- Outer lumen

A Thrombosed False Lumen versus a Mural Thrombus

A mural thrombus tends to be circumferential in relation to the aortic lumen; thrombosed false lumen will spiral longitudinally. Intimal calcification if present is peripheral to mural thrombus. Mural thrombus tends to have an irregular internal border, whereas the internal border of a false lumen is typically smooth.[3]

Aortic Dissection, Intramural Hematoma, and Penetrating Atherosclerotic Ulcer

An aortic dissection, intramural hematoma, and penetrating atherosclerotic ulcer (PAU) differ in clinical and radiographic presentation.[4] In an aortic dissection, a flap traverses the aortic lumen. An intramural hematoma and a PAU do not have flaps. Intramural hematomas can occur as a primary event where there is spontaneous bleeding from the vasa vasorum into the media, or a PAU can cause an intramural hematoma. Patients with an intramural hematoma and a PAU are usually in the seventh to ninth decades of life; they are typically older than patients who have had aortic dissections. An intramural hematoma and a PAU usually typically occur in patients with hypertension. A PAU is usually associated with severe aortic atherosclerosis. Both intramural hematoma and PAU typically occur in the descending aorta. Specifically, a PAU occurs in the middle and distal third of the descending thoracic aorta. The following features are helpful in differentiating an intramural hematoma and a PAU from other entities.

Intramural Hematoma versus Mural Thrombus

Intramural hematomas may occasionally be difficult to differentiate from mural thrombus. Intramural hematoma is hyperdense on unenhanced computed tomography (CT). Intramural hematomas are subintimal, whereas mural thrombus lies on top of the intima.[5]

Intramural Hematoma versus Thrombosed False Lumen

An intramural hematoma tends to be circumferential in relation to the aortic lumen, whereas a thrombosed false lumen will spiral longitudinally. If there is very slow flow in the false lumen, this can sometimes be detected by cine magnetic resonance imaging (MRI).[3,5]

Penetrating Atherosclerotic Ulcer versus Ulcerated Atheromatous Plaque

An ulcerated atheromatous plaque can resemble a penetrating atherosclerotic ulcer. However, the ulceration in an atheromatous plaque does not extend beyond the intima. The PAU will have associated findings not seen in an ulcerated atheromatous plaque. These may include intramural hematoma, focal outpouching of the aortic wall, and thickening and contrast enhancement of the peripheral aortic wall.[1,6]

Penetrating Atherosclerotic Ulcer versus Branch Artery Pseudoaneurysm Accompanying Aortic Dissection

Pseudoaneurysms are sometimes seen in the thrombosed false lumen of an aortic dissection. These are collections of contrast which are related to branch artery origins and that do not communicate with the aortic lumen.[7] However, these can resemble PAUs. Branch artery pseudoaneurysms typically do not involve the lateral pleural wall of the aorta. PAUs typically do not occur near the origins of aortic branch arteries.

References

1. Batra P, Bigoni B, Manning J, et al. Pitfalls in the diagnosis of thoracic aortic dissection at CT angiography. Radiographics 2000;20:309–320
2. Lepage MA, Quint LE, Sonnad SS, Deeb GM, Williams DM. Aortic dissection: CT features that distinguish true lumen from false lumen. AJR Am J Roentgenol 2001;177:207–211
3. Castaner E, Andreu M, Gallardo X, Mata JM, Cabezeulo MA, Pallardo Y. CT in nontraumatic acute thoracic aortic disease: typical and atypical features and complications. Radiographics 2003;23:S93–S110
4. Coady MA, Rizzo JA, Elefteriades JA. Pathologic variants of thoracic aortic dissections. Penetrating atherosclerotic ulcers and intramural hematomas. Cardiol Clin 1999;17: 637–657

5. Macura KJ, Corl FM, Fishman EK, Bluemke DA. Pathogenesis in acute aortic syndromes: aortic dissection, intramural hematoma, and penetrating atherosclerotic ulcer. AJR Am J Roentgenol 2003;181: 309–316

6. Bhalla S, West OC. CT of nontraumatic thoracic aortic emergencies. Semin Ultrasound CT MR 2005;26: 281–304

7. Williams DM, Cronin P, Dasika N, et al. Aortic branch artery pseudoaneurysms accompanying aortic dissection. Part II. Distinction from penetrating atherosclerotic ulcers. J Vasc Interv Radiol 2006;17: 773–781

66

Cardiac Aneurysms and Abnormalities

True versus False Left Ventricular Aneurysm

A false aneurysm of the left ventricle is a rare complication of myocardial infarction. A false aneurysm is a contained rupture; the wall does not contain myocardial elements. It is important to differentiate a false aneurysm from a true aneurysm, which has a wall containing myocardial elements, as a false aneurysm can rupture at any age and requires surgical repair.

Features of False Left Ventricular Aneurysms[1]

- Inferior or inferolateral wall location
- Narrow ostium connecting aneurysm sac to ventricle
- Delayed pericardial enhancement on magnetic resonance imaging (MRI)

Atrial Myxoma versus Thrombus

MRI signal characteristics are typically not useful in differentiating atrial myxomas from thrombus, as they can both be heterogeneous in signal intensity on spin echo images and hypointense on gradient echo images. However, myxomas tend to be more heterogeneous in attenuation than thrombi on computed tomography (CT).[2] Location is helpful as thrombi typically arise from the posterior and lateral atrial walls and the atrial appendages. Myxomas typically arise from the interatrial septum, in particular, the fossa ovalis. Myxomas usually have a thin stalk; however, this typically cannot be demonstrated by MRI. A narrow base of attachment suggests a myxoma.[3] Enhancement is seen in myxomas but not thrombus.

Features of Atrial Myxomas

- Enhancement
- Arise from interatrial septum
- Narrow base of attachment

Delayed Myocardial Enhancement

Delayed myocardial contrast enhancement during MRI is a sign of scarring after myocardial infarction. However, there are many other etiologies of delayed myocardial enhancement besides infarction.[4] When delayed enhancement occurs in nonischemic myocardial disease, it is typically not in an arterial distribution and occurs in the mid-wall (compared with transmural or subendocardial enhancement in infarction).

Etiologies of Delayed Myocardial Enhancement

- Myocardial infarction
- Myocarditis
- Vasculitis
- Sarcoidosis

- Cardiomyopathy–dilated, restrictive, or hypertrophic
- Arrhythmogenic right ventricular dysplasia
- Muscular dystrophy

Atrial Septal Defect versus Fossa Ovalis

A fossa ovalis can sometimes be confused with an ostium secundum atrial septal defect on MRI. The atrial septal defect should have increased thickness of the septum at the margins of the defect. In a fossa ovalis, the septum at the margin of the defect is thin. Cine MRI may demonstrate a flow void from a left-to-right shunt in an atrial septal defect.

References

1. Konen E, Merchant N, Gutierrez C, et al. True vs. false left ventricular aneurysm: differentiation with MR imaging – initial experience. Radiology 2005;236:65–70
2. Grebenc ML, Rosado de Christenson ML, Burke AP, Green CE, Galvin JR. Primary cardiac and pericardial neoplasms: radiologic-pathologic correlation. Radiographics 2000;20:1073–1103
3. Araoz PA, Mulvagh SL, Tazelaar HD, Julsrud PR, Breen JF. CT and MRI imaging of benign primary cardiac neoplasms with echocardiographic correlation. Radiographics 2000;20:1303–1319
4. Vogel-Claussen J, Rochitte CE, Wu KC, et al. Delayed enhancement MR imaging: utility in myocardial assessment. Radiographics 2006;26:795–810

IV   Abdomen

67

Overview of Liver Lesions

Hemangioma

Demographics

- More common in women

Classic Imaging Appearance

- Enhancement: Peripheral nodular discontinuous enhancement progressing centripetally, persistent enhancement equal to the vessels
- Magnetic resonance imaging (MRI):
  - T1-weighted: Hypointense
  - T2-weighted: Hyperintense

Differentiating Features

Hemangioma versus Hypervascular Metastasis or Hepatocellular Carcinoma

- Enhancement in hemangiomas is equal to the vessels.
- Hemangiomas have persistent enhancement on delayed images.
- Hemangiomas have a greater degree of T2-weighted MRI (T2WI) hyperintensity.
- Hemangiomas may have perilesional enhancement (however, this can be seen in hepatocellular carcinoma [HCC]).

Cholangiocarcinoma versus Hemangioma

- Peripheral enhancement in cholangiocarcinoma is less than in the vessels and usually continuous rather than nodular and discontinuous.
- Both lesions can have capsular retraction.

Focal Nodular Hyperplasia

Demographics

- Young to middle-aged women

Classic Imaging Features

- Central scar
- Enhancement: Homogeneous arterial phase enhancement, delayed enhancement of central scar
- Computed tomography (CT):
  - Noncontrast: Isodense or hypodense
  - Arterial phase: Hyperdense
  - Portal phase: Isodense or hypodense
  - Delayed phase: Isodense, central scar hyperdense
- MRI:
  - T1-weighted: Isointense or hypointense
  - T2-weighted: Isointense or hyperintense

Differentiating Features

- Central scar
- Homogeneity
- Arterial phase enhancement

Focal Nodular Hyperplasia versus Adenoma

- Greater degree of arterial phase enhancement than adenoma
- More likely to be isodense in the portal phase than adenoma
- More homogeneous than adenoma
- Central scar very rarely seen in adenoma
- Hemorrhage very rarely seen in focal nodular hyperplasia (FNH)
- Macroscopic fat can be seen in adenomas, but is rare in FNH
- Delayed gadobenate dimeglumine (Gd-BOPTA; Multihance, Bracco Imaging, Milan, Italy) uptake is seen in FNH, but not adenomas
- Subcapsular feeding arteries more likely in adenoma

Focal Nodular Hyperplasia versus Fibrolamellar Hepatocellular Carcinoma

- In FNH, the central scar is hyperintense on T2WI, hypointense in fibrolamellar HCC.
- Delayed enhancement of central scar is seen in FNH, but not fibrolamellar HCC.
- Scar is smaller in FNH.
- Intracellular lipid detectable by chemical shift MRI is more commonly seen in FNH.
- Fibrolamellar HCC is larger, more lobulated, and more heterogeneous.
- Calcifications are very rare in FNH, but common in fibrolamellar HCC.

Hepatic Adenoma

Demographics

- Young and middle-aged women
- Oral contraceptive use
- Men – anabolic steroids or glycogen storage disease

Classic Imaging Features

- Enhancement: Arterial phase enhancement, often heterogeneous

- CT:
  - Noncontrast: Isodense or hypodense
  - Arterial phase: Hyperdense, often heterogeneous
  - Portal phase: Hyperdense, isodense, or hypodense
  - Delayed phase: Isodense or hypodense
- MRI:
  - T1-weighted: Hypointense, often heterogeneous
  - T2-weighted: Hyperintense, often heterogeneous

Differentiating Features

- Arterial phase enhancement
- Heterogeneity
- Hemorrhage
- Macroscopic and microscopic fat

Adenoma versus Focal Nodular Hyperplasia

- Lesser degree of arterial phase enhancement than FNH
- More likely to be hyperdense in the portal phase than FNH
- More heterogeneous than FNH
- Central scar is very rarely seen in adenoma.
- Hemorrhage is very rarely seen in FNH.
- Macroscopic fat can be seen in adenomas, but is rare in FNH.
- Delayed Gd-BOPTA (Multihance) uptake is seen in FNH, but not adenomas.
- Subcapsular feeding arteries more likely in adenoma

Hepatocellular Carcinoma

Demographics

- Cirrhotic livers
- Usually after 30 years of age, later onset in lower incidence areas
- More common in men, particularly in high incidence areas

Classic Imaging Appearance

- Enhancement: Heterogeneous arterial phase enhancement
- CT:
  - Noncontrast: Hypodense
  - Arterial phase: Hyperdense, heterogeneous
  - Portal phase: Hypodense, heterogeneous
  - Delayed phase: Hypodense
- MRI:
  - T1-weighted: Hypointense
  - T2-weighted: Hyperintense

Differentiating Features

- Cirrhotic liver
- Hypervascular
- Rapid washout, lack of delayed enhancement
- Heterogeneous
- T2WI hyperintense
- Capsule

HCC versus Regenerating or Dysplastic Nodule

- HCC has arterial phase enhancement (rarely regenerating or dysplastic nodules may enhance)
- HCC is hyperintense on T2WI.
- HCC is more heterogeneous.
- HCC is hypoattenuating or hypointense on portal and delayed images.
- HCC may have a peripheral enhancing capsule.

Hepatocellular Carcinoma versus Pseudolesion (from Arterioportal Shunt)

- HCCs have early enhancement with rapid central washout. Pseudolesions usually enhance later and the enhancement persists longer.
- HCCs may have coronal enhancement surrounding the lesion.
- A rounded configuration is more likely in HCC.
- Bulging of the capsule is only seen in HCC.

- Pseudolesions are isointense to liver on T1WI and T2WI.

Small Hepatocellular Carcinoma versus Small Hemangioma

- Enhancement in HCC is usually less than in the vessels.
- HCC does not have persistent enhancement on delayed images.
- HCC is usually less hyperintense on T2WI.

Fibrolamellar Hepatocellular Carcinoma

Demographics

- Most common in young adults; no sex predilection

Classic Imaging Features

- Central scar
- Enhancement: Heterogeneous arterial phase enhancement
- CT:
  - Noncontrast: Heterogeneous, calcification common
  - Arterial phase: Hyperdense, heterogeneous
  - Portal phase: Isodense or hypodense
  - Delayed phase: Isodense
- MRI:
  - T1-weighted: Hypointense
  - T2-weighted: Hyperintense, heterogeneous

Differentiating Features

- Arterial phase enhancement
- Central scar
- Calcification
- Large size
- Heterogeneity

Fibrolamellar Hepatocellular Carcinoma versus Focal Nodular Hyperplasia

- Central scar is T2WI hypointense in fibrolamellar HCC, hyperintense in FNH.

- Delayed enhancement of central scar is seen in FNH, but not fibrolamellar HCC.
- Scar is larger in fibrolamellar HCC.
- Intracellular lipid detectable by chemical shift MRI is more commonly seen in FNH.
- Fibrolamellar HCC is larger, more lobulated, and more heterogeneous.
- Calcifications are common in fibrolamellar HCC, but rare in FNH.

Cholangiocarcinoma (Peripheral)

Demographics

- Older than 50 years of age

Classic Imaging Appearance

- Enhancement: Peripheral enhancement progressing centripetally, delayed enhancement
- MRI:
  - T1-weighted: Hypointense, heterogeneous
  - T2-weighted: Heterogeneous, particularly centrally

Differentiating Features

- Peripheral enhancement progressing centripetally
- Delayed enhancement
- Capsular retraction
- Bile duct dilatation peripheral to tumor

Cholangiocarcinoma versus Hemangioma

- Peripheral enhancement in cholangiocarcinoma is less than in the vessels and is usually continuous rather than nodular and discontinuous.
- Both lesions can have capsular retraction.

Biliary Hamartoma

Demographics

- No sex or age predilection

Classic Imaging Features

- Multiple small cystic-appearing nodules
- Enhancement: Possible rim enhancement
- CT:
  - Noncontrast: Hypodense, fluid density
- MRI:
  - T1-weighted: Hypointense
  - T2-weighted: Hyperintense

Differentiating Features

- Irregular in shape
- Less than 1.5 cm in size
- Adjacent to medium-size portal tracts
- Scattered throughout entire liver, including subcapsular region
- Best seen on enhanced CT and T2WI
- Very hyperintense on T2WI
- No enhancement or slight rim enhancement

Hepatic Angiomyolipoma

Demographics

- Marked female predominance
- Age range 30–70 years
- Associated with tuberous sclerosis

Classic Imaging Features

- Enhancement: Arterial phase enhancement that persists on delayed images
- CT:
  - Noncontrast: Heterogeneous, areas of fat density
- MRI:
  - T1-weighted: Heterogeneous, high T1WI signal from fat
  - T2-weighted: Heterogeneous

Differentiating Features

- Fat component
- Arterial phase enhancement
- Prolonged enhancement
- Central feeding vessels

Hepatic Angiomyolipoma versus Hepatocellular Carcinoma

- Angiomyolipoma has greater fat component.
- Both lesions enhance on arterial phase, but angiomyolipoma peaks later.
- Angiomyolipoma has prolonged enhancement, which is rare in HCC.
- HCC often has a capsule, which is not seen in angiomyolipoma.
- The feeding vessels in an angiomyolipoma are central, in HCC they are peripheral.

Epithelioid Hemangioendothelioma

Demographics

- Adults, average age 45 years old, slight female predominance

Classic Imaging Appearance

- Peripheral nodules that can coalesce into large confluent peripheral masses
- Enhancement: Target appearance – hypodense center with peripheral enhancing rim and hypodense halo around the enhancing rim
- CT:
  - Noncontrast: Hypodense
- MRI:
  - T1-weighted: Hypointense
  - T2-weighted: Hyperintense

Differentiating Features

- Peripheral location
- Target enhancement pattern
- Capsular retraction

Peliosis Hepatis

Demographics

- Associated with malignancies, chronic infections, acquired immune deficiency syndrome, drugs (e.g., oral contraceptives, anabolic steroids)
- No sex predilection

Classic Imaging Appearance

- Multiple lesions, size ranges from 1 mm to several centimeters
- Enhancement: Peripheral enhancement progressing centripetally, or central enhancement progressing centrifugally – persists on delayed images
- CT:
  - Noncontrast: Hypodense
- MRI:
  - T1-weighted: Hypointense, may have areas of hyperintensity from hemorrhage
  - T2-weighted: Hyperintense

Differentiating Features

- Lack of mass effect
- Multiplicity
- Progressive enhancement pattern starting centrally or peripherally
- Prolonged enhancement

Hemangioma versus Peliosis Hepatis

- Peliosis lacks mass effect
- If peliosis has peripheral enhancement, it is typically continuous rather than nodular and discontinuous.

Noncirrhotic Regenerative Nodules

Demographics

- Associated with disorders that impair hepatic blood flow, e.g., Budd-Chiari, autoimmune disease, autoimmune hepatitis, lympho- and myeloproliferative disorders, steroids, and antineoplastic medications

Classic Imaging Appearance

- Enhancement: Arterial phase enhancement

- CT:
  - Noncontrast: Isodense
- MRI:
  - T1-weighted: Often hyperintense
  - T2-weighted: Isointense or hypointense

- Noncirrhotic regenerative nodules are often hypervascular
- Noncirrhotic regenerative nodules are often hyperintense on T1WI
- Larger noncirrhotic regenerative nodules often have central scars

Differentiating Features

- Noncirrhotic regenerative nodules versus cirrhotic regenerative nodules

Additional Readings

1. Ahmadi T, Itai Y, Takahashi M, et al. Angiomyolipoma of the liver: significance of CT and MR dynamic study. Abdom Imaging 1998;23:520–526
2. Brancatelli G, Federle MP, Grazioli L, Golfieri R, Lencioni R. Benign regenerative nodules in Budd-Chiari syndrome and other vascular disorders of the liver: radiologic-pathologic and clinical correlation. Radiographics 2002;22:847–862
3. Federle MP, Jeffrey RB, Desser TS, et al. Diagnostic Imaging: Abdomen. Salt Lake City, UT:Amirsys;2004
4. Freeny PC, Grossholz M, Kaakaji K, Schmiedl UP. Significance of hyperattenuating and contrast-enhancing hepatic nodules detected in the cirrhotic liver during arterial phase helical CT in pre-liver transplant patients: radiologic-histopathologic correlation of explanted livers. Abdom Imaging 2003; 28:333–346
5. Gouya H, Vignaux O, Legmann P, de Pigneux G, Bonnin A. Peliosis hepatis: triphasic helical CT and dynamic MRI findings. Abdom Imaging 2001;26: 507–509
6. Ito K, Fujita T, Shimizu A, et al. Multiarterial phase dynamic MRI of small early enhancing hepatic lesions in cirrhosis or chronic hepatitis: differentiating between hypervascular hepatocellular carcinomas and pseudolesions. AJR Am J Roentgenol 2004;183:699–705
7. Kim T, Federle MP, Baron RL, Peterson MS, Kawamori Y. Discrimination of small hepatic hemangiomas from hypervascular malignant tumors smaller than 3 cm with three-phase helical CT. Radiology 2001; 219:699–706
8. Luo TY, Itai Y, Eguchi N, et al. Von Meyenburg complexes of the liver: imaging findings. J Comput Assist Tomogr 1998;22:372–378
9. Maetani Y, Itoh K, Egawa H, et al. Benign hepatic nodules in Budd-Chiari syndrome: radiologic-pathologic correlation with emphasis on the central scar. AJR Am J Roentgenol 2002;178:869–875
10. Miller WJ, Dodd GD III, Federle MP, Baron RL. Epithelioid hemangioendothelioma of the liver: imaging findings with pathologic correlation. AJR Am J Roentgenol 1992;159:53–57
11. Mortele B, Mortele K, Seynaeve P, Vandevelde D, Kunnen M, Ros PR. Hepatic bile duct hamartomas (von Meyenburg Complexes): MR and MR cholangiography findings. J Comput Assist Tomogr 2002;26:438–443
12. Outwater EK, Ito K, Siegelman E, Martin CE, Bhatia M, Mitchell DG. Rapidly enhancing hepatic hemangiomas at MRI: distinction from malignancies with T2-weighted images. J Magn Reson Imaging 1997;7: 1033–1039
13. Qayyum A, Graser A, Westphalen A, et al. CT of benign hypervascular liver nodules in autoimmune hepatitis. AJR Am J Roentgenol 2004;183:1573–1576
14. Steinke K, Terraciano L, Wiesner W. Unusual cross-sectional imaging findings in hepatic peliosis. Eur Radiol 2003;13:1916–1919
15. Yan F, Zeng M, Zhou K, et al. Hepatic angiomyolipoma: various appearances on two-phase contrast scanning of spiral CT. Eur J Radiol 2002;41:12–18
16. Yang DM, Yoon MH, Kim HS, Kim HS, Chung JW. Capsular retraction in hepatic giant hemangioma: CT and MR features. Abdom Imaging 2001;26:36–38

68

Hypervascular Liver Lesions

The primary etiologies of hypervascular liver lesions are the hypervascular primary liver lesions and hypervascular metastases. Renal cell cancer, breast cancer, thyroid cancer, melanoma, carcinoid, islet cell, and sarcomas are the most common hypervascular liver metastases.[1] Small hemangiomas that demonstrate flash filling during early phase imaging can sometimes appear as small hypervascular lesions. The most common etiologies for a solitary large hypervascular mass in the absence of a primary malignancy are focal nodular hyperplasia (FNH), hepatic adenoma and hepatocellular carcinoma (HCC). Many HCCs can be differentiated on the basis of aggressive features and clinical setting. FNH and adenomas both occur in young and middle-aged women and adenomas are seen in

the setting of oral contraceptive use. Multiple imaging features are helpful for differentiating the two lesions (**Table 68.1**). A FNH with a central scar may be difficult to differentiate from a fibrolamellar carcinoma (see Chapter 70) and hepatic adenomas usually cannot be differentiated from low-grade HCCs.

Specific magnetic resonance imaging (MRI) contrast agents may be helpful in differential diagnosis. Gadobenate dimeglumine (Multihance, Bracco Imaging, Milan, Italy) differs from conventional gadolinium-based agents as 3 to 5% of the dose is eliminated through the hepatobiliary pathway. As hepatic adenomas lack bile ducts they are hypointense on delayed (1 to 3 hours) images after gadobenate dimeglumine images. Focal nodular hyperplasia contains

Table 68.1 Focal Nodular Hyperplasia versus Hepatic Adenoma[3,19–21]

	FNH	Adenoma
Central scar	+	−
Heterogeneous enhancement	−	+
Heterogeneous intensity	−	+
Subcapsular feeding arteries	−	+
Degree of arterial phase enhancement*	>	<
Hemorrhage	−	+/−
T1WI hyperintensity	+/−	+/−
Delayed gadobenate dimeglumine uptake	+	−

Abbreviations: FNH, focal nodular hyperplasia; T1WI, T1-weighted magnetic resonance imaging.

* FNH has a greater degree of enhancement than adenoma in the arterial phase. FNH has an enhancement ratio of >1.6 (arterial phase attenuation compared with noncontrast attenuation) compared <1.6 for adenomas. However, in the portal phase FNH is often isodense; adenomas are often hyperdense.[20]

malformed biliary ductules and almost all lesions will be hyperintense or isointense to liver on delayed images.[2] Gadobenate dimeglumine is superior to superparamagnetic iron oxide (SPIO) particles for characterizing FNH,[3] as FNH and adenomas may have a comparable degree of SPIO uptake.[4]

Features of Specific Hypervascular Liver Lesions

Regenerative Nodules in Budd–Chiari Syndrome

Benign regenerative hepatic nodules have been described in Budd–Chiari syndrome, which are multiple, small, and hypervascular. These are likely a result of insufficient blood supply to portions of the liver that will atrophy, with compensatory nodular hyperplasia in areas of the liver with adequate blood supply. These nodules have also been reported in other systemic disorders, which impair hepatic blood flow, such as autoimmune disease, lympho- and myeloproliferative disorders, and after treatment with steroids and antineoplastic medications.[5] Similar nodules have also been described in autoimmune hepatitis.[6] These regenerative nodules are distinct from nodular regenerative hyperplasia (see Chapter 73)[7] in which there is no fibrosis between the nodules. These nodules can have central scars, especially if >1 cm in size. The lesions are sometimes hyperintense on T1-weighted imaging (T1WI) and usually isointense to hypointense on T2-weighted imaging (T2WI). Like focal nodular hyperplasia, they can demonstrate delayed gadobenate dimeglumine uptake. The multiplicity of these nodules is helpful in distinguishing them from other hypervascular liver lesions. The regenerative nodules in Budd–Chiari syndrome differ from regenerative nodules secondary to cirrhosis in these respects:[8]

- More often hyperintense on T1WI
- Usually enhance on arterial-phase images
- Larger lesions (>1 cm) often have central scars

Hepatic Angiosarcoma

The enhancement in hepatic angiosarcomas usually does not resemble that of hemangiomas. Focal areas of enhancement in angiosarcomas have less attenuation than the aorta and have irregular shapes, and could be central or ring-shaped. There is usually progressive enhancement on delayed images, which helps distinguish angiosarcoma from HCC. In addition, the presence of splenic metastases that is common in angiosarcoma aids in differentiation from HCC.[9]

Peliosis Hepatis

Multiple blood-filled cysts of varying size in the liver characterize peliosis hepatis. It is associated with malignancies, chronic infections, acquired immune deficiency syndrome (AIDS) and various drugs such as oral contraceptives and anabolic steroids. Reported enhancement patterns include peripheral enhancement progressing centripetally (mimicking a hemangioma) and central enhancement progressing centrifugally (more common).[10,11] Typically, the lesions lack mass effect, which is helpful in distinguishing them from other liver lesions. There is usually prolonged enhancement on delayed images, which is helpful in distinguishing peliosis from other hypervascular liver lesions.

Cholangiocarcinoma

Hypervascular intrahepatic cholangiocarcinomas are rare.[12] They have prolonged enhancement on delayed images, which helps differentiate them from HCC.

Hemangioma versus Hypervascular Tumors

Hemangiomas can usually be differentiated from other lesions on the basis of a globular, peripheral, progressive enhancement pattern. However, small hemangiomas can enhance homogeneously on arterial or portal phase images, and thus be difficult to distinguish from other hypervascular lesions. Some ways to distinguish a hemangioma in this case are[13,14]

- Degree of enhancement: The degree of enhancement of a hemangioma is equal to the aorta in the arterial phase and blood pool in the portal phase; other hypervascular lesions have a less degree of enhancement.
- Prolonged enhancement: On delayed imaging, hemangiomas will continue to have attenuation similar to blood pool, while other lesions will have washed out and become hypodense relative to the liver.
- T2WI: Hemangiomas are more hyperintense on heavily T2WI than other hypervascular lesions
- Perilesional enhancement: Hemangiomas sometimes demonstrate perilesional enhancement in the arterial phase (transient hepatic attenuation difference) (see Chapter 77). However, this finding is also seen in HCC.

Hypervascular Liver Lesions in Cirrhosis

HCC should be strongly considered when a hypervascular liver lesion is seen in the setting of cirrhosis. However, in some cases hypervascular pseudolesions and regenerating and dysplastic nodules can be difficult to differentiate from HCC.

Hepatocellular carcinomas are hypervascular and hyperintense on T2WI, which usually differentiates them from regenerating and dysplastic nodules. However, in rare cases regenerating and dysplastic nodules can be hypervascular.[15,16] In these atypical cases, some features of HCC that can be helpful in differentiating between HCC and regenerating or dysplastic nodules are

- Lesion heterogeneity
- Hypoattenuation or hypointensity on portal and delayed images
- Peripheral enhancing capsule
- T2WI hyperintensity

In patients with cirrhosis or chronic hepatitis, small hypervascular pseudolesions can be seen of uncertain etiology (arterioportal shunts may be one cause). These can be difficult to differentiate from small HCCs.

Some features of HCCs that can be helpful in differentiation from pseudolesions are[17]

- Rapid central washout: HCCs have early enhancement with rapid central washout. Pseudolesions usually enhance later and the enhancement persists longer.
- Coronal enhancement surrounding the lesion: This finding is not seen in pseudolesions.
- A rounded configuration is more likely in HCC.
- Bulging of the capsule is only seen in HCC.
- Pseudolesions are isotense to liver on T1WI and T2WI.

Another potentially hypervascular lesion seen in cirrhosis is confluent hepatic fibrosis.[18] However, it is rare for confluent hepatic fibrosis to enhance in the arterial phase; there is usually delayed enhancement. Confluent hepatic fibrosis is usually hyperintense on T2WI and if it is also hypervascular, it could potentially be confused with HCC. Confluent hepatic fibrosis can usually be easily distinguished from HCC by these features:

- Characteristic location in the anterior right and medial left lobes
- Wedge shape
- Capsular retraction
- Vessels pass directly through; lack of vascular invasion

Types of Hypervascular Liver Lesions[9,11,12,15,19]

- Focal nodular hyperplasia
- Hepatic adenoma
- Hepatocellular carcinoma
- Fibrolamellar HCC
- Hypervascular metastases
- Hemangiomas (small)
- Regenerative nodules in Budd–Chiari syndrome (and other vascular disorders)
- Angiomyolipoma
- Angiosarcoma
- Peliosis hepatis
- Cholangiocarcinoma (rare)
- Dysplastic nodules in cirrhosis (rare)
- Regenerating nodules in cirrhosis (rare)

References

1. Oliver JH III, Baron RL. Helical biphasic contrast-enhanced CT of the liver: technique, indications, interpretation, and pitfalls. Radiology 1996;201:1–14
2. Grazioli L, Morana G, Kirchin MA, Schneider G. Accurate differentiation of focal nodular hyperplasia from hepatic adenoma at gadobenate dimeglumine-enhanced MR imaging: prospective study. Radiology 2005;236:166–177
3. Grazioli L, Morana G, Kirchin MA, et al. MRI of focal nodular hyperplasia (FNH) with gadobenate dimeglumine (Gd-BOPTA) and SPIO (ferumoxides): an intra-individual comparison. J Magn Reson Imaging 2003;17:593–602
4. Grandin C, Van Beers BE, Robert A, Gigot JF, Geubel A, Pringot J. Benign hepatocellular tumors: MRI after superparamagnetic iron oxide administration. J Comput Assist Tomogr 1995;19:412–418
5. Brancatelli G, Federle MP, Grazioli L, Golfieri R, Lencioni R. Benign regenerative nodules in Budd-Chiari syndrome and other vascular disorders of the liver: radiologic-pathologic and clinical correlation. Radiographics 2002;22:847–862
6. Qayyum A, Graser A, Westphalen A, et al. CT of benign hypervascular liver nodules in autoimmune hepatitis. AJR Am J Roentgenol 2004;183:1573–1576
7. Clouet M, Boulay I, Boudiaf M, et al.. Imaging features of nodular regenerative hyperplasia of the liver mimicking hepatic metastases. Abdom Imaging 1999;24: 258–261
8. Maetani Y, Itoh K, Egawa H, et al. Benign hepatic nodules in Budd-Chiari syndrome: radiologic-pathologic correlation with emphasis on the central scar. AJR Am J Roentgenol 2002;178:869–875
9. Koyama T, Fletcher JG, Johnson CD, Kuo MS, Notohara K, Burgart LJ. Primary hepatic angiosarcoma: findings at CT and MR imaging. Radiology 2002;222:667–673
10. Gouya H, Vignaux O, Legmann P. de PG, Bonnin A. Peliosis hepatis: triphasic helical CT and dynamic MRI findings. Abdom Imaging 2001;26:507–509
11. Steinke K, Terraciano L, Wiesner W. Unusual cross-sectional imaging findings in hepatic peliosis. Eur Radiol 2003;13:1916–1919
12. Yoshida Y, Imai Y, Murakami T, et al. Intrahepatic cholangiocarcinoma with marked hypervascularity. Abdom Imaging 1999;24:66–68
13. Kim T, Federle MP, Baron RL, Peterson MS, Kawamori Y. Discrimination of small hepatic hemangiomas from hypervascular malignant tumors smaller than 3 cm with three-phase helical CT. Radiology 2001;219: 699–706
14. Outwater EK, Ito K, Siegelman E, Martin CE, Bhatia M, Mitchell DG. Rapidly enhancing hepatic hemangiomas at MRI: distinction from malignancies with T2-weighted images. J Magn Reson Imaging 1997;7: 1033–1039
15. Freeny PC, Grossholz M, Kaakaji K, Schmiedl UP. Significance of hyperattenuating and contrast-enhancing hepatic nodules detected in the cirrhotic liver during arterial phase helical CT in pre-liver transplant patients: radiologic-histopathologic correlation of explanted livers. Abdom Imaging 2003;28: 333–346
16. Krinsky GA, Theise ND, Rofsky NM, Mizrachi H, Tepperman LW, Weinreb JC. Dysplastic nodules in cirrhotic liver: arterial phase enhancement at CT and MR imaginga case report. Radiology 1998;209: 461–464
17. Ito K, Fujita T, Shimizu A, et al. Multiarterial phase dynamic MRI of small early enhancing hepatic lesions in cirrhosis or chronic hepatitis: differentiating between hypervascular hepatocellular carcinomas and pseudolesions. AJR Am J Roentgenol 2004; 183: 699–705
18. Ohtomo K, Baron RL, Dodd GD III, et al. Confluent hepatic fibrosis in advanced cirrhosis: appearance at CT. Radiology 1993;188:31–35
19. Casillas VJ, Amendola MA, Gascue A, Pinnar N, Levi JU, Perez JM. Imaging of nontraumatic hemorrhagic hepatic lesions. Radiographics 2000;20:367–378
20. Ruppert-Kohlmayr AJ, Uggowitzer MM, Kugler C, Zebedin D, Schaffler G, Ruppert GS. Focal nodular hyperplasia and hepatocellular adenoma of the liver: differentiation with multiphasic helical CT. AJR Am J Roentgenol 2001;176:1493–1498
21. Hussain SM, Terkivatan T, Zondervan PE, Lanjouw E. de RS, Ijzermans JN, de Man RA. Focal nodular hyperplasia: findings at state-of-the-art MR imaging, US, CT, and pathologic analysis. Radiographics 2004;24: 3–17

69

Liver Lesions with Delayed/ Prolonged Enhancement

Lesions with delayed enhancement have prominent enhancement occurring after the arterial phase. Delayed enhancement in a liver lesion usually corresponds to fibrotic tissue.[1] Some lesions (e.g., cavernous hemangiomas) have prolonged enhancement. This is early enhancement that persists on delayed images.

Features of Specific Lesions with Delayed/Prolonged Enhancement

Hepatocellular Carcinoma

Capsular enhancement in hepatocellular carcinoma (HCC) can be delayed or prolonged.[2] Central prolonged enhancement in HCC is rare, but is sometimes seen in scirrhous HCCs. (Due to the higher contrast resolution of magnetic resonance imaging (MRI), this is seen more often on MRI than on computed tomography [CT].)[3]

Metastases

Delayed enhancement in metastases is most commonly seen in metastatic colorectal adenocarcinoma. This delayed enhancement occurs in the central portion of the lesion.[2]

Confluent Hepatic Fibrosis

Confluent hepatic fibrosis is seen in advanced cirrhosis. It is wedge-shaped and usually involves the anterior and medial segments. It is associated with capsular retraction.[4]

Inflammatory Pseudotumor

Inflammatory pseudotumor is a rare benign tumorlike lesion. The liver is the second most common site after the lung. Delayed peripheral rim-like or septal enhancement can be seen in these lesions.[5]

Peliosis Hepatis

Multiple blood-filled cysts of varying size in the liver characterize peliosis hepatis. It is associated with malignancies, chronic infections, acquired immune deficiency syndrome (AIDS), and various drugs such as oral contraceptives and anabolic steroids. Reported enhancement patterns include peripheral enhancement progressing centripetally (mimicking a hemangioma) and central enhancement progressing centrifugally.[6,7] Typically, there is lack of mass effect, which helps differentiate peliosis from other hepatic lesions.

Adenomatosis

Liver adenomatosis occurs most often in young women and has three pathologic forms: steatotic, peliotic, and mixed. Multifocal lesions are noted which are iso- to hyperintense on T1-weighted MRI and hyperintense on T2-weighted MRI. The peliotic form does not have signal dropout on fat-suppressed images and has arterial enhancement that persists on delayed phases. The steatotic form has signal dropout on fat-suppressed images and has arterial enhancement without delayed enhancement.[8]

Liver Lesions with Prolonged/Delayed Enhancement[2,3,5,7]

- Cavernous hemangioma
- Cholangiocarcinoma (intrahepatic)
- Focal nodular hyperplasia (central scar)

- Hepatocellular carcinoma (usually capsular enhancement)
- Metastases
- Confluent hepatic fibrosis
- Lymphoma
- Abscess
- Epithelioid hemangioendothelioma
- Peliosis hepatitis
- Inflammatory pseudotumor
- Adenomatosis (peliotic and mixed forms)

References

1. Yoshikawa J, Matsui O, Kadoya M, Gabata T, Arai K, Takashima T. Delayed enhancement of fibrotic areas in hepatic masses: CT-pathologic correlation. J Comput Assist Tomogr 1992;16:206–211
2. Itoh K, Nishimura K, Togashi K, et al. Hepatocellular carcinoma: MR imaging. Radiology 1987;164: 21–25
3. Gabata T, Matsui O, Kadoya M, et al. Delayed MR imaging of the liver: correlation of delayed enhancement of hepatic tumors and pathologic appearance. Abdom Imaging 1998;23:309–313
4. Ohtomo K, Baron RL, Dodd GD III, et al. Confluent hepatic fibrosis in advanced cirrhosis: appearance at CT. Radiology 1993;188:31–35
5. Nishimura R, Mogami H, Teramoto N, Tanada M, Kurita A. Inflammatory pseudotumor of the liver in a patient with early gastric cancer: CT-histopathological correlation. Jpn J Clin Oncol 2005;35:218–220
6. Steinke K, Terraciano L, Wiesner W. Unusual cross-sectional imaging findings in hepatic peliosis. Eur Radiol 2003;13:1916–1919
7. Gouya H, Vignaux O, Legmann P, de Pigneux G, Bonnin A. Peliosis hepatis: triphasic helical CT and dynamic MRI findings. Abdom Imaging 2001;26:507–509
8. Lewin M, Handra-Luca A, Arrive L, et al. Liver adenomatosis: classification of MR imaging features and comparison with pathologic findings. Radiology 2006; 241:443–440

70

Liver Lesions with Central Scar

The most common lesions with a central scar are focal nodular hyperplasia (FNH), fibro-lamellar hepatocellular carcinoma (HCC), and hemangiomas. Hemangiomas can usually be differentiated by the characteristic enhancement pattern. FNH and fibrolamellar HCC can be more difficult to differentiate as they are both hypervascular tumors with central scars seen in young patients. Many imaging features can be helpful in differentiation of these two lesions (**Table 70.1**).

Patients with Budd–Chiari syndrome may have multiple hypervascular lesions with central scars. Benign regenerative hepatic nodules have been described in Budd–Chiari syndrome, which are multiple, small, and hypervascular. These are likely a result of insufficient blood supply to portions of the liver that will atrophy,

Table 70.1 Focal Nodular Hyperplasia versus Fibrolamellar Carcinoma[6,7,8]

	FNH	Fibrolamellar HCC
Sex	Female	No sex predilection
Size >5 cm	-	+
Surface Lobulation	-	+
Heterogeneity	-	+
Calcifications	-	±
Capsular Retraction	-	Rare
Scar Size	<2 cm	>2 cm
Scar Intensity	T2WI hyperintense	T2WI hypointense
Delayed Scar Enhancement	+	-
Capsule*	-	±
Pseudocapsule†	±	±
Intracellular Lipid	+	-
Malignant Features‡	-	±

Abbreviations: FNH, focal nodular hyperplasia; HCC, hepatocellular carcinoma; T1WI, T1-weighted magnetic resonance images; T2WI, T2-weighted magnetic resonance images.

* HCCs can have a true capsule, which is hypointense on T1WI and T2WI and demonstrates delayed or prolonged enhancement.[9]

† The pseudocapsule in FNH may be secondary to compression of surrounding vessels and parenchyma. It is hyperintense on T2WI and may have delayed enhancement. HCCs can also have a pseudocapsule. If this is seen in conjunction with a true capsule, it would appear as a ring of hypointensity surrounded by hyperintensity on T2WI.[10]

‡ Invasion of hepatic vessels and bile ducts, adenopathy, extrahepatic lesions.

with compensatory nodular hyperplasia in areas of the liver with adequate blood supply. These nodules have also been reported in other systemic disorders that impair hepatic blood flow, such as autoimmune disease, lymphoproliferative and myeloproliferative disorders, and after treatment with steroids and antineoplastic medications.[1] Similar nodules have also been described in autoimmune hepatitis.[2] These regenerative nodules are distinct from nodular regenerative hyperplasia (see Chapter 73)[3] in which there is no fibrosis between the nodules. These nodules can have central scars, especially if >1 cm in size. The nodules are sometimes hyperintense on T1-weighted magnetic resonance imaging (T1WI) and usually isointense to hypointense on T2-weighted magnetic resonance imaging (T2WI). The multiplicity of these nodules is helpful in distinguishing them from other hypervascular liver lesions. The regenerative

nodules in Budd–Chiari syndrome differ from regenerative nodules secondary to cirrhosis in these respects:[4]

- More often hyperintense on T1WI
- Usually enhance on arterial-phase images
- Larger lesions (>1 cm) often have central scars

Liver Lesions with Central Scar[4,5,6]

- Focal nodular hyperplasia
- Fibrolamellar hepatocellular carcinoma
- Hemangiomas (large)
- Hepatocellular carcinoma
- Cholangiocarcinoma
- Metastases
- Regenerative nodules in Budd–Chiari syndrome (and other vascular disorders)
- Hepatic adenoma (rare)

References

1. Brancatelli G, Federle MP, Grazioli L, Golfieri R, Lencioni R. Benign regenerative nodules in Budd-Chiari syndrome and other vascular disorders of the liver: radiologic-pathologic and clinical correlation. Radiographics 2002;22:847–862
2. Qayyum A, Graser A, Westphalen A, et al. CT of benign hypervascular liver nodules in autoimmune hepatitis. AJR Am J Roentgenol 2004;183:1573–1576
3. Clouet M, Boulay I, Boudiaf M, et al.. Imaging features of nodular regenerative hyperplasia of the liver mimicking hepatic metastases. Abdom Imaging 1999;24:258–261
4. Maetani Y, Itoh K, Egawa H, et al. Benign hepatic nodules in Budd-Chiari syndrome: radiologic-pathologic correlation with emphasis on the central scar. AJR Am J Roentgenol 2002;178:869–875
5. Grazioli L, Federle MP, Brancatelli G, Ichikawa T, Olivetti L, Blachar A. Hepatic adenomas: imaging and pathologic findings. Radiographics 2001;21:877–892
6. Rummeny E, Weissleder R, Sironi S, et al. Central scars in primary liver tumors: MR features, specificity, and pathologic correlation. Radiology 1989;171: 323–326
7. Ichikawa T, Federle MP, Grazioli L, Madariaga J, Nalesnik M, Marsh W. Fibrolamellar hepatocellular carcinoma: imaging and pathologic findings in 31 recent cases. Radiology 1999;213:352–361
8. Blachar A, Federle MP, Ferris JV, et al. Radiologists' performance in the diagnosis of liver tumors with central scars using specific CT criteria. Radiology 2002;223: 532–539
9. Hussain SM, Terkivatan T, Zondervan PE, Lanjouw E. de RS, Ijzermans JN, de Man RA. Focal nodular hyperplasia: findings at state-of-the-art MR imaging, US, CT, and pathologic analysis. Radiographics 2004;24: 3–17
10. Itoh K, Nishimura K, Togashi K, et al. Hepatocellular carcinoma: MR imaging. Radiology 1987;164:21–25

71

Cystic Liver Lesions

A broad range of liver lesions can appear cystic. Hepatocellular carcinoma and hemangioma are the primary liver lesions which are most likely to appear as cystic lesions. Fluid-fluid levels in a lesion are nonspecific and seen in both benign and malignant lesions.[1] They are usually secondary to hemorrhage.

Less Common Etiologies of Hepatic Cysts

Ciliated Hepatic Foregut Cyst

Ciliated hepatic foregut cysts are histologically similar to mediastinal foregut cysts. They are usually solitary and are most commonly seen in a subcapsular location in the medial segment of the left lobe. The contents of the cysts are variable; the cysts can contain serous fluid, lipid, and mucoid material. On magnetic resonance imaging (MRI), they are hyperintense on T2-weighted magnetic resonance imaging (T2WI), but can have a variable signal intensity on T1-weighted magnetic resonance imaging (T1WI). On computed tomography (CT), they can have high attenuation numbers. The appearance can mimic a solid lesion, but they can be differentiated by their lack of enhancement and characteristic location.[2]

Undifferentiated Embryonal Cell Sarcoma

Undifferentiated embryonal cell sarcoma is a rare malignant hepatic tumor, usually occurring in older children and adolescents. The tumors usually have abundant myxoid stroma, which makes the tumors appear cystic on imaging although they are usually predominately solid. The tumors usually appear as very large, solitary, well-defined lesions with heterogeneous enhancement.[3]

Biliary Hamartoma

One cause of multiple small cystic-appearing lesions is biliary hamartomas. Multiple biliary hamartomas present as multiple small cystic-appearing lesions throughout the liver (Von Meyenburg complex). These can be difficult to differentiate from multiple simple cysts, microabscesses, Caroli's disease, or metastases. The following features of biliary hamartomas are helpful in diagnosis:[4,5]

- Irregular in shape
- <1.5 cm in size
- Adjacent to medium-size portal tracts
- Scattered throughout entire liver, including subcapsular region
- Best seen on enhanced CT and T2WI
- Very hyperintense on T2WI
- No enhancement or slight rim enhancement

Types of Cystic Liver Lesions[3]

- Simple cyst
- Polycystic liver disease
- Ciliated hepatic foregut cyst

- Cystic primary neoplasms
- Biliary cystadenoma/cystadenocarcinoma
- Hemangioma
- Hepatocellular carcinoma
- Undifferentiated embryonal sarcoma
- Cystic metastases – hypervascular metastases with necrosis and cystic degeneration, or cystic

- metastases (e.g., mucinous adenocarcinomas)
- Infectious – abscess, echinococcal cyst
- Hematoma
- Biloma
- Caroli's disease
- Biliary hamartoma
- Extrapancreatic pseudocyst

References

1. Soyer P, Bluemke DA, Fishman EK, Rymer R. Fluid-fluid levels within focal hepatic lesions: imaging appearance and etiology. Abdom Imaging 1998;23:161–165
2. Fang SH, Dong DJ, Zhang SZ. Imaging features of ciliated hepatic foregut cyst. World J Gastroenterol 2005;11:4287–4289
3. Mortele KJ, Ros PR. Cystic focal liver lesions in the adult: differential CT and MR imaging features. Radiographics 2001;21:895–910
4. Luo TY, Itai Y, Eguchi N, et al. Von Meyenburg complexes of the liver: imaging findings. J Comput Assist Tomogr 1998;22:372–378
5. Mortele B, Mortele K, Seynaeve P, Vandevelde D, Kunnen M, Ros PR. Hepatic bile duct hamartomas (von Meyenburg Complexes): MR and MR cholangiography findings. J Comput Assist Tomogr 2002;26: 438–443

Calcified Liver Lesions

Calcification in hepatic lesions is nonspecific and can be seen in a wide range of infectious lesions and primary and metastatic tumors. In certain cases, the presence of calcification is helpful in narrowing the differential diagnosis. For example, in a liver lesion with a central scar, the presence of calcification suggests fibrolamellar hepatocellular carcinoma rather than focal nodular hyperplasia.

Features of Specific Tumors with Calcification

Fibrolamellar Hepatocellular Carcinoma

Fibrolamellar hepatocellular carcinoma has a reported incidence of calcification as high as 68%.[1] The calcification(s) are usually small and located centrally in the fibrous scar.

Hemangioma

Calcification in hemangiomas can appear as multiple spotty calcifications (phleboliths) or large, usually central, areas of calcification.[2]

Cholangiocarcinoma

Calcification can be seen secondary to mucous secretions. Calcification is more common in cholangiocarcinoma than in untreated hepatocellular carcinoma.[3]

Hepatocellular Adenoma

Calcifications are often located eccentrically, and may be seen in cystic areas related to hemorrhage or necrosis.[2,4]

Focal Nodular Hyperplasia

Calcification in focal nodular hyperplasia is rare (1.4%).[5]

Hepatoblastoma

Hepatoblastoma is the most common symptomatic liver tumor occurring under the age of 5 years. There is a male sex predilection. Calcification is common. A dense or coarse calcification pattern suggests hepatoblastoma rather than infantile hemangioendothelioma.[6]

Infantile Hemangioendothelioma

Infantile hemangioendothelioma usually presents in the first 6 months of life. There is a female sex predilection. Calcifications are common (seen histopathologically in 50% of cases). The calcifications in infantile hemangioendothelioma are usually more fine and granular than in hepatoblastoma.[7]

Calcified Hepatic Lesions[2]

- Infectious – Tuberculosis, histoplasmosis, echinococcus, schistosomiasis, chronic pyogenic or amebic abscess

- Metastases – Mucinous tumors (colon, breast, stomach, ovary), osteosarcoma, chondrosarcoma
- Primary liver lesions
  - Fibrolamellar hepatocellular carcinoma
  - Intrahepatic cholangiocarcinoma
  - Hemangioma
- Hepatocellular carcinoma
- Hepatocellular adenoma
- Focal nodular hyperplasia (rare)
- Biliary cystadenoma/cystadenocarcinoma
- Hepatic epithelioid hemangioendothelioma
- Hepatoblastoma
- Infantile hemangioendothelioma

Additional Readings

1. Ichikawa T, Federle MP, Grazioli L, Madariaga J, Nalesnik M, Marsh W. Fibrolamellar hepatocellular carcinoma: imaging and pathologic findings in 31 recent cases. Radiology 1999;213:352–361
2. Stoupis C, Taylor HM, Paley MR, et al. The Rocky liver: radiologic-pathologic correlation of calcified hepatic masses. Radiographics 1998;18:675–685
3. Ros PR, Buck JL, Goodman ZD, Ros AM, Olmsted WW. Intrahepatic cholangiocarcinoma: radiologic-pathologic correlation. Radiology 1988;167:689–693
4. Grazioli L, Federle MP, Brancatelli G, Ichikawa T, Olivetti L, Blachar A. Hepatic adenomas: imaging and pathologic findings. Radiographics 2001;21:877–892
5. Caseiro-Alves F, Zins M, Mahfouz A-E, et al. Calcification in focal nodular hyperplasia: a new problem for differentiation from fibrolamellar hepatocellular carcinoma. Radiology 1996;198:889–892
6. Dachman AH, Pakter RL, Ros PR, Fishman EK, Goodman ZD, Lichtenstein JE. Hepatoblastoma: radiologic-pathologic correlation in 50 cases. Radiology 1987;164:15–19
7. Roos JE, Pfiffner R, Stallmach T, Stuckmann G, Marincek B, Willi U. Infantile hemangioendothelioma. Radiographics 2003;23:1649–1655

73

Hemorrhagic Liver Lesions

Liver hemorrhage without trauma can be seen in conditions such as amyloidosis, HELLP (hemolysis, elevated liver enzymes, and low platelet count) syndrome, and vasculitis.[1] The most common liver lesions to hemorrhage are hepatic adenomas and hepatocellular carcinomas.

Rare Hemorrhagic Liver Lesions

Hepatic Angiosarcoma

The enhancement in hepatic angiosarcomas usually does not resemble that of hemangiomas. Focal areas of enhancement in angiosarcomas have less attenuation than the aorta and have irregular shapes, and could be central or ring-shaped. There is usually progressive enhancement on delayed images, which helps distinguish angiosarcoma from hepatocellular carcinoma. In addition, the presence of splenic metastases, which are common in angiosarcoma, aids in differentiation from hepatocellular carcinoma.[2]

Nodular Regenerative Hyperplasia

Nodular regenerative hyperplasia is characterized by diffuse hyperplastic nodules composed of cells resembling normal hepatocytes, without fibrosis around the nodules. Nodular regenerative hyperplasia is of uncertain etiology. It can be associated with myeloproliferative or lymphoproliferative disorders.[3] It has an equal sex predilection and is seen in a wide range of ages. Patients can be asymptomatic or present with noncirrhotic portal hypertension. Computed tomography (CT) and magnetic resonance imaging (MRI) of the liver can be normal, can show multiple nodules mimicking metastatic disease, or rarely have a cirrhotic appearance.[4] The lack of fibrosis between the nodules in nodular regenerative hyperplasia distinguishes it from the regenerative nodules seen in Budd–Chiari[5] syndrome, where fibrosis can develop between the nodules. Hemorrhage in this condition is rare.

Hemorrhagic Liver Lesions[1–3,6–8]

- Hepatocellular carcinoma
- Hepatic adenoma
- Metastases: Lung cancer, renal cell cancer, melanoma most common
- Hemangioma
- Angiosarcoma
- Focal nodular hyperplasia
- Nodular regenerative hyperplasia
- Hepatic angiomyolipoma

References

1. Casillas VJ, Amendola MA, Gascue A, Pinnar N, Levi JU, Perez JM. Imaging of nontraumatic hemorrhagic hepatic lesions. Radiographics 2000;20:367–378

2. Koyama T, Fletcher JG, Johnson CD, Kuo MS, Notohara K, Burgart LJ. Primary hepatic angiosarcoma: findings at CT and MR imaging. Radiology 2002;222:667–673

3. Dachman AH, Ros PR, Goodman ZD, Olmsted WW, Ishak KG. Nodular regenerative hyperplasia of the liver: clinical and radiologic observations. AJR Am J Roentgenol 1987;148:717–722

4. Clouet M, Boulay I, Boudiaf M, et al. Imaging features of nodular regenerative hyperplasia of the liver mimicking hepatic metastases. Abdom Imaging 1999;24:258–261

5. Brancatelli G, Federle MP, Grazioli L, Golfieri R, Lencioni R. Benign regenerative nodules in Budd-Chiari syndrome and other vascular disorders of the liver: radiologic-pathologic and clinical correlation. Radiographics 2002;22:847–862

6. Graham E, Cohen AW, Soulen M, Faye R. Symptomatic liver hemangioma with intra-tumor hemorrhage treated by angiography and embolization during pregnancy. Obstet Gynecol 1993;81:813–816

7. Becker YT, Raiford DS, Webb L, Wright JK, Chapman WC, Pinson CW. Rupture and hemorrhage of hepatic focal nodular hyperplasia. Am Surg 1995;61:210–214

8. Guidi G, Catalano O, Rotondo A. Spontaneous rupture of a hepatic angiomyolipoma: CT findings and literature review. Eur Radiol 1997;7:335–337

74

Liver Lesions with Macroscopic Fat

The most common solitary tumors containing fat are hepatocellular carcinoma and hepatic adenoma.[1] Fatty change in adenomatosis is more frequent compared with a solitary adenoma. Macroscopic fat in a focal nodular hyperplasia is very rare.[2]

Metastases that contain macroscopic fat are rare, but include metastatic ovarian dermoid, teratoma, liposarcoma, and Wilms' tumor.[3]

A less common lesion with macroscopic fat is hepatic angiomyolipoma.[3,4] Angiomyolipomas are rare benign hepatic tumors, which are found predominately in women. They have been associated with tuberous sclerosis and renal angiomyolipomas. Three patterns can be seen on imaging: approximately equal portions of fat, vessels, and smooth muscle; a predominance of fat component, and a minimal fat component. Angiomyolipomas with approximately equal portions of fat, vessels, and smooth muscle have the most characteristic appearance. Angiomyolipomas with a predominance of fat are usually not distinguishable from myelolipomas or lipomas. Lesions with minimal fat are often difficult to distinguish from hepatocellular carcinoma (HCC) with fatty change. Both angiomyolipomas with minimal fat and HCCs with fatty change can appear as hypervascular masses with areas of fat. Numerous features are helpful in distinguishing the two lesions (**Table 74.1**).

Liver Lesions with Macroscopic Fat[3,4,5]

- Hepatocellular carcinoma (HCC)
- Hepatic adenoma/adenomatosis
- Angiomyolipoma
- Metastases
- Focal nodular hyperplasia
- Lipoma
- Liposarcoma
- Myelolipoma
- Lipopeliosis
- Adrenal rest tumor

Table 74.1 Hepatic Angiomyolipoma versus Hepatocellular Carcinoma[6,7]

	Angiomyolipoma	Hepatocellular Carcinoma
Fat Component	Greater	Lesser
Early Enhancement	+ (Peaks later)	+
Persistent Enhancement	+	−
Capsule	−	+
Feeding Vessels	Central	Peripheral

- Pericaval fat
- Extramedullary hematopoiesis
- Hepatic teratoma

- Langerhans cell histiocytosis
- Hydatid cyst
- Pseudolipoma of Glisson capsule

References

1. Valls C, Iannacconne R, Alba E, et al. Fat in the liver: diagnosis and characterization. Eur Radiol 2006;16: 2292–2308
2. Stanley G, Jeffrey RB Jr, Feliz B. CT findings and histopathology of intratumoral steatosis in focal nodular hyperplasia: case report and review of the literature. J Comput Assist Tomogr 2002;26: 815–817
3. Basaran C, Karcaaltincaba M, Akata D, et al. Fat-containing lesions of the liver: cross-sectional imaging findings with emphasis on MRI. AJR Am J Roentgenol 2005;184:1103–1110
4. Prasad SR, Wang H, Rosas H, et al. Fat-containing lesions of the liver: radiologic-pathologic correlation. Radiographics 2005;25:321–331
5. Savoye-Collet C, Goria O, Scotte M, Hemet J. MR imaging of hepatic myelolipoma. AJR Am J Roentgenol 2000; 174:574–575
6. Yan F, Zeng M, Zhou K, et al. Hepatic angiomyolipoma: various appearances on two-phase contrast scanning of spiral CT. Eur J Radiol 2002;41:12–18
7. Ahmadi T, Itai Y, Takahashi M, et al. Angiomyolipoma of the liver: significance of CT and MR dynamic study. Abdom Imaging 1998;23:520–526

75

Liver Lesions with Microscopic Fat

Liver lesions may contain microscopic fat, which can be detected as signal loss on opposed-phase chemical shift magnetic resonance imaging (MRI). Some of these lesions such as hepatocellular carcinoma and hepatic adenoma can also contain macroscopic fat.

Microscopic Fat-Containing Liver Lesions[1,2]

- Focal hepatic steatosis
- Hepatocellular carcinoma: fat distribution tends to be more patchy than in adenomas

- Hepatic adenoma
- Focal nodular hyperplasia (rare)
- Regenerating nodules (rare)
- Metastases: e.g., from primaries containing microscopic fat such as clear cell renal carcinoma (rare)

References

1. Basaran C, Karcaaltincaba M, Akata D, et al. Fat-containing lesions of the liver: cross-sectional imaging findings with emphasis on MRI. AJR Am J Roentgenol 2005;184:1103–1110

2. Valls C, Iannacconne R, Alba E, et al. Fat in the liver: diagnosis and characterization. Eur Radiol 2006;16: 2292–2308

76

Liver Lesions with Hyperintensity on T1-Weighted Magnetic Resonance Imaging

Hyperintensity on T1-weighted magnetic resonance images (T1WI) in a liver lesion could be secondary to macroscopic fat or hemorrhage, but some hepatic lesions can be hyperintense without hemorrhage or macroscopic fat. This could be secondary to microscopic fat, copper, protein, mucin, or melanin.[1,2]

Regenerative nodules in cirrhosis are usually hypointense on T1WI (unlike dysplastic nodules, which are typically hyperintense). Rarely, regenerative nodules can be hyperintense.[3]

Benign regenerative hepatic nodules have been described in Budd–Chiari syndrome as multiple, small, and hypervascular. These are likely a result of insufficient blood supply to portions of the liver, which will atrophy, with compensatory nodular hyperplasia in areas of the liver with adequate blood supply. These nodules have also been reported in other systemic disorders that impair hepatic blood flow, such as autoimmune disease and lymphoproliferative and myeloproliferative disorders; they can occur after treatment with steroids and antineoplastic medications as well.[4] Similar nodules have also been described in autoimmune hepatitis.[5] These regenerative nodules are distinct from nodular regenerative hyperplasia (see Chapter 73),[6] in which there is no fibrosis between the nodules. These nodules can have central scars, especially if >1 cm in size. The lesions are sometimes hyperintense on T1WI

and are usually isointense to hypointense on T2WI.[4] The multiplicity of these nodules is helpful in distinguishing them from other hypervascular liver lesions. The regenerative nodules in Budd–Chiari syndrome differ from regenerative nodules secondary to cirrhosis in three respects:[7]

- More often hyperintense on T1WI
- Usually enhance on arterial-phase images
- Larger lesions (>1 cm) often have central scars

Liver Lesions with T1WI Hyperintensity[2,3,7,8]

- Lesions with macroscopic fat (see Chapter 74)
- Lesions with hemorrhage (see Chapter 73)
- Focal hepatic steatosis
- Hepatic adenoma
- Focal nodular hyperplasia
- Hepatocellular carcinoma
- Metastases: Hemorrhagic lesions, melanoma, colon, ovarian, pancreatic mucinous cystic, myeloma
- Dysplastic nodule in cirrhosis
- Regenerative nodule in cirrhosis (rare)
- Regenerative nodules in Budd–Chiari syndrome (and other vascular disorders)
- Biliary cystadenoma/cystadenocarcinoma: From mucin, protein, hemorrhage

References

1. Lee MJ, Hahn PF, Saini S, Mueller PR. Differential diagnosis of hyperintense liver lesions on T1-weighted MR images. AJR Am J Roentgenol 1992;159:1017–1020
2. Mathieu D, Paret M, Mahfouz AE, et al. Hyperintense benign liver lesions on spin-echo T1-weighted MR images: pathologic correlations. Abdom Imaging 1997;22:410–417
3. Krinsky GA, Israel G. Nondysplastic nodules that are hyperintense on T1-weighted gradient-echo MR imaging: frequency in cirrhotic patients undergoing transplantation. AJR Am J Roentgenol 2003;180:1023–1027
4. Brancatelli G, Federle MP, Grazioli L, Golfieri R, Lencioni R. Benign regenerative nodules in Budd-Chiari syndrome and other vascular disorders of the liver: radiologic-pathologic and clinical correlation. Radiographics 2002;22:847–862
5. Qayyum A, Graser A, Westphalen A, et al. CT of benign hypervascular liver nodules in autoimmune hepatitis. AJR Am J Roentgenol 2004;183:1573–1576
6. Clouet M, Boulay I, Boudiaf M, et al. Imaging features of nodular regenerative hyperplasia of the liver mimicking hepatic metastases. Abdom Imaging 1999;24: 258–261
7. Maetani Y, Itoh K, Egawa H, et al. Benign hepatic nodules in Budd-Chiari syndrome: radiologic-pathologic correlation with emphasis on the central scar. AJR Am J Roentgenol 2002;178:869–875
8. Kelekis NL, Semelka RC, Woosley JT. Malignant lesions of the liver with high signal intensity on T1-weighted MR images. J Magn Reson Imaging 1996;6:291–294

77

Liver Lesions with Hypointensity on T2-Weighted Magnetic Resonance Imaging

Liver lesions can contain areas of T2-weighted magnetic resonance imaging (T2WI) hypointensity secondary to hemorrhage or calcification. Other etiologies include fibrosis, desmoplastic stroma, cellular necrosis, mucin, and iron deposition.[1,2] Lesions can be diffusely hypointense (e.g., a siderotic regenerating nodule), have heterogeneous areas of hypointensity (e.g., from hemorrhage), or central hypointensity (e.g., a fibrotic central scar in cholangiocarcinoma).

Liver Lesions with Hypointensity on T2WI[2–7]

- Hemorrhagic lesions (see Chapter 73)
- Calcified lesions (see Chapter 72)
- Regenerating nodules in cirrhosis

- Regenerating nodules in Budd–Chiari syndrome
- Dysplastic nodules in cirrhosis
- Hepatocellular carcinoma (HCC): Rare, HCC is usually hyperintense on T2WI
- Melanoma metastases
- Tuberculosis (fibrous stage)
- Echinococcus alveolaris: Infiltrative
- Wilson's disease

Liver Lesions with Central T2WI Hypointensity[1,2,8,9]

- Fibrosis/scar in tumors (fibrolamellar HCC, hemangioma, cholangiocarcinoma, angiosarcoma)
- Metastases: Colorectal

References

1. Maetani Y, Itoh K, Watanabe C, et al. MR imaging of intrahepatic cholangiocarcinoma with pathologic correlation. AJR Am J Roentgenol 2001;176:1499–1507
2. Outwater E, Tomaszewski JE, Daly JM, Kressel HY. Hepatic colorectal metastases: correlation of MR imaging and pathologic appearance. Radiology 1991; 180:327–332
3. Hussain HK, Syed I, Nghiem HV, et al. T2-weighted MR imaging in the assessment of cirrhotic liver. Radiology 2004;230:637–644
4. Yu RS, Zhang SZ, Wu JJ, Li RF. Imaging diagnosis of 12 patients with hepatic tuberculosis. World J Gastroenterol 2004;10:1639–1642
5. Etlik O, Bay A, Arslan H, et al. Contrast-enhanced CT and MRI findings of atypical hepatic *Echinococcus*

alveolaris infection. Pediatr Radiol 2005;35: 546–549
6. Marti-Bonmati L. MR imaging characteristics of hepatic tumors. Eur Radiol 1997;7:249–258
7. Kozic D, Svetel M, Petrovic I, Sener RN, Kostic VS. Regression of nodular liver lesions in Wilson's disease. Acta Radiol 2006;47:624–627
8. Koyama T, Fletcher JG, Johnson CD, Kuo MS, Notohara K, Burgart LJ. Primary hepatic angiosarcoma: findings at CT and MR imaging. Radiology 2002;222: 667–673
9. Ros PR, Lubbers PR, Olmsted WW, Morillo G. Hemangioma of the liver: heterogeneous appearance on T2-weighted images. AJR Am J Roentgenol 1987; 149:1167–1170

78

Transient Hepatic Attenuation Difference

A transient hepatic attenuation difference (THAD) or transient hepatic intensity difference (THID) is seen during biphasic liver computed tomography (CT) or magnetic resonance imaging (MRI). It refers to an area of nontumorous increased or decreased attenuation on arterial phase images, which becomes isoattenuating on portal-phase images. In most cases, the attenuation in a THAD is increased rather than decreased. Typically, the THAD has no mass effect with vessels coursing through the area, and a wedge-shaped appearance with straight margins.

When encountering a THAD, the interpreter should search for an associated lesion (causing arterioportal shunting) deep to the THAD and portal vein obstruction. Portal vein obstruction results in increased compensatory arterial flow and decreased unopacified portal flow. A similar phenomenon is seen from hepatic parenchymal compression, which decreases portal flow.

Interpretation of THADs in cirrhotic livers can be difficult as cirrhotic livers can contain small nontumorous arterioportal shunts, but also can develop hepatocellular carcinomas (HCC) with arterioportal shunts.[1] Thus, it is important to search for a HCC deep to any THAD seen in cirrhotic patient.

Causes of Transient Hepatic Attenuation Difference[2-5]

- Arterioportal shunts: Associated with a lesion, iatrogenic or idiopathic
  - Hepatocellular carcinoma
  - Hemangioma
  - Cholangiocarcinoma
  - Hypervascular metastases
  - Interventional procedures
  - Cirrhosis
- Portal vein obstruction
- Inflammatory (e.g., secondary to cholecystitis or abscess)
- Aberrant blood supply: Systemic venous circulation may drain into the liver via vascular variants such as the accessory cystic vein and capsular veins. As this systemic venous flow may be opacified when the portal venous flow is unopacified, a hyperattenuating area on arterial phase images may result. This is most common in the subscapular region, anterior to the porta hepatitis, and adjacent to the gallbladder fossa and falciform ligament.
- Steal phenomenon from hypervascular tumors: The steal phenomenon could result in an area of hyperattenuation or hypoattenuation. For example, a focal nodular hyperplasia has been

reported to be associated with a transient area of hypoattenuation.[5] If the THAD is hyperattenuating, it usually involves the entire lobe containing the lesion.[3]

- Hepatic parenchymal compression (e.g., adjacent to rib compression, peritoneal implant)
- Idiopathic
- Hepatic arterial obstruction (rare)
- Hepatic venous obstruction (rare)

References

1. Oliver JH III, Baron RL. Helical biphasic contrast-enhanced CT of the liver: technique, indications, interpretation, and pitfalls. Radiology 1996;201:1–14
2. Chen WP, Chen JH, Hwang JI, et al. Spectrum of transient hepatic attenuation differences in biphasic helical CT. AJR Am J Roentgenol 1999;172:419–424
3. Colagrande S, Centi N, La VG, Villari N. Transient hepatic attenuation differences. AJR Am J Roentgenol 2004; 183:459–464
4. Kitade M, Yoshiji H, Yamao J, et al. Intrahepatic cholangiocarcinoma associated with central calcification and arterio-portal shunt. Intern Med 2005;44: 825–828
5. Kim HJ, Kim AY, Kim TK, et al. Transient hepatic attenuation differences in focal hepatic lesions: dynamic CT features. AJR Am J Roentgenol 2005;184: 83–90

79

Hepatic Capsular Retraction

Retraction of the liver capsule can be associated with an adjacent hepatic tumor, but can also be seen without a hepatic tumor. It is a nonspecific sign. If associated with a tumor it may be secondary to necrosis and desmoplastic reaction within the tumor.

One rare tumor that is typically associated with capsular retraction is hepatic epithelioid hemangioendothelioma. Hepatic epithelioid hemangioendothelioma is a low-grade malignant vascular liver tumor that is intermediate in clinical course between cavernous hemangioma and angiosarcoma. The lesions occur only in adults with a mean age of 45 years and a slight female sex predilection. In addition to capsular retraction, other imaging findings include peripheral nodules, which can coalesce into large confluent peripheral masses. A characteristic pattern of enhancement is a target appearance of a hypodense center with enhancing peripheral rim and a hypodense halo around the enhancing peripheral rim.[1]

A cause of capsular retraction not related to a tumor is confluent hepatic fibrosis, which is seen in advanced cirrhosis. Confluent hepatic fibrosis is wedge-shaped and usually involves the anterior and medial segments.[2]

Retraction of the Liver Capsule Associated with a Liver Tumor[3,4]

- Metastases: Can occur both pre- and post-treatment, and with both an increase and decrease in size of the lesions[5]
- Cholangiocarcinoma
- Epithelioid hemangioendothelioma
- Hemangioma: Hemangiomas that cause capsular retraction are usually >4 cm in size[6]
- Hepatocellular carcinoma
- Fibrolamellar hepatocellular carcinoma
- Focal nodular hyperplasia[7]

Retraction of the Liver Capsule Not Caused by a Liver Tumor

- Confluent hepatic fibrosis
- Biliary obstruction
- Primary sclerosing cholangitis
- Trauma
- Recurrent pyogenic cholangitis
- Bile duct necrosis

Additional Readings

1. Miller WJ, Dodd GD III, Federle MP, Baron RL. Epithelioid hemangioendothelioma of the liver: imaging findings with pathologic correlation. AJR Am J Roentgenol 1992;159:53–57

2. Ohtomo K, Baron RL, Dodd GD III, et al. Confluent hepatic fibrosis in advanced cirrhosis: appearance at CT. Radiology 1993;188:31–35

3. Mortele KJ, Praet M, Van Vlierberghe H, de Hemptinne B, Zou K, Ros PR. Focal nodular hyperplasia of the liver: detection and characterization with plain and dynamic-enhanced MRI. Abdom Imaging 2002;27:700–707

4. Yang DM, Kim HS, Cho SW, Kim HS. Pictorial review: various causes of hepatic capsular retraction: CT and MR findings. Br J Radiol 2002;75:994–1002

5. Fennessy FM, Mortele KJ, Kluckert T, et al. Hepatic capsular retraction in metastatic carcinoma of the breast occurring with increase or decrease in size of subjacent metastasis. AJR Am J Roentgenol 2004;182: 651–655

6. Yang DM, Yoon MH, Kim HS, Kim HS, Chung JW. Capsular retraction in hepatic giant hemangioma: CT and MR features. Abdom Imaging 2001;26:36–38

7. Ko KR, Lee DH, Park JS, et al. Focal nodular hyperplasia with retraction of liver capsule: a case report. Korean J Radiol 2003;4:66–69

80

Periportal Halo

The appearance of a periportal low-attenuation halo is usually related to altered hepatic lymphatic flow, most often lymphatic fluid overload or hepatic lymphatic obstruction.[1]

A periportal halo has been described on magnetic resonance imaging (MRI) in primary biliary cirrhosis. Unlike the most periportal halos, which are hyperintense on T2-weighted MR images (T2WI), the halo in primary biliary cirrhosis is hypointense on both T1-weighted MR images and T2WI and likely related to fibrosis rather than edema or inflammation.[2]

In liver transplants, a periportal halo is most commonly seen in recently transplanted allografts and with ascites. There is a questionable correlation with acute rejection, but the presence of a periportal halo cannot be used to diagnose acute rejection.[3]

Possible Causes of a Periportal Halo[1-5]

- Trauma
  - Hepatic laceration: Hemorrhage dissecting in periportal tissue
  - Elevated central venous pressure (e.g., vigorous intravenous fluid administration, pericardial tamponade)
- Cirrhosis
- Hepatitis
- Hepatic tumors
- Biliary obstruction
- Porta hepatis masses (e.g., adenopathy)
- Right-sided heart failure
- Liver transplants
- Bone marrow transplant (microvenous occlusive disease)
- Acute pyelonephritis
- Mucinous cholangiocarcinoma
- Primary biliary cirrhosis

References

1. Aspestrand F, Schrumpf E, Jacobsen M, Hanssen L, Endresen K. Increased lymphatic flow from the liver in different intra-and extrahepatic diseases demonstrated by CT. J Comput Assist Tomogr 1991;15:550–554
2. Wenzel JS, Donohoe A, Ford KL III, Glastad K, Watkins D, Molmenti E. Primary biliary cirrhosis: MR imaging findings and description of MR imaging periportal halo sign. AJR Am J Roentgenol 2001;176:885–889
3. Stevens SD, Heiken JP, Brunt E, Hanto DW, Flye MW. Low-attenuation periportal collar in transplanted liver is not reliable CT evidence of acute allograft rejection. AJR Am J Roentgenol 1991;157:1195–1198
4. Zissin R, Kots E, Rachmani R, Hadari R, Shapiro-Feinberg M. Hepatic periportal tracking associated with severe acute pyelonephritis. Abdom Imaging 2000;25:251–254
5. Mizukami Y, Ohta H, Arisato S, et al. Case report: mucinous cholangiocarcinoma featuring a multicystic appearance and periportal collar in imaging. J Gastroenterol Hepatol 1999;14:1223–1226

81

Liver Lesions with Supraparamagnetic Iron Oxide Uptake

Uptake of supraparamagnetic iron oxide (SPIO) particles reflects reticuloendothelial system activity. Uptake of SPIO agents in the liver is detected as signal loss on T2*- or T2-weighted magnetic resonance imaging (T2WI).

Most focal nodular hyperplasias and adenomas have detectable SPIO uptake, but less than normal liver.[1,2] However, the degree of signal loss in these lesions can be comparable[2] making differentiation between the two lesions by SPIO imaging difficult.

Well-differentiated hepatocellular carcinomas (HCCs) can have SPIO uptake, but the degree of uptake is substantially less than for the other lesions. Moderate to poorly differentiated HCC can show a minimal degree of uptake.[3]

Hemangiomas are the only lesion to show an increase in signal intensity on T1WI after SPIO administration, due to the T1 effect of SPIO particles in the blood pool.[4]

Liver Lesions with Supraparamagnetic Iron Oxide Uptake[1–4]

- Focal nodular hyperplasia
- Hepatic adenoma
- Low-grade hepatocellular carcinoma
- Hemangioma
- Dysplastic nodule

References

1. Takeshita K, Nagashima I, Frui S, et al. Effect of superparamagnetic iron oxide-enhanced MRI of the liver with hepatocellular carcinoma and hyperplastic nodule. J Comput Assist Tomogr 2002;26:451–455
2. Grandin C, Van Beers BE, Robert A, Gigot JF, Geubel A, Pringot J. Benign hepatocellular tumors: MRI after superparamagnetic iron oxide administration. J Comput Assist Tomogr 1995;19:412–418
3. Grazioli L, Morana G, Kirchin MA, et al. MRI of focal nodular hyperplasia (FNH) with gadobenate dimeglumine (Gd-BOPTA) and SPIO (ferumoxides): an intraindividual comparison. J Magn Reson Imaging 2003; 17:593–602
4. Montet X, Lazeyras F, Howarth N, et al. Specificity of SPIO particles for characterization of liver hemangiomas using MRI. Abdom Imaging 2004;29:60–70

82

Diffuse Liver Disease

Conditions Associated with a Hyperdense Liver[1-3]

- Amiodarone administration
- Iron overload
- Hemochromatosis
- Hemosiderosis
- Wilson's disease
- Glycogen storage disease
- Gold treatment
- Thorotrast

Conditions Associated with a Hypodense Liver[4-6]

- Diffuse steatosis: A steatotic liver will exhibit a lower mean attenuation than the spleen on noncontrast images.[4]

- Active alcoholic cirrhosis: Low density is not seen in acute viral hepatitis, viral cirrhosis, or inactive alcoholic cirrhosis.[5]
- Nonalcoholic hepatic steatosis: Compared with patients with simple steatosis, the liver is larger in craniocaudal dimension, and the caudate-to-right-lobe ratio is greater.[6]

Central Increased Liver Density

- Budd–Chiari syndrome
- Primary sclerosing cholangitis: Secondary to caudate lobe pseudotumor[7]

References

1. Mortele KJ, Ros PR. Imaging of diffuse liver disease. Semin Liver Dis 2001;21:195–212
2. De Maria M, De Simone G, Laconi A, Mercadante G, Pavone P, Rossi P. Gold storage in the liver: appearance on CT scans. Radiology 1986;159:355–366
3. Patrick D, White FE, Adams PC. Long-term amiodarone therapy: a cause of increased hepatic attenuation on CT. Br J Radiol 1984;57:573–576
4. Piekarski J, Goldberg HI, Royal SA, Axel L, Moss AA. Difference between liver and spleen CT numbers in the normal adult: its usefulness in predicting the presence of diffuse liver disease. Radiology 1980;137:727–729
5. Fritz GA, Schoellnast H, Deutschmann HA, et al. Density histogram analysis of unenhanced hepatic computed tomography in patients with diffuse liver diseases. J Comput Assist Tomogr 2006;30:201–205
6. Oliva MR, Mortele KJ, Segatto E, et al. Computed tomography features of nonalcoholic steatohepatitis with histopathologic correlation. J Comput Assist Tomogr 2006;30:37–43
7. Dodd GD, Baron RL, Oliver JH, Federle MP. End-stage primary sclerosing cholangitis: CT findings of hepatic morphology. Radiology 1999;211:357–362

83

Cirrhosis

The imaging features of cirrhosis sometimes differ depending on the etiology. In particular, primary sclerosis cholangitis and primary biliary cirrhosis have features, which can suggest the etiology. Imaging features can also aid in differentiating alcoholic from viral cirrhosis.

Alcoholic versus Viral Cirrhosis[1]

Alcoholic Cirrhosis

There is more frequent caudate enlargement and right posterior hepatic notch (indentation in medial surface of right posterior lobe) visualization in alcoholic cirrhosis.

Viral Cirrhosis

Regenerative nodules are usually larger in viral cirrhosis.

Primary Sclerosing Cholangitis[2]

Primary sclerosing cholangitis (PSC) occurs more commonly in men and usually has an onset between 30 and 60 years of age. However, it can also be seen in children. The etiology is unknown, but it is associated with ulcerative colitis. Biliary dilatation in conjunction with cirrhosis suggests PSC as the etiology. The following hepatic findings are more common in primary sclerosing cholangitis than in other etiologies of cirrhosis.[3]

- Lobulated contour
- Caudate lobe pseudotumor: Severe hypertrophy with increased attenuation
- Focal atrophy of the left lateral or right posterior segments
- Large regenerative nodules[4]
- Peripheral increased enhancement on arterial phase images: Increased enhancement is more commonly segmental in other etiologies of cirrhosis[5]

Primary Biliary Cirrhosis

Primary biliary cirrhosis is a slowly progressive autoimmune disease that primarily affects women. The peak incidence is in the fifth decade; it is rarely seen in persons below 25 years of age.[6] The following findings are more common in primary biliary cirrhosis than in other etiologies of cirrhosis.[3]

- Diffuse hypertrophy
- Specific patterns of fibrosis: Thin perilobular fibrous bands (lacelike pattern), or perivascular cuffing (hepatic veins surrounded by fibrosis)
- Periportal halo sign: Seen on magnetic resonance imaging, low signal intensity on T1-and T2-weighted images centered around portal venous branches[7]

References

1. Okazaki H, Ito K, Fujita T, Koike S, Takano K, Matsunaga N. Discrimination of alcoholic from virus-induced cirrhosis on MR imaging. AJR Am J Roentgenol 2000;175: 1677–1681
2. Dodd GD III, Baron RL, Oliver JH III, Federle MP. End-stage primary sclerosing cholangitis: CT findings of hepatic morphology in 36 patients. Radiology 1999; 211:357–362
3. Dodd GD III, Baron RL, Oliver JH III, Federle MP. Spectrum of imaging findings of the liver in end-stage cirrhosis: part I, gross morphology and diffuse abnormalities. AJR Am J Roentgenol 1999;173: 1031–1036
4. Bader TR, Beavers KL, Semelka RC. MR imaging features of primary sclerosing cholangitis: patterns of cirrhosis in relationship to clinical severity of disease. Radiology 2003;226:675–685
5. Ito K, Mitchell DG, Outwater EK, Blasbalg R. Primary sclerosing cholangitis: MR imaging features. AJR Am J Roentgenol 1999;172:1527–1533
6. Kaplan MM, Gershwin ME. Primary biliary cirrhosis. N Engl J Med 2005;353:1261–1273
7. Wenzel JS, Donohoe A, Ford KL III, Glastad K, Watkins D, Molmenti E. Primary biliary cirrhosis: MR imaging findings and description of MR imaging periportal halo sign. AJR Am J Roentgenol 2001;176:885–889

84

Mimics of Cirrhosis

The appearance of the liver can mimic cirrhosis in several conditions. This has been referred to as pseudocirrhosis. Pseudocirrhosis can be seen after chemotherapy, in livers both with and without metastatic disease. In patients with metastatic disease to the liver treated with chemotherapy, the appearance of pseudocirrhosis can evolve over 1 to 3 months. Pathologically, nodular regenerative hyperplasia is usually seen (rather than scar formation at the site of treated metastases). The appearance of pseudocirrhosis may make imaging evaluation difficult, as these patients often have residual disease in the cirrhotic-appearing liver.[1]

Nodular regenerative hyperplasia is characterized by diffuse hyperplastic nodules composed of cells resembling normal hepatocytes, without fibrosis around the nodules. It has an equal sex predilection and is seen in wide age range. Nodular regenerative hyperplasia is of uncertain etiology. It can be associated with myeloproliferative or lymphoproliferative disorders.[2] Patients can be asymptomatic or present with noncirrhotic portal hypertension. Computed tomography and magnetic resonance imaging of the liver can be normal, can show multiple nodules mimicking metastatic disease, or rarely have a cirrhotic appearance.[3] The lack of fibrosis between the nodules in nodular regenerative hyperplasia distinguishes it from the regenerative nodules seen in Budd–Chiari[4] syndrome where fibrosis can develop between the nodules.

Mimics of Cirrhosis[5,6]

- Chemotherapy treated liver metastases
- Chemotherapy induced hepatotoxicity
- Metastatic disease
- Regeneration after hepatic necrosis
- Nodular regenerative hyperplasia

References

1. Young ST, Paulson EK, Washington K, Gulliver DJ, Vredenburgh JJ, Baker ME. CT of the liver in patients with metastatic breast carcinoma treated by chemotherapy: findings simulating cirrhosis. AJR Am J Roentgenol 1994; 163:1385–1388
2. Dachman AH, Ros PR, Goodman ZD, Olmsted WW, Ishak KG. Nodular regenerative hyperplasia of the liver: clinical and radiologic observations. AJR Am J Roentgenol 1987;148:717–722
3. Clouet M, Boulay I, Boudiaf M, et al. Imaging features of nodular regenerative hyperplasia of the liver mimicking hepatic metastases. Abdom Imaging 1999;24: 258–261
4. Brancatelli G, Federle MP, Grazioli L, Golfieri R, Lencioni R. Benign regenerative nodules in Budd-Chiari syndrome and other vascular disorders of the liver: radiologic-pathologic and clinical correlation. Radiographics 2002;22:847–862
5. Gupta AA, Kim DC, Krinsky GA, Lee VS. CT and MRI of cirrhosis and its mimics. AJR Am J Roentgenol 2004;183:1595–1601
6. Schreiner SA, Gorman B, Stephens DH. Chemotherapy-related hepatotoxicity causing imaging findings resembling cirrhosis. Mayo Clin Proc 1998;73: 780–783

85

Magnetic Resonance Cholangiopancreatography Pitfalls

The following pitfalls can mimic calculi on magnetic resonance cholangiopancreatography.

Susceptibility Artifact

This can be secondary to air, clips, calcium, or stents. Intraluminal air can usually be differentiated from a calculus as air is non-dependent.

Flow Void

On T2-weighted magnetic resonance images (T2WI) with a relatively short echo time, a flow void can occasionally be seen in a dilated duct with both rapid and slow flow. It can also be seen at the point of insertion of a prominent cystic duct.[1] The characteristic location is central in the lumen. The flow void will resolve on heavily T2WI (e.g., with an echo time greater than 1100 ms).[2,3]

Vascular Impression

Pseudoobstruction of the extrahepatic bile duct can result from arterial pulsatile compression. This typically has a linear appearance traversing the duct and does not cause proximal dilatation. The common hepatic duct is the most common site of pseudoobstruction (typically from a crossing right hepatic artery), followed by the left hepatic duct, proximal common bile duct, and right hepatic duct.[4]

Sphincter Contraction

Forceful contraction of the sphincter of Oddi can result in retrograde invagination and a "pseudocalculus" sign in the distal common bile duct. This can be differentiated from a calculus, as only the superior margin will be outlined by high-signal intensity bile.[1] In addition, a filling defect from sphincter contraction usually does not persist on all images.[3]

References

1. Irie H, Honda H, Kuroiwa T, et al. Pitfalls in MR cholangiopancreatographic interpretation. Radiographics 2001;21:23–37
2. Sugita R, Sugimura E, Itoh M, Ohisa T, Takahashi S, Fujita N. Pseudolesion of the bile duct caused by flow effect: a diagnostic pitfall of MR cholangiopancreatography. AJR Am J Roentgenol 2003;180:467–471
3. Van Hoe L, Mermuys K, Vanhoenacker P. MRCP pitfalls. Abdom Imaging 2004;29:360–387
4. Watanabe Y, Dohke M, Ishimori T, et al. Pseudo-obstruction of the extrahepatic bile duct due to artifact from arterial pulsatile compression: a diagnostic pitfall of MR cholangiopancreatography. Radiology 2000;214: 856–860

86

Cystic Pancreatic Lesions

Differential Diagnosis of Pancreatic Cystic Lesions

Types of Cystic Pancreatic Masses

- Pseudocyst
- Serous cystadenoma
- Mucinous cystic neoplasm
- Intraductal papillary mucinous tumor

Rare Cystic Pancreatic Masses

- Solid and pseudopapillary epithelial neoplasms
- Cystic islet cell tumors: May have a hypervascular rim and cyst in cyst appearance[8]
- Simple cysts (rare in adults)

Pancreatic Cyst Mimics

Mimics of pancreatic cystic masses, such as duodenal diverticula, should first be excluded.

History of Pancreatitis

The most important clinical question is whether there has been prior pancreatitis. With a history of pancreatitis, pseudocyst is the most likely diagnosis in most cases.

Duct Communication/Dilatation

If communication with the pancreatic duct can be demonstrated, or if the duct is dilated, the differential is pseudocyst/chronic pancreatitis and intraductal papillary mucinous tumor (IPMT). Mucinous cystic neoplasm and serous cystadenoma rarely communicate with the duct. In the majority of cases, the main pancreatic duct will be dilated in an IPMT. A main duct IPMT will cause pancreatic ductal dilatation and may mimic the appearance of chronic pancreatitis. A combined (main and side-branch) IPMT can result in both a cystic mass and pancreatic ductal dilatation and can mimic the appearance of chronic pancreatitis and pseudocyst. A side-branch IPMT often is similar in appearance to a combined IPMT because there is often dilatation of the main pancreatic duct due to impaired drainage. If a side-branch IPMT presents without main duct dilatation, the differential diagnosis also might include serous cystadenoma and mucinous cystic neoplasm (however, these entities usually do not communicate with the duct).

A history of prior pancreatitis is the primary differentiating factor between a pseudocyst/chronic pancreatitis and IPMT. IPMT often has internal nodularity, which is not seen in pseudocysts. The appearance of the pancreatic duct can also be helpful in differential diagnosis (**Table 86.1**).

No Duct Communication/Dilatation

If there is no communication with the duct or duct dilatation, then serous cystadenoma and mucinous cystic neoplasm are the primary considerations (**Table 86.2**).

Table 86.1 Pancreatic Duct in Intraductal Papillary Mucinous Tumor (IPMT) versus Chronic Pancreatitis[1,9]

	IPMT	Chronic Pancreatitis
Duct Strictures	−	+
Duct Nodularity*	+	−
Papillary Bulging[†]	+	−
Stability	−	+
Branch Dilatation	Uncinate, tail	+

*Secondary to papillary tumor, mucin globs

[†]More common in malignant IPMT

Table 86.2 Mucinous Cystic Neoplasm versus Serous Cystadenoma[10,11,12]

	Mucinous	Serous
Cyst Size >2 cm	+	−
Cysts ≤6	+	−
Calcification	Peripheral	Central
External Contour	Smooth	Lobulated
Wall Enhancement	+	−
Internal Nodularity	+	−
Age	40–60	60+
M:F	1:9	1:2–3

Imaging Features of Specific Cystic Pancreatic Neoplasms

Mucinous Tumors

IPMT and mucinous cystic neoplasm are distinct entities. Radiologically the primary difference is that IPMT communicates with the pancreatic duct, but they also differ in clinical presentation (**Table 86.3**).

Side-Branch IPMT versus Serous Cystadenoma

A microcystic side-branch IPMT can have an appearance of small cysts in the 1 to 2 cm range, mimicking a serous cystadenoma. The "cysts" in a side-branch IPMT will have a configuration of tubes and arcs if examined closely as they represent dilated ducts.[1] This has also been described as a pleomorphic or clubbed fingerlike shape.[2] In addition, nodularity in the cysts (ducts) may be seen.

Unilocular Macrocystic Serous Cystadenoma versus Mucinous Cystic Neoplasm and IPMT

Rarely serous cystadenoma can be macrocystic and unilocular. It can still be differentiated from mucinous cystic neoplasm by the features in **Table 86.4**. IPMT can be differentiated by its pleomorphic or clubbed fingerlike shape. A macrocystic serous cystadenoma will have proximal main pancreatic duct dilatation, whereas IPMT will have dilatation of the distal or entire main pancreatic duct.[2] A pseudocyst can resemble a unilocular serous cystadenoma, but the serous cystadenoma is more likely to have a lobulated contour.

Table 86.3 Intraductal Papillary Mucinous Tumor (IPMT) versus Mucinous Cystic Neoplasm[1]

	IPMT	Mucinous Cystic Neoplasm
Location	Head, uncinate	Body, tail
Age	60 +	40–60
M:F	2:1	1:9
Presentation	Pain, pancreatitis	Often asymptomatic

Table 86.4 Unilocular Serous Cystadenoma versus Mucinous Cystic Neoplasm[10]

	Unilocular Serous Cystadenoma	Mucinous Cystic Neoplasm
Location	Head	Body, tail
Lobulated Contour	+	−
Wall Enhancement	−	+

Radiographic Characteristics of Malignant Intraductal Papillary Mucinous Tumor[3–6]

- Main pancreatic duct involvement
- Papillary bulging
- Main pancreatic duct dilatation >10 mm
- Diffuse or multifocal
- Solid mass
- Dense or calcified intraluminal content
- Mural nodularity >5 mm
- Size >5 cm (combined or branch duct type)
- Common bile duct or common hepatic duct dilatation ≥15 mm

- Presence of biliary stent for obstructive jaundice

Radiographic Characteristics of Solid and Pseudopapillary Epithelial Neoplasms[7]

Compared with the lesions discussed above, these tumors present in a younger age group (mean age 25 years) and usually in women. They are well-encapsulated and more complex in appearance containing solid components, hemorrhage, and fluid-debris levels. Calcification is sometimes seen.

References

1. Grogan JR, Saeian K, Taylor AJ, Quiroz F, Demeure MJ, Komorowski RA. Making sense of mucin-producing pancreatic tumors. AJR Am J Roentgenol 2001;176: 921–929
2. Kim SY, Lee JM, Kim SH, et al. Macrocystic neoplasms of the pancreas: CT differentiation of serous oligocystic adenoma from mucinous cystadenoma and intraductal papillary mucinous tumor. AJR Am J Roentgenol 2006;187(5):1192–1198
3. Fukukura Y, Fujiyoshi F, Sasaki M, Inoue H, Yonezawa S, Nakajo M. Intraductal papillary mucinous tumors of the pancreas: thin-section helical CT findings. AJR Am J Roentgenol 2000;174:441–447
4. Taouli B, Vilgrain V, Vullierme MP, et al. Intraductal papillary mucinous tumors of the pancreas: helical CT with histopathologic correlation. Radiology 2000; 217:757–764
5. Kawai M, Uchiyama K, Tani M, et al. Clinicopathological features of malignant intraductal papillary mucinous tumors of the pancreas: the differential diagnosis from benign entities. Arch Surg 2004;139:188–192
6. Kawamoto S, Lawler LP, Horton KM, Eng J, Hruban RH, Fishman EK. MDCT of intraductal papillary mucinous neoplasm of the pancreas: evaluation of features predictive of invasive carcinoma. AJR Am J Roentgenol 2006;186(3):687–695
7. Buetow PC, Buck JL, Pantongrag-Brown L, Beck KG, Ros PR, Adair CF. Solid and papillary epithelial neoplasm of the pancreas: imaging-pathologic correlation on 56 cases. Radiology 1996;199:707–711
8. Ligneau B, Lombard-Bohas C, Partensky C, et al. Cystic endocrine tumors of the pancreas: clinical, radiologic, and histopathologic features in 13 cases. Am J Surg Pathol 2001;25(6):752–760
9. Procacci C, Megibow AJ, Carbognin G, et al. Intraductal papillary mucinous tumor of the pancreas: a pictorial essay. Radiographics 1999;19: 1447–1463
10. Cohen-Scali F, Vilgrain V, Brancatelli G, et al. Discrimination of unilocular macrocystic serous cystadenoma from pancreatic pseudocyst and mucinous cystadenoma with CT: initial observations. Radiology 2003;228:727–733
11. Johnson CD, Stephens DH, Charboneau JW, Carpenter HA, Welch TJ. Cystic pancreatic tumors: CT and sonographic assessment. AJR Am J Roentgenol 1988;151: 1133–1138
12. Friedman AC, Lichtenstein JE, Dachman AH. Cystic neoplasms of the pancreas. Radiological-pathological correlation. Radiology 1983;149:45–50

87

Hypervascular Pancreatic Lesions

Islet cell tumors are by far the most common hypervascular mass in the pancreas. However, other etiologies are possible. Hypervascular pancreatic metastases are usually from renal cell carcinoma.[1] Hypervascular pancreatic metastases from breast cancer have also been reported.[2]

The solid variant of serous cystadenomas is very rare, and these lesions can be hypervascular and mimic islet cell tumors. In cases of solid serous cystadenomas, magnetic resonance imaging can occasionally identify tiny cystic components, even if no cystic components are identified by computed tomography.[3]

Hypervascular Pancreatic Lesions[1–3]

- Islet Cell Tumors
- Metastases
- Solid serous cystadenoma
- Splenosis

References

1. Ng CS, Loyer EM, Iyer RB, David CL, DuBrow RA, Charnsangavej C. Metastases to the pancreas from renal cell carcinoma: findings on three-phase contrast-enhanced helical CT. AJR Am J Roentgenol 1999;172: 1555–1559
2. Boudghene FP, Deslandes PM, LeBlanche AF, Bigot JM. US and CT imaging features of intrapancreatic metastases. J Comput Assist Tomogr 1994;18:905–910
3. Takeshita K, Kutomi K, Takada K, et al. Unusual imaging appearances of pancreatic serous cystadenoma: correlation with surgery and pathologic analysis. Abdom Imaging 2005;30:610–615

88

Focal Chronic Pancreatitis versus Pancreatic Cancer

Focal chronic pancreatitis can appear as a mass and is difficult to differentiate from pancreatic carcinoma (**Table 88.1**). Both focal chronic pancreatitis and pancreatic carcinoma enhance less than normal pancreatic tissue. The degree and time of enhancement does not distinguish between the two.[1] Infiltration of the fat around the superior mesenteric artery is suspicious for pancreatic carcinoma, but this is not specific and can also be seen in chronic pancreatitis.[2]

Table 88.1 Focal Chronic Pancreatitis versus Pancreatic Cancer[3,4]

	Pancreatic Cancer	Focal Chronic Pancreatitis
Calcification	−	+
Duct Dilatation	Smooth, beaded	Irregular
Duct Caliber	Larger	Smaller
Gland Caliber	Smaller	Larger
Double Duct Sign	+	−
SMA to SMV Ratio	> 1	< 1

Abbreviations: SMA, superior mesenteric artery; SMV, superior mesenteric vein.

References

1. Johnson PT, Outwater EK. Pancreatic carcinoma versus chronic pancreatitis: dynamic MR imaging. Radiology 1999;212:213–218
2. Schulte SJ, Baron RL, Freeny PC, Patten RM, Gorell HA, Maclin ML. Root of the superior mesenteric artery in pancreatitis and pancreatic carcinoma: evaluation with CT. Radiology 1991;180:659–662
3. Elmas N, Oran I, Oyar O, Ozer H. A new criterion in differentiation of pancreatitis and pancreatic carcinoma: artery-to-vein ratio using the superior mesenteric vessels. Abdom Imaging 1996;21:331–333
4. Karasawa E, Goldberg HI, Moss AA, Federle MP, London SS. CT pancreatogram in carcinoma of the pancreas and chronic pancreatitis. Radiology 1983;148:489–493

89

Pancreatic Lymphoma versus Carcinoma

Primary pancreatic lymphoma is a rare manifestation of B-cell non-Hodgkin's lymphoma. The differentiation between pancreatic lymphoma and adenocarcinoma is important as a patient with suspected lymphoma could have a nonsurgical biopsy rather than surgical biopsy and staging. Lymphoma can be treated by chemotherapy without surgical staging and a palliative Whipple's procedure, and has a better prognosis than adenocarcinoma. The following findings suggest pancreatic lymphoma rather than adenocarcinoma[1]:

- Lack of pancreatic ductal dilatation even with pancreatic invasion
- Adenopathy below the level of the renal veins

References

1. Merkle EM, Bender GN, Brambs HJ. Imaging findings in pancreatic lymphoma: differential aspects. AJR Am J Roentgenol 2000;174:671–675

Splenic Lesions

The differential diagnosis of splenic lesions is broad, but can be more easily approached if divided into solitary and multiple lesions. The next consideration is whether the lesion(s) are cystic, solid and nonvascular, or vascular. The vascular lesions can be distinguished from the solid nonvascular lesions by a greater degree of enhancement.

Cystic Splenic Lesions

Lymphangioma

Lymphangiomas are more common in children. They usually appear as single or multiple cystic lesions, sometimes multiloculated, which are often subcapsular in location. Curvilinear peripheral mural calcifications can be seen. Lymphangiomas are usually hypointense on T1-weighted magnetic resonance images (T1WI), but may be hyperintense from hemorrhage or proteinaceous material. They do not enhance.[1]

Echinococcal Cyst

Daughter cysts can be seen either peripherally or throughout the lesion, resulting in a multilocular appearance. These daughter cysts can appear less dense on computed tomography (CT) and more hypointense on T1WI relative to fluid in the parent cyst. Other possible differentiating features include collapsed parasitic membranes within the cyst, a low-intensity rim around the cyst secondary to a fibrous capsule, and cyst wall calcification.[2]

Cystic Metastasis

Splenic metastases, which are necrotic or mucinous, can appear cystic. Serosal implants from ovarian cancer can appear as peripheral cystic lesions.

Vascular Splenic Lesions

Hemangioma

Hemangiomas are the most common benign primary neoplasm of the spleen, and the second most common focal lesion (after cysts). They are most often seen in patients between the ages of 30 and 50. There may be a slight male predilection. Splenic hemangiomas have been associated with Klippel–Trenaunay–Weber syndrome (the presence of phleboliths in or adjacent to the spleen suggests a visceral angiomatosis syndrome).[3] Most hemangiomas are smaller than 2 cm. There is occasional calcification. Hemangiomas are usually homogeneously hyperintense on T2-weighted magnetic resonance images (T2WI; more homogeneous than hamartomas). Hemangiomas have a variable enhancement pattern. They can have a similar enhancement pattern to liver hemangiomas (progressive centripetal enhancement with persistent delayed enhancement), but differ from liver hemangiomas in that most do not have peripheral enhancing nodules. Some hemangiomas demonstrate mottled enhancement. Smaller hemangiomas may enhance homogeneously.[1,4]

Hamartoma

Splenic hamartomas are rare lesions composed of malformed red pulp elements. They can be seen in any age and have no sex predilection. They are associated with tuberous sclerosis. Hamartomas usually have well-defined margins and occasionally contain calcification and fatty components. They are usually heterogeneously hyperintense on T2WI (but sometimes can be hypointense on T2WI if fibrous). The enhancement pattern of hamartomas can be helpful in differentiating hamartomas from other lesions. Hamartomas often demonstrate diffuse heterogeneous early contrast enhancement and homogeneous prolonged enhancement.[1,5] Compared with hemangiomas, hamartomas have greater heterogeneity on T2WI and more heterogeneous[4] enhancement on early contrast-enhanced images. The presence of prolonged enhancement is helpful for differentiating hamartomas from other solid lesions such as lymphoma.[1]

Hemangioendothelioma

A splenic hemangioendothelioma may represent an intermediate entity between a hemangioma and angiosarcoma. They occur more frequently in young adults without a gender predilection. Imaging features are not specific and can mimic angiosarcoma.[1]

Hemangiopericytoma

Hemangiopericytomas have a high rate of local recurrence and can metastasize. A reported appearance is a large multilobulated mass with multiple other smaller lesions throughout the spleen. The appearance can mimic angiosarcoma.

Angiosarcoma

Angiosarcomas occur in the age range of 50 to 79 years with a slight male sex predilection. Unlike hepatic angiosarcoma, there is no association with exposure to vinyl chloride or other chemicals. The diagnosis can usually be suggested by imaging due the aggressive appearance of the mass and presence of metastases. Angiosarcoma does not usually metastasize to abdominal lymph nodes, which may be helpful in differentiating it from splenic lymphoma or metastasis (which could mimic an avascular angiosarcoma).[6]

Solid, Nonvascular Splenic Lesions

Lymphoma

Splenic lymphoma can appear as diffuse enlargement, multiple nodules, or a solitary mass. The lesions are typically isotense on T1WI and T2WI. Occasionally, lymphoma can be hypointense on T2WI, which is helpful in distinguishing lymphoma from other lesions.[2]

Inflammatory Pseudotumor

These rare lesions can be hypointense on T2WI and demonstrate delayed contrast enhancement.[7]

Solitary Splenic Lesions[1,2,8]

- Cystic
  - Posttraumatic cyst
  - Congenital cyst
  - Pancreatic pseudocyst
  - Echinococcal cyst
  - Abscess
  - Lymphangioma
  - Cystic metastasis
- Vascular
  - Hemangioma
  - Hamartoma
  - Hemangiopericytoma

- ○ Hemangioendothelioma
- ○ Angiosarcoma
- Solid, nonvascular
  - ○ Lymphoma
  - ○ Metastases
  - ○ Sarcoid
  - ○ Inflammatory pseudotumor

Multiple Nodules

There is a broad differential diagnosis for multiple splenic nodules. The most common etiologies, broken up by clinical presentation are[9]

- Symptomatic, no known malignancy: Lymphoma, infection (immunocompromised), sarcoid
- Asymptomatic: Benign tumor (e.g., hemangiomatosis, littoral cell angioma, remote infection), sarcoid, nonlymphomatous metastatic disease

Nodule size may be helpful in differentiation. Lymphoma usually has large nodules, which are variable in size. Infection usually has small nodules, which are uniform in size. The nodules in sarcoid are intermediate in size.

The presence of adenopathy is often not helpful. Abdominal adenopathy is seen in 40 to 70% of cases of splenic lymphoma, but is commonly seen in all the disorders noted above except benign tumor. The nodes in lymphoma are usually larger than those in sarcoid; they tend to be more confluent, have greater involvement of the retrocrural space.[3]

T2WI hypointensity of the lesions may be helpful for differential diagnosis. Both lymphoma and sarcoid can be hypointense on T2WI, although sarcoid is more commonly so.

One unusual cause of multiple T2WI hypointense splenic lesions is littoral cell angioma. Littoral cell angioma is rare vascular tumor unique to the spleen composed of multiple blood-filled vascular channels. It has no definite sex predilection. There is usually laboratory evidence of hypersplenism. The most common imaging appearance is splenomegaly with innumerable masses, which are hypodense on portal phase images. On delayed images, the lesions may become isoattenuating to the spleen, which is helpful in differentiation from other lesions. The lesions can be hypointense on both T1WI and T2WI due to hemosiderin deposition.[1,10]

Patients with portal hypertension can have multiple hypointense T2WI foci, secondary to hemosiderin deposition in the spleen. These are known as Gamma–Gandy bodies.[3]

Another cause of multiple T2WI hypointense splenic lesions is Gaucher's disease. In Gaucher's disease, glucocerebrosides accumulate in the phagocytic cells of the reticuloendothelial system. Imaging manifestations include splenomegaly and less commonly multiple nodules.[3] Lymphoma, sarcoid, and littoral cell angioma should also be considered in the setting of splenomegaly and multiple T2WI hypointense nodules.

Splenic Lesions that Are Hypointense on T2-Weighted Magnetic Resonance Imaging[2,3,7]

- Lymphoma (atypical)
- Sarcoid
- Hamartoma (atypical)
- Inflammatory pseudotumor
- Littoral cell angioma
- Gamma-Gandy bodies
- Gaucher's disease

References

1. Abbott RM, Levy AD, Aguilera NS, Gorospe L, Thompson WM. From the archives of the AFIP: primary vascular neoplasms of the spleen: radiologic-pathologic correlation. Radiographics 2004;24: 1137–1163
2. Warshauer DM, Hall HL. Solitary splenic lesions. Semin Ultrasound CT MR 2006;27:370–388
3. Kamaya A, Weinstein S, Desser TS. Multiple lesions of the spleen: differential diagnosis of cystic and solid lesions. Semin Ultrasound CT MR 2006;27:389–403
4. Luna A, Ribes R, Caro P, Luna L, Aumente E, Ros PR. MRI of focal splenic lesions without and with dynamic gadolinium enhancement. AJR Am J Roentgenol 2006;186:1533–1547

5. Yu RS, Zhang SZ, Hua JM. Imaging findings of splenic hamartoma. World J Gastroenterol 2004;10:2613–2615
6. Thompson WM, Levy AD, Aguilera NS, Gorospe L, Abbott RM. Angiosarcoma of the spleen: imaging characteristics in 12 patients. Radiology 2005;235: 106–115
7. Irie H, Honda H, Kaneko K, et al. Inflammatory pseudo-tumors of the spleen: CT and MRI findings. J Comput Assist Tomogr 1996;20:244–248
8. Urrutia M, Mergo PJ, Ros LH, Torres GM, Ros PR. Cystic masses of the spleen: radiologic-pathologic correlation. Radiographics 1996;16:107–129
9. Warshauer DM, Molina PL, Worawattanakul S. The spotted spleen: CT and clinical correlation in a tertiary care center. J Comput Assist Tomogr 1998;22: 694–702
10. Levy AD, Abbott RM, Abbondanzo SL. Littoral cell angioma of the spleen: CT features with clinicopathologic comparison. Radiology 2004;230:485–490

91

Adrenal Adenoma versus Metastasis

Adrenal adenomas are the most common adrenal lesions. As an incidental finding, a small homogeneous adrenal lesion is highly likely to be an adenoma. In patients with cancer, it is often important to determine whether an adrenal lesion is an adenoma or metastasis. The methods below should be only applied to relatively homogeneous adrenal lesions. Adrenal adenomas generally cannot be diagnosed by imaging in masses with substantial areas of necrosis or hemorrhage.[1]

Diagnosis of Lipid-Rich Adrenal Adenomas

Adrenal adenomas have intracytoplasmic lipid that is not present in metastases. Detection of lipid content differentiates adenomas from metastases. This can be evaluated by noncontrast computed tomography (CT) or chemical shift magnetic resonance imaging (MRI).

Noncontrast Computed Tomography

Adenomas have lower attenuation values than metastases. Using a threshold attenuation value of 10 Hounsfield units (HU), the sensitivity is 71% and the specificity 98%.[2]

Chemical Shift Magnetic Resonance Imaging

Adenomas demonstrate signal loss on opposed phased chemical shift imaging. Both visual and quantitative analysis can be used to evaluate whether there is signal loss. Two quantitative parameters that have been used to diagnose lipid content are

1. Lesion signal loss >20% on opposed phase imaging
2. Adrenal-to-spleen ratio ≤ 0.70:[3] The adrenal-to-spleen ratio is the adrenal mass-to-spleen signal intensity ratio on opposed phase images divided by the adrenal mass-to-spleen signal intensity ratio in phase images.

Diagnosis of Lipid-Poor Adrenal Adenomas

Ten to 40% of adrenal adenomas will be lipid poor[4] and cannot be diagnosed as adenomas on noncontrast CT. Although adenomas can have noncontrast CT attenuation values >10, a non-calcified nonhemorrhagic adrenal lesion measuring >43 HU is suspicious for malignancy.[5] In lesions with an attenuation value >10 but < 43 on noncontrast CT, chemical shift MRI and contrast-enhanced CT may be helpful for diagnosis.

Chemical Shift Magnetic Resonance Imaging

Even if the adenoma appears lipid poor on noncontrast CT, chemical shift MRI may still detect lipid and can (in 62% of cases) definitively characterize the lesion as an adenoma.[6]

Contrast-Enhanced Computed Tomography

Although adenomas enhance, they will have a faster rate of contrast washout than metastases. This is true of both lipid-rich and lipid-poor adenomas. If a delayed 15-min postcontrast scan is obtained, the contrast washout from an adrenal lesion can be assessed. The percentage of enhancement washout can be calculated: $[(E-D)/(E-U)] \times 100$, where E is the enhanced attenuation value, D is the delayed value, and U is the unenhanced value. A threshold washout ratio of 60% can be used to differentiate adenomas from metastases. If unenhanced scans are not available, the enhanced value only can be used as the denominator $[(E-D)/E] \times 100$, with 40% as the threshold value.[4] If delayed imaging is performed at 10 min rather than 15 min, washout values of 52% and 37.5% (without an unenhanced scan) can be used.[5]

Pheochromocytomas versus Adenomas

Pheochromocytomas can have low attenuation values on noncontrast CT and mimic adenomas (pheochromocytomas can have microscopic and even macroscopic fat).[7] The incidence of this finding is unknown, but it is likely rare.[8] A pheochromocytoma will usually have a slower rate of washout than an adenoma.[3] However, in some cases, a pheochromocytoma can have rapid washout and mimic an adenoma on delayed washout CT exams.[9]

Adrenal Lesions with Low Density on Unenhanced Computed Tomography

- Adenoma
- Hyperplasia
- Cyst
- Myelolipoma
- Pheochromocytoma
- Adrenocortical carcinoma

Adrenal Lesions with Signal Loss on Chemical Shift Magnetic Resonance Imaging

- Adenoma
- Hyperplasia
- Myelolipoma
- Pheochromocytoma
- Adrenocortical carcinoma[10]
- Adrenal metastasis: Clear cell renal carcinoma, hepatocellular carcinoma[11,12]

References

1. Dunnick NR, Korobkin M. Imaging of adrenal incidentalomas: current status. AJR Am J Roentgenol 2002;179:559–568
2. Boland GW, Lee MJ, Gazelle GS, Halpern EF, McNicholas MM, Mueller PR. Characterization of adrenal masses using unenhanced CT: an analysis of the CT literature. AJR Am J Roentgenol 1998;171:201–204
3. Sahdev A, Reznek RH. Imaging evaluation of the nonfunctioning indeterminate adrenal mass. Trends Endocrinol Metab 2004;15:271–276
4. Caoili EM, Korobkin M, Francis IR, Cohan RH, Dunnick NR. Delayed enhanced CT of lipid-poor adrenal adenomas. AJR Am J Roentgenol 2000;175:1411–1415
5. Blake MA, Kalra MK, Sweeney AT, et al. Distinguishing benign from malignant adrenal masses: multi-detector row CT protocol with 10-minute delay. Radiology 2006;238:578–585
6. Israel GM, Korobkin M, Wang C, Hecht EN, Krinsky GA. Comparison of unenhanced CT and chemical shift MRI in evaluating lipid-rich adrenal adenomas. AJR Am J Roentgenol 2004;183:215–219
7. Blake MA, Krishnamoorthy SK, Boland GW, et al. Low-density pheochromocytoma on CT: a mimicker of adrenal adenoma. AJR Am J Roentgenol 2003;181:1663–1668
8. Motta-Ramirez GA, Remer EM, Herts BR, Gill IS, Hamrahian AH. Comparison of CT findings in symptomatic and incidentally discovered pheochromocytomas. AJR Am J Roentgenol 2005;185:684–688
9. Park BK, Kim B, Ko K, Jeong SY, Kwon GY. Adrenal masses falsely diagnosed as adenomas on unenhanced and delayed contrast-enhanced computed tomography: Pathological correlation. Eur Radiol 2006;16:642–647

10. Yamada T, Saito H, Moriya T, et al. Adrenal carcinoma with a signal loss on chemical shift magnetic resonance imaging. J Comput Assist Tomogr 2003;27:606–608

11. Shinozaki K, Yoshimitsu K, Honda H, et al. Metastatic adrenal tumor from clear-cell renal carcinoma: a pitfall of chemical shift MR imaging. Abdom Imaging 2001;26:439–442

12. Sydow BD, Rosen MA, Siegelman ES. Intracellular lipid within metastatic hepatocellular carcinoma of the adrenal gland: A potential diagnostic pitfall of chemical shift imaging of the adrenal gland. AJR Am J Roentgenol 2006;187:W550–1

92

Adrenal Lesions with Macroscopic Fat

The vast majority of adrenal lesions containing macroscopic fat are myelolipomas. Some lesions contain macroscopic fat, but rarely occur in the adrenals. Other adrenal lesions very rarely contain macroscopic fat.

Adrenal Lesions with Macroscopic Fat[1–5]

- Myelolipoma
- Lipoma
- Teratoma
- Angiomyolipoma
- Liposarcoma
- Pheochromocytoma
- Adrenocortical carcinoma
- Adenoma
- Hyperplasia

References

1. Lam KY, Lo CY. Adrenal lipomatous tumours: a 30 year clinicopathological experience at a single institution. J Clin Pathol 2001;54:707–712
2. Ramsay JA, Asa SL, Van Nostrand AW, Hassaram ST, de Harven EP. Lipid degeneration in pheochromocytomas mimicking adrenal cortical tumors. Am J Surg Pathol 1987;11:480–486
3. Heye S, Woestenborghs H, Van Kerkhove F, Oyen R. Adrenocortical carcinoma with fat inclusion: case report. Abdom Imaging 2005;30:641–643
4. Papotti M, Sapino A, Mazza E, Sandrucci S, Volante M, Bussolati G. Lipomatous changes in adrenocortical adenomas. Report of two cases. Endocr Pathol 1996;7:223–228
5. Finch C, Davis R, Truong LD. Extensive lipomatous metaplasia in bilateral macronodular adrenocortical hyperplasia. Arch Pathol Lab Med 1999;123:167–169

93

Cushing Syndrome

Endogenous Cushing syndrome is usually adrenocorticotropic hormone (ACTH)-dependent (80 to 85%), and less likely ACTH-independent (15 to 20%). ACTH-dependent Cushing syndrome is usually secondary to a pituitary adenoma. ACTH-independent Cushing syndrome is usually secondary to a hyperfunctioning adrenal adenoma. Rarely, bilateral adrenal disease (ACTH-independent macronodular hyperplasia or primary pigmented nodular adrenal disease) can cause Cushing syndrome.[1]

The presence of an adrenal nodule in Cushing syndrome does not always indicate a hyperfunctioning nodule. An ACTH-dependent macronodular hyperplasia with a dominant nodule, or a nonhyperfunctioning adenoma can also cause this appearance. ACTH-producing adenomas will usually result in atrophy of the remaining adrenal tissue. Thus, in a patient with Cushing disease and an adrenal nodule with normal or hyperplastic adrenal limbs, the possibility of an ACTH-dependent hyperplasia (with an incidental non-hyperfunctioning nodule) or ACTH-dependent macronodular hyperplasia should be considered.[2]

Bilateral adrenal disease is a rare cause of Cushing syndrome. ACTH-independent macronodular hyperplasia is a rare disease of uncertain pathogenesis. It is distinct from the much more common form of macronodular hyperplasia secondary to ACTH stimulation. Patients present at a later age than those with functioning adenomas (mean age of 51 years in one series) and sex predilection has been reported to be even or more frequent in males. The adrenal glands are massively enlarged with numerous nodules >4 cm. The nodules are hyperintense to liver on T2-weighted magnetic resonance images (T2WI) unlike the nodules in ACTH-dependent macronodular hyperplasia, which are similar in intensity to liver.[1,3]

Another rare bilateral adrenal disease that can cause Cushing's syndrome is primary pigmented nodular adrenocortical disease. Approximately 50% of cases are sporadic. The other half is familial, associated with the Carney complex (myxomas, spotty skin pigmentation, schwannomas, and other endocrine and nonendocrine tumors). It usually presents in younger female patients. The adrenal gland is usually not enlarged. The adrenal cortex can be atrophic with small nodules forming a string-of-beads appearance. On MRI, the nodules can be less intense than adjacent cortical tissue on both T1-weighted magnetic resonance images (T1WI) and on T2WI.[1,3]

Etiologies of Cushing Syndrome[1]

ACTH-dependent Cushing Syndrome

- Pituitary adenoma
- Ectopic ACTH source

ACTH-independent Cushing Syndrome

- Unilateral adrenal disease
- Hyperfunctioning adrenal adenoma
- Adrenal carcinoma

Bilateral Adrenal Disease (Rare)

- ACTH-independent macronodular hyperplasia
- Primary pigmented nodular adrenocortical disease

References

1. Rockall AG, Babar SA, Sohaib SA, et al. CT and MR imaging of the adrenal glands in ACTH-independent cushing syndrome. Radiographics 2004;24:435–452
2. Choyke PL, Doppman JL. Case 18: adrenocorticotropic hormone-dependent Cushing syndrome. Radiology 2000;214:195–198
3. Lacroix A, Bourdeau I. Bilateral adrenal Cushing's syndrome: macronodular adrenal hyperplasia and primary pigmented nodular adrenocortical disease. Endocrinol Metab Clin North Am 2005;34:441–458

94

Hyperaldosteronism

Primary hyperaldosteronism (Conn's syndrome) can be secondary to an aldosterone-producing adenoma or less likely, a bilateral adrenal hyperplasia. However, identification of an adrenal nodule in a patient with Conn's syndrome does not always indicate an aldosterone-producing adenoma. Other etiologies are a dominant nodule in macronodular hyperplasia and a nonhyperfunctioning adenoma. Thus, it is important to determine whether an adrenal nodule in a patient with Conn's syndrome is the etiology of the disease. The size of the adrenal gland limbs is helpful in these cases.

Size of Adrenal Limbs in Hyperaldosteronism[1,2]

The adrenal gland limbs will be larger in patients with bilateral adrenal hyperplasia than in aldosterone-producing adenoma. The limbs will enlarge more than the body. Measurement of limb width can be helpful in differential diagnosis:

1. Limb width ≥5 mm: Adrenal hyperplasia
2. Limb width ≤3 mm: Adrenal hyperplasia excluded
3. Limb width between 3 and 5 mm with multiple nodules: Macronodular hyperplasia
4. Limb width between 3 and 5 mm with one nodule: This could be secondary to an aldosterone-producing adenoma or a bilateral adrenal hyperplasia with a coincidental nonhyperfunctioning adenoma. Adrenal vein sampling could be considered in this situation.

References

1. Lingam RK, Sohaib SA, Vlahos I, et al. CT of primary hyperaldosteronism (Conn's syndrome): the value of measuring the adrenal gland. AJR Am J Roentgenol 2003;181:843–849

2. Sohaib SA, Peppercorn PD, Allan C, et al. Primary hyperaldosteronism (Conn syndrome): MR imaging findings. Radiology 2000;214:527–531

95

Hyperdense Renal Lesions

Hyperdense renal lesions can be seen on unenhanced or enhanced computed tomography (CT).

Noncontrast Computed Tomography

Some renal lesions are hyperdense (greater in attenuation than normal renal parenchyma) on unenhanced images. Renal cell carcinomas are usually isoattenuating or hypoattenuating on unenhanced images. A minority (13% in one study)[1] are hyperattenuating. A rare cause of a hyperdense renal lesion is focal chronic tubulointerstitial inflammation. This is a nonspecific response to persistent tubular injury, which causes the tubules to become filled with concentrated proteinaceous fluid.[2]

Hyperdense Renal Lesions on Unenhanced Computed Tomography

Common Lesions

- Hyperdense cysts

Uncommon Lesions

- Renal cell carcinoma

Rare Cases[1,2]

- Angiomyolipoma with minimal fat
- Oncocytoma
- Metanephric adenoma
- Focal chronic tubulointerstitial inflammation

Portal-Phase Contrast-Enhanced Computed Tomography

High attenuation renal lesions are commonly seen on portal-phase contrast-enhanced CT images. An attenuation >70 Hounsfield units (HU) and internal heterogeneity suggests renal cell carcinoma rather than hyperdense cyst on portal-phase CT images.[3]

References

1. Kim JK, Park SY, Shon JH, Cho KS. Angiomyolipoma with minimal fat: differentiation from renal cell carcinoma at biphasic helical CT. Radiology 2004;230:677–684
2. Choi DJ, Shandar S, Stachurski D, Banner DF. Nonneoplastic hyperdense enhancing renal mass: CT findings and pathologic correlation. AJR Am J Roentgenol 2005;184:1597–1599
3. Suh M, Coakley FV, Qayyum A, Yeh BM, Breiman RS, Lu Y. Distinction of renal cell carcinomas from high-attenuation renal cysts at portal venous phase contrast-enhanced CT. Radiology 2003;228:330–334

96

Renal Lesions with Fat

Almost all fat-containing renal masses are angiomyolipomas. Fat density has been reported in renal cell carcinomas, but this is extremely rare. However, a mass that contains both fat and calcification is suspicious for renal cell carcinoma as angiomyolipomas rarely contain calcification.[1] Fat density without calcification has been reported in papillary renal cell carcinoma, secondary to adipose tissue[1] and cholesterol necrosis.[2] Papillary renal cell carcinomas tend to be more homogeneous and enhance less than clear cell carcinomas.[3] Clear cell renal carcinomas often have intracytoplasmic fat, which can be detected by chemical shift magnetic resonance imaging (MRI),[4] but do not have macroscopic fat detectable by computed tomography (CT).

Although the vast majority of fat-containing renal masses are angiomyolipomas, a renal cell carcinoma should be considered if[2,5]

1. Calcification is seen in addition to fat.
2. There are signs of local invasion and/or adenopathy.
3. Large areas of necrosis in the lesion are seen.
4. Fat is seen in conjunction with a homogeneous and hypovascular lesion (possible papillary subtype renal carcinoma).

Renal Lesions with Macroscopic Fat[1,5]

- Angiomyolipoma
- Papillary cell renal carcinoma
- Lipoma
- Liposarcoma
- Fat-containing oncocytoma
- Wilms' tumor

References

1. Schuster TG, Ferguson MR, Baker DE, Schaldenbrand JD, Solomon MH. Papillary renal cell carcinoma containing fat without calcification mimicking angiomyolipoma on CT. AJR Am J Roentgenol 2004;183:1402–1404
2. Lesavre A, Correas JM, Merran S, Grenier N, Vieillefond A, Helenon O. CT of papillary renal cell carcinomas with cholesterol necrosis mimicking angiomyolipomas. AJR Am J Roentgenol 2003;181:143–145
3. Herts BR, Coll DM, Novick AC, et al. Enhancement characteristics of papillary renal neoplasms revealed on triphasic helical CT of the kidneys. AJR Am J Roentgenol 2002;178:367–372
4. Yoshimitsu K, Honda H, Kuroiwa T, et al. MR detection of cytoplasmic fat in clear cell renal cell carcinoma utilizing chemical shift gradient-echo imaging. J Magn Reson Imaging 1999;9:579–585
5. Helenon O, Merran S, Paraf F, et al. Unusual fat-containing tumors of the kidney: a diagnostic dilemma. Radiographics 1997;17:129–144

97

Angiomyolipomas with Minimal Fat

A threshold value of ≤ -10 Hounsfield units (HU) can be used to differentiate renal angiomyolipoma (AML) from other renal lesions.[1] However, intratumoral fat in AMLs may not be detectable on computed tomography (CT) in 4.5% of cases.[2] In these cases, it is often not possible to distinguish an AML from a renal cell carcinoma. Features that suggest the diagnosis of AML with minimal fat in these cases are[2-4]

1. Homogeneous enhancement
2. Prolonged enhancement pattern: Minimal difference in attenuation between corticomedullary and early excretory phase images

3. Homogeneous high attenuation on nonenhanced images: However, ~13% of renal cell carcinomas are also high attenuation
4. Quantification of intratumoral fat can be performed with chemical shift gradient echo magnetic resonance imaging (MRI). Although other renal tumors such as clear cell renal carcinoma contain intratumoral fat, AMLs with minimal fat have more fat content, which can be detected with quantitative parameters. A threshold signal intensity index [(in phase tumor signal intensity – out of phase tumor signal intensity)/(in phase tumor signal intensity)] $\times$ 100 of >25% is accurate for a diagnosis of AML with minimal fat.[2]

References

1. Simpson E, Patel U. Diagnosis of angiomyolipoma using computed tomography-region of interest, or = −10 HU or 4 adjacent pixels < or = −10 HU are recommended as the diagnostic thresholds. Clin Radiol 2006;61:410–416
2. Kim JK, Kim SH, Jang YJ, et al. Renal angiomyolipoma with minimal fat: differentiation from other neoplasms at double-echo chemical shift FLASH MR imaging. Radiology 2006;239:174–180
3. Jinzaki M, Tanimoto A, Narimatsu Y, et al. Angiomyolipoma: imaging findings in lesions with minimal fat. Radiology 1997;205:497–502
4. Kim JK, Park SY, Shon JH, Cho KS. Angiomyolipoma with minimal fat: differentiation from renal cell carcinoma at biphasic helical CT. Radiology 2004;230:677–684

98

Renal Parenchyma with Hypointensity on T2-Weighted Magnetic Resonance Imaging

On T2-weighted magnetic resonance images (T2WI) the kidneys normally have moderately high signal intensity with no difference between the cortex and the medulla. Low signal intensity in the renal parenchyma could be secondary to hemosiderin, hemorrhage, calcification, or fibrosis. Three main categories of disease that result in renal parenchymal T2WI hypointensity are intravascular hemolysis, infection, and vascular disease. In extravascular hemolysis iron is deposited in the liver and spleen. In intravascular hemolysis, when direct release of hemosiderin in the plasma exceeds the binding capacity of plasma haptoglobin, hemoglobin is filtered in the glomerulus and stored in the proximal convoluted tubule as hemosiderin. Intravascular hemolysis does not result in hemosiderin accumulation outside the kidney.[1,2] Intravascular hemolysis can be seen with mechanical shear (most commonly from a prosthetic valve), paroxysmal nocturnal hemoglobinuria, and rarely sickle cell anemia.

Paroxysmal nocturnal hemoglobinuria is an acquired stem cell disorder caused by increased sensitivity to complement.[1] Hemolysis, thrombosis, and deficient hematopoiesis are possible sequela.

Patients with sickle cell anemia usually do not have hemosiderin deposition in the renal cortex as the hemolysis is extravascular. However, in acute hemolytic crises and severe disease, intravascular hemolysis can occur resulting in low T2WI signal in the renal cortex. Unlike paroxysmal nocturnal hemoglobinuria or mechanical hemolysis, in these cases the spleen will usually be hypointense on T2WI as well.

Renal cortical necrosis is a cause of cortical T2WI hypointensity without intravascular hemolysis. In renal cortical necrosis, the cortical T2WI hypointensity can be seen even if there is no cortical calcification.[3,4]

Renal medullary T2WI hypointensity is rare. One cause is hemorrhagic fever with renal syndrome, which was formerly known as Korean hemorrhagic fever. It is caused by a rodent-transmitted Hantavirus and occurs primarily in Asia and Europe. Disease manifestations include fever, visceral hemorrhage, and renal failure. Hemorrhage occurs in the renal medulla, right atrium, and anterior pituitary gland.[1] In both hemorrhagic fever with renal syndrome and renal vein thrombosis, the T2WI hypointensity predominately involves the outer portion of the medulla.[5]

Renal Cortex with Hypointensity on T2-Weighted Magnetic Resonance Imaging[1]

- Paroxysmal nocturnal hemoglobinuria
- Mechanical hemolysis (prosthetic valve)
- Sickle cell disease (severe disease and acute hemolytic crisis)
- Renal cortical necrosis

Renal Medulla with Hypointensity on T2-Weighted Magnetic Resonance Imaging[1]

- Hemorrhagic fever with renal syndrome
- Renal vein thrombosis

References

1. Jeong JY, Kim SH, Lee HJ, Sim JS. Atypical low-signal-intensity renal parenchyma: causes and patterns. Radiographics 2002;22:833–846
2. Roubidoux MA. MR imaging of hemorrhage and iron deposition in the kidney. Radiographics 1994;14:1033–1044
3. Francois M, Tostivint I, Mercadl L, Bellin MF, Izzedine H, Deray G. MR imaging features of acute bilateral renal cortical necrosis. Am J Kidney Dis 2000;35:745–748
4. Kim SH, Han MC, Kim S, Lee JS. MR imaging of acute renal cortical necrosis. A case report. Acta Radiol 1992;33:431–433
5. Kim SH, Kim S, Lee JS, et al. Hemorrhagic fever with renal syndrome: MR imaging of the kidney. Radiology 1990;175:823–825

99

Renal Infarction versus Pyelonephritis

Renal infarction and pyelonephritis can occasionally be difficult to differentiate by imaging as they can both cause wedge-shaped areas of decreased renal enhancement.

The cortical rim sign is seen in renal infarction and not pyelonephritis. The cortical rim sign refers to perfusion of an intact subcapsular renal cortex (2 to 4 mm) supplied by collateral capsular circulation. However, the cortical rim sign is only seen in ~50% of infarcts.[1] It is also not seen immediately after infarction. In posttraumatic renal infarction, the earliest appearance is within 8 h and the median time to appearance is 7 days.[2] The cortical rim sign is not exclusive to renal infarction and has also been reported in renal vein thrombosis and acute tubular necrosis.[3]

Another sign of renal infarction is "flip-flop" enhancement.[4] This refers to a hyperdense region on delayed computed tomography (CT) images in the same region as a hypodense region on nephrographic phase images. However, this finding is also seen in renal infection.[5] The finding of flip-flop enhancement would be more useful to differentiate an infarct or infection from a mass.

References

1. Wong WS, Moss AA, Federle MP, Cochran ST, London SS. Renal infarction: CT diagnosis and correlation between CT findings and etiologies. Radiology 1984;150: 201–205
2. Kamel IR, Berkowitz JF. Assessment of the cortical rim sign in posttraumatic renal infarction. J Comput Assist Tomogr 1996;20:803–806
3. Hann L, Pfister FC. Renal subcapsular rim sign: new etiologies and pathogenesis. AJR Am J Roentgenol 1982;138:51–54
4. Suzer O, Shirkhoda A, Jafri SZ, Madrazo BL, Bis KG, Mastromatteo JF. CT features of renal infarction. Eur J Radiol 2002;44:59–64
5. Dalla-Palma L, Pozzi-Mucelli F, Pozzi-Mucelli RS. Delayed CT findings in acute renal infection. Clin Radiol 1995;50:364–370

100

Imaging Signs of the Bowel

Target Sign

A stratified pattern of enhancement in the bowel wall is seen when inner and outer layers of high attenuation surround a central submucosal area of low attenuation. If the submucosal low density is fat attenuation, this is referred to as the *fat halo sign*. If the submucosal low density is higher than fat density, this can be referred to as the *target sign*. This is a nonspecific finding that usually indicates inflammation or ischemia. Conditions in which it has been noted include inflammatory bowel disease, infectious enterocolitis, ischemia, radiation enteritis, intramural hemorrhage, and bowel edema in cirrhotic patients.[1,2] The primary value of this finding is that it usually indicates a nonneoplastic etiology for bowel wall thickening, although rarely an infiltrating scirrhous carcinoma can have this appearance.[1]

Fat Halo Sign

Submucosal fat deposition in the bowel wall has been called the fat halo sign.[3] This manifests as a three-layered target sign in the bowel wall with fat density in the middle layer. The fat can usually be distinguished from edema by a lower attenuation, but it is of higher attenuation than mesenteric fat. The fat halo sign usually indicates a chronic process, most likely chronic inflammatory bowel disease.[4] It is more common

in ulcerative colitis than Crohn's disease. However, it can be seen acutely in graft-versus-host disease and after cytoreductive therapy.[5] It is also sometimes a normal variant, particularly in the terminal ileum and colon. Normal variant submucosal fat is most commonly seen when the bowel lumen is collapsed, and may be related to obesity.[4]

Bowel Wall Submucosal Fat (Fat Halo Sign)[4–7]

- Chronic inflammatory bowel disease
- Normal variant
- Cytoreductive therapy
- Graft-versus-host disease
- Chronic radiation enteritis

Accordion Sign

The accordion sign is seen when edematous haustral folds separated by contrast material between the folds simulate the appearance of an accordion. This was originally described as specific for pseudomembranous colitis, but it is a nonspecific sign of severe colonic edema and has also been reported in non-C difficile infectious colitis, inflammatory and ischemic colitis, and edema related to cirrhosis.[8] The presence of severe wall thickening in conjunction with the accordion sign suggests pseudomembranous colitis because pseudomembranous colitis and Crohn's disease are associated with the most severe degrees of wall thickening among all types of colitis.[9]

Pseudomembranous colitis can be differentiated from Crohn's disease by the presence of ascites and a more irregular wall in pseudomembranous colitis.

References

1. Macari M, Balthazar EJ. CT of bowel wall thickening: significance and pitfalls of interpretation. AJR Am J Roentgenol 2001;176:1105–1116
2. Ahualli J. The target sign: bowel wall. Radiology 2005; 234:549–550
3. Wittenberg J, Harisinghani MG, Jhaveri K, Varghese J, Mueller PR. Algorithmic approach to CT diagnosis of the abnormal bowel wall. Radiographics 2002;22:1093–1107
4. Philpotts LE, Heiken JP, Westcott MA, Gore RM. Colitis: use of CT findings in differential diagnosis. Radiology 1994;190:445–449
5. Muldowney SM, Balfe DM, Hammerman A, Wick MR. "Acute" fat deposition in bowel wall submucosa: CT appearance. J Comput Assist Tomogr 1995;19:390–393
6. Harisinghani MG, Wittenberg J, Lee W, Chen S, Gutierrez AL, Mueller PR. Bowel wall fat halo sign in patients without intestinal disease. AJR Am J Roentgenol 2003;181:781–784
7. Chen S, Harisinghani MG, Wittenberg J. Small bowel CT fat density target sign in chronic radiation enteritis. Australas Radiol 2003;47:450–452
8. Macari M, Balthazar EJ, Megibow AJ. The accordion sign at CT: a nonspecific finding in patients with colonic edema. Radiology 1999;211:743–746
9. Thoeni RF, Cello JP. CT imaging of colitis. Radiology 2006;240:623–638

101

Diverticulitis versus Colon Cancer

Diverticulitis and colon cancer can sometimes be difficult to differentiate by computed tomography (CT) **(Table 101.1)**. The most helpful differentiating findings seen in diverticulitis are:

- The presence of noninflamed and inflamed diverticula
- Mild degree of enhancement
- Target enhancement pattern
- Pericolonic inflammation
- Abscess formation
- Free air
- Length >10 cm[1,2]

The most helpful differentiating findings seen in colon cancer are presence of pericolonic lymph nodes and a luminal mass. Pericolonic inflammation out of portion to the degree of bowel thickening is the most specific finding for diverticulitis. In right-sided diverticulitis, the most helpful findings in differentiating the disease from colon cancer are preserved wall enhancement and inflamed diverticula.[3] Arrowhead-shaped wall thickening is a sign of diverticulitis, but is also seen in appendicitis.

Table 101.1 Diverticulitis versus Colon Cancer[1–5]

	Diverticulitis	Colon Cancer
Pericolonic inflammation (out of proportion to bowel wall thickening)	+	−
Pericolonic edema	+	−
Fluid at root of mesentery	+	−
Length >10 cm	+	−
Extraluminal air or fluid	+	−
Mesenteric vascular engorgement	+	−
Sawtooth haustral thickening	+	−
Arrowhead-shaped wall thickening	+	−
Inflamed diverticula	+	−
Preserved wall enhancement pattern	+	−
Luminal mass	−	+
Pericolonic lymph nodes	−	+
Shoulder formation	−	+
Length <5 cm	±	+
Degree of enhancement	<	>
Target enhancement pattern	+	−

Additional Readings

1. Chintapalli KN, Chopra S, Ghiatas AA, Esola CC, Fields SF, Dodd GD III. Diverticulitis versus colon cancer: differentiation with helical CT findings. Radiology 1999; 210:429–435

2. Shen SH, Chen JD, Tiu CM, et al. Differentiating colonic diverticulitis from colon cancer: the value of computed tomography in the emergency setting. J Chin Med Assoc 2005;68:411–418

3. Jang HJ, Lim HK, Lee SJ, Lee WJ, Kim EY, Kim SH. Acute diverticulitis of the cecum and ascending colon: the value of thin-section helical CT findings in excluding colonic carcinoma. AJR Am J Roentgenol 2000;174:1397–1402

4. Rao PM, Rhea JT. Colonic diverticulitis: evaluation of the arrowhead sign and the inflamed diverticulum for CT diagnosis. Radiology 1998;209:775–779

5. Padidar AM, Jeffrey RB Jr, Mindelzun RE, Dolph JF. Differentiating sigmoid diverticulitis from carcinoma on CT scans: mesenteric inflammation suggests diverticulitis. AJR Am J Roentgenol 1994;163:81–83

102

Perforated Appendicitis

It is sometimes difficult to differentiate perforated from nonperforated appendicitis. Abscess and extraluminal air are the most specific findings for perforated appendicitis, but have low sensitivity. Periappendiceal inflammatory stranding and focal defect in the enhancing appendiceal wall are more sensitive, but less specific. Partial volume averaging is often misinterpreted as a focal defect in the appendiceal wall. The visualization of appendicoliths increases the probability of perforation. The presence of one or more appendicoliths in association with periappendiceal inflammation is highly suspicious for perforation.[1,2]

Findings Suggestive of Perforated Appendicitis[1,3–5]

- Extraluminal air
- Abscess
- Moderate or severe periappendiceal inflammatory stranding
- Focal defect in enhancing appendiceal wall
- Larger appendical diameter (mean 15 mm in perforated appendicitis)
- Phlegmon
- Terminal ileal thickening
- Extraluminal appendicolith
- Ileus

References

1. Foley TA, Earnest F, Nathan MA, Hough DM, Schiller HJ, Hoskin TL. Differentiation of nonperforated from perforated appendicitis: accuracy of CT diagnosis and relationship of CT to length of hospital stay. Radiology 2005;235:89–96
2. Pinto Leite N, Pereira JM, Cunha R, Pinto P, Sirlin C. CT evaluation of appendicitis and its complications: imaging techniques and key diagnostic findings. AJR Am J Roentgenol 2005;185:406–417
3. Horrow MM, White DS, Horrow JC. Differentiation of perforated from nonperforated appendicitis at CT. Radiology 2003;227:46–51
4. Oliak D, Sinow R, French S, Udani VM, Stamos MJ. Computed tomography scanning for the diagnosis of perforated appendicitis. Am Surg 1999;65:959–964
5. Bixby SD, Lucey BC, Soto JA, Theyson JM, Ozonoff A, Varghese JC. Perforated versus nonperforated acute appendicitis: accuracy of multidetector CT detection. Radiology 2006;241:780–786

103

Epiploic Appendagitis versus Omental Infarction

Epiploic appendices are small adipose protrusions from the serosal surface of the colon. The appendices can undergo torsion with resulting ischemia/infarction. Epiploic appendagitis can occur anywhere there is an epiploic appendage, but the majority (53%) of cases are in the sigmoid colon region. Epiploic appendagitis can mimic diverticulitis or appendicitis clinically, but can be differentiated from appendicitis and diverticulitis on computed tomography (CT), with characteristic findings of a 1- to 4-cm fat attenuation mass (often with a hyperattenuating rim), periappendiceal fat stranding, and thick-ened visceral peritoneal lining. A central area ("central dot") of high attenuation can be seen in slightly more than half of cases, possibly secondary to a thrombosed vein.[1] Omental infarction most commonly affects the right side, and is likely due to congenitally tenuous blood supply of the right omentum with subsequent torsion. Epiploic appendagitis and omental infarction are both forms of intraabdominal focal fat infarction, but can often be differentiated by imaging (**Table 103.1**). However, both entities have a benign course and can be treated conservatively.[2]

Table 103.1 Epiploic Appendagitis versus Omental Infarction[3,4]

	Epiploic Appendagitis	Omental Infarction
Age	Adults	15% in pediatric patients
Size	< 5 cm	Can be >5 cm
Location	Adjacent to sigmoid	Adjacent to cecum, ascending colon
Hyperattenuating Rim	+	−
Central Dot	+	−
Lobulated Appearance	+	−

References

1. Singh AK, Gervais DA, Hahn PF, Rhea J, Mueller PR. CT appearance of acute appendagitis. AJR Am J Roentgenol 2004;183:1303–1307
2. van Breda Vriesman AC. de Mol van Otterloo AJ, Puylaert JB. Epiploic appendagitis and omental infarction. Eur J Surg 2001;167:723–727
3. Singh AK, Gervais DA, Hahn PF, Sagar P, Mueller PR, Novelline RA. Acute epiploic appendagitis and its mimics. Radiographics 2005;25:1521–1534
4. Ng KS, Tan AG, Chen KK, Wong SK, Tan HM. CT features of primary epiploic appendagitis. Eur J Radiol 2006; 59:284–288

104

Solid Peritoneal Masses

Because the differential diagnosis of solid peritoneal masses is very broad, it is useful to divide the differential in masses that diffusely involve the peritoneal space and those that are confined to the mesentery.

Diffuse Peritoneal Masses

The most likely etiology is peritoneal carcinomatosis, most commonly from an ovarian, colon, or stomach primary site. This is often seen in conjunction with ascites. There are many other possible etiologies, which are rare and overlap in appearance.

Peritoneal Tuberculosis

Peritoneal tuberculosis can resemble peritoneal carcinomatosis. Certain imaging finding are helpful in differentiating tuberculous peritonitis from peritoneal carcinomatosis (**Table 104.1**).

Peritoneal Lymphomatosis

Peritoneal lymphomatosis is rare and usually cannot be distinguished from peritoneal carcinomatosis. Ascites with loculation or septation and a diffuse distribution of enlarged lymph nodes may suggest the diagnosis.[1]

Peritoneal Leiomyosarcomatosis

The gastrointestinal tract is the most common primary site in peritoneal dissemination of leiomyosarcomas, but other primary sites such as the mesentery, retroperitoneum, genitourinary tract and soft tissues are also possible. Features suggesting peritoneal leiomyosarcomatosis are necrosis, liver metastases, and minimal or absent ascites.[2]

Table 104.1 Peritoneal Carcinomatosis versus Tuberculous Peritonitis[13]

	Carcinomatosis	Tuberculosis
Irregular peritoneal infiltration	More common	Less common
Mesenteric Changes	Less common	More common
Macronodules >5 mm in diameter	Less common	More common
Low density center in masses[*]	Less common	More common
Calcification[†]	Less common	More common
Thin omental line covering infiltrated omentum	Less common	More common

[*] Can be seen in treated lymphoma, Burkitt's lymphoma, metastases, abscess, and Whipple's disease
[†] Can be seen in implants from ovarian serous adenocarcinoma

Peritoneal Amyloidosis

Peritoneal amyloidosis is a rare manifestation of systemic amyloidosis. Calcification and poor or absent enhancement of the amyloid deposits may be helpful in suggesting the diagnosis.[3]

Peritoneal Sarcoidosis

Peritoneal sarcoidosis is rare and usually presents with ascites.[4] However, ascites in the setting of sarcoidosis is more likely related to cardiac or hepatic disease rather than peritoneal involvement.[5]

Desmoplastic Small Round Cell Tumor

Desmoplastic small round cell tumor is an aggressive malignancy seen primarily in young adults or adolescents. There may be a male sex predilection. It should be considered when there are peritoneal masses with absence of an organ-based primary site. A large retrovesical mass is sometimes seen.[6] Hemorrhage, necrosis, and punctate calcifications in the masses can occasionally be seen.[7]

Serous Surface Papillary Carcinoma of the Peritoneum

Serous surface papillary carcinoma of the peritoneum occurs in postmenopausal women. It is histologically indistinguishable from ovarian serous papillary carcinoma, but does not involve the ovaries. It presents most commonly with ascites, omental caking, and peritoneal nodules.[8]

Solid Diffuse Peritoneal Disease[5]

- Peritoneal carcinomatosis
- Tuberculosis peritonitis
- Peritoneal mesothelioma
- Peritoneal lymphomatosis
- Peritoneal leiomyosarcomatosis
- Amyloidosis
- Sarcoidosis
- Desmoplastic small round cell tumor
- Serous surface papillary carcinoma of the peritoneum

Mesenteric Lesions

Although the diffuse peritoneal lesions discussed above can cause mesenteric masses, they are not typically confined to the mesentery. Masses centered in the mesentery have a different differential diagnosis. If a mesenteric lesion is spiculated, the differential diagnosis is usually carcinoid and sclerosing mesenteritis. Otherwise, lymphoma, metastases, sarcoma, desmoid, and gastrointestinal stromal tumor (GIST) are considerations. Several features are helpful for distinguishing these entities (**Table 104.2**).

Table 104.2 Features of Solid Mesenteric Masses[9–11,14]

	Lymphoma	Carcinoid	Sclerosing Mesenteritis	Desmoid	GIST	Sarcoma
Spiculated margin	−	+	+	−	−	−
Preservation of fat halo around vessels	−	−	+	−	−	−
Calcification	+ (Treated)	+	+	−	−	−
Adjacent bowel involvement	−	+	−	+	−	−
Bowel mass or wall thickening	−	+	−	−	−	−
Aneurysmal bowel dilatation	+	−	−	−	+	−
Necrosis, hemorrhage	−	−	−	−	+	+
Location in jejunal mesentery	−	−	+	−	−	−

Malignant Fibrous Histiocytoma

Malignant fibrous histiocytoma (MFH) is the most common sarcoma, but MFH would usually not be confined to the mesentery.

Mesenteric Fibromatosis

Mesenteric fibromatosis is the spectrum of deep fibromatoses, which include intraabdominal, abdominal wall, and extraabdominal fibromatoses. The most common site of an intraabdominal fibromatosis is the mesentery. Unlike abdominal wall fibromatoses which are most commonly seen in young women, mesenteric fibromatosis has no gender predilection and is seen in a wide range of ages. A minority of cases are associated with the Gardner syndrome variant of familial adenomatous polyposis (FAP). Most patients with FAP and mesenteric fibromatosis also have a history of abdominal surgery.[9]

Sclerosing Mesenteritis

Sclerosing mesenteritis is an idiopathic disorder in which varied degrees of fibrosis, fat necrosis, and inflammation are seen histologically. It is also known as retractile mesenteritis and mesenteric panniculitis (when acute inflammation and necrosis are present). Unlike mesenteric fibromatosis, it does not involve the muscularis propria of the bowel wall.[9] There is wide range in age of presentation with a male gender predilection. The appearance can vary from subtle increased attenuation in the mesenteric fat to a solid mass.[10]

Gastrointestinal Stromal Tumor

Gastrointestinal stromal tumors can present as a mesenteric mass if there is an exophytic mass from the bowel, or rarely, if there is a primary mesenteric GIST. Primary mesenteric GISTs are usually very large with extensive areas of low attenuation.[11]

Plexiform Neurofibroma

Plexiform neurofibromas of the mesentery are often of relatively low density on computed tomography (CT) and can mimic the adenopathy seen in lymphoma, tuberculosis, or Whipples disease. A characteristic feature on magnetic resonance imaging is a ring-like or septated fascicular pattern, which is not seen in adenopathy.[12]

Inflammatory Pseudotumor

Inflammatory pseudotumor most commonly occurs in the pediatric or young adult populations. It is more common in the lung and orbit.[9]

Extrapleural Solitary Fibrous Tumor

Extrapleural solitary fibrous tumors are tumors of mesothelial origin, which most commonly arise in the pleura. The mean age of presentation is 54 years and there is a slight male sex predilection.[9]

Solid Mesenteric Lesions[9]

- Lymphoma
- Metastases
- Sclerosing mesenteritis
- Carcinoid tumor
- Desmoid (mesenteric fibromatosis)
- Sarcoma
- Gastrointestinal stromal tumor (GIST)
- Neurofibromatosis
- Inflammatory pseudotumor
- Extrapleural solitary fibrous tumor

References

1. Kim Y, Cho O, Song S, Lee H, Rhim H, Koh B. Peritoneal lymphomatosis: CT findings. Abdom Imaging 1998; 23:87–90

2. Rha SE, Ha HK, Kim AY, et al. Peritoneal leiomyosarcomatosis originating from gastrointestinal leiomyosarcomas: CT features. Radiology 2003;227:385–390

3. Horger M, Vogel M, Brodoefel H, Schimmel H, Claussen C. Omental and peritoneal involvement in systemic amyloidosis: CT with pathologic correlation. AJR Am J Roentgenol 2006;186:1193–1195

4. Uthman IW, Bizri AR, Shabb NS, Khury MY, Khalifeh MJ. Peritoneal sarcoidosis: case report and review of the literature. Semin Arthritis Rheum 1999;28: 351–354

5. Pickhardt PJ, Bhalla S. Unusual nonneoplastic peritoneal and subperitoneal conditions: CT findings. Radiographics 2005;25:719–730

6. Bellah R, Suzuki–Bordalo L, Brecher E, Ginsberg JP, Maris J, Pawel BR. Desmoplastic small round cell tumor in the abdomen and pelvis: report of CT findings in 11 affected children and young adults. AJR Am J Roentgenol 2005;184:1910–1914

7. Pickhardt PJ, Fisher AJ, Balfe DM, Dehner LP, Huettner PC. Desmoplastic small round cell tumor of the abdomen: radiologic–histopathologic correlation. Radiology 1999;210:633–638

8. Morita H, Aoki J, Taketomi A, Sato N, Endo K. Serous surface papillary carcinoma of the peritoneum: clinical, radiologic, and pathologic findings in 11 patients. AJR Am J Roentgenol 2004;183:923–928

9. Levy AD, Rimola J, Mehrotra AK, Sobin LH. From the archives of the AFIP: benign fibrous tumors and tumorlike lesions of the mesentery: radiologic-pathologic correlation. Radiographics 2006;26: 245–264

10. Horton KM, Lawler LP, Fishman EK. CT findings in sclerosing mesenteritis (panniculitis): spectrum of disease. Radiographics 2003;23:1561–1567

11. Kim HC, Lee JM, Kim SH, et al. Primary gastrointestinal stromal tumors in the omentum and mesentery: CT findings and pathologic correlations. AJR Am J Roentgenol 2004;182:1463–1467

12. Levy AD, Patel N, Dow N, Abbott RM, Miettinen M, Sobin LH. From the archives of the AFIP: abdominal neoplasms in patients with neurofibromatosis type 1: radiologic-pathologic correlation. Radiographics 2005;25:455–480

13. Ha HK, Jung JI, Lee MS, et al. CT differentiation of tuberculous peritonitis and peritoneal carcinomatosis. AJR Am J Roentgenol 1996;167:743–748

14. Daskalogiannaki M, Voloudaki A, Prassopoulos P, et al. CT evaluation of mesenteric panniculitis: prevalence and associated diseases. AJR Am J Roentgenol 2000;174:427–431

105

Cystic Peritoneal and Retroperitoneal Masses

Cystic Peritoneal Masses

The differential diagnosis of cystic peritoneal masses is broad. Mesenteric, omental, and retroperitoneal cysts derive from the same embryologic structures. The term *mesenteric cyst* is often used to refer to cysts that do not connect to the retroperitoneum. Two frequent types of mesenteric cysts are of lymphatic and mesothelial origin. These differ in mode of presentation.

Lymphangiomas

Lymphangiomas predominate in boys. They can present with acute abdominal pain and often are attached to adjacent structures such as bowel. Unlike simple lymphatic cysts, they can be aggressive and recur if incompletely resected. They are more common in the mesentery in childhood and occur in the retroperitoneum during adulthood. Internal septations are usually present. The wall and the septations usually enhance. Lymphangiomas could be of similar density, less dense or more dense than fluid on computed tomography (CT). On magnetic resonance imaging (MRI), they are occasionally hyperintense on T1-weighted magnetic resonance images (T1WI) secondary to hemorrhage or fat.[1-3]

Mesothelial Cysts

Cysts of mesothelial origin are seen more commonly in young and middle-aged women, presenting with indolent symptoms. Mesothelial cysts differ from lymphangiomas in that they have no internal septations and are never hyperintense on T1WI.[3] Benign cystic mesothelioma (also known as peritoneal inclusion cyst) often arises from the pelvis, and is associated with a history of pelvic surgery, endometriosis, or pelvic inflammatory disease. It is not associated with asbestos exposure. Benign cystic mesothelioma is typically multiloculated in appearance. Unlike simple mesothelial cysts, they can be aggressive and recur if incompletely resected.[2,4]

Enteric Cysts

Peritoneal cysts can also be of enteric or urogenital origin. Enteric cysts have a thin wall lined with gastrointestinal mucosa; duplication cysts are thick-walled and contain all normal bowel wall layers.[2]

Urogenital Cysts

Urogenital cysts are derived from vestigial remnants of the Wolffian or Mullerian ducts. They are usually in the adnexal region. Mullerian cysts often occur in obese patients with menstrual irregularities.[2,4]

Etiology of Cystic Peritoneal Masses[2]

- Lymphatic origin: Simple lymphatic cyst, lymphangioma
- Nonpancreatic pseudocyst

- Enteric origin: Enteric duplication cyst, enteric cyst
- Mesothelial origin: Simple mesothelial cyst, benign cystic mesothelioma, malignant cystic mesothelioma
- Mucinous cystadenoma and cystadenocarcinoma: Ovarian or nonovarian
- Cystic teratoma: Ovarian or nonovarian
- Pseudomyxoma peritonei
- Urogenital cyst
- Hydatid cyst

Cystic Masses Containing Fat[5]

- Cystic teratoma
- Lymphangioma
- Lymphocele

Cystic Retroperitoneal Masses

The differential diagnosis of cystic retroperitoneal masses includes the entities in the differential diagnosis of cystic peritoneal masses with a few additional entities.

In the proper clinical setting, lymphoceles, urinomas, and hematomas should be considered. Bronchogenic cysts usually occur in the mediastinum, but can rarely occur in the retroperitoneum. Primary retroperitoneal cystic teratomas are seen mostly in female patients and often diagnosed in newborns. Rarely, primary mucinous cystadenomas can be seen in women with normal ovaries. Certain solid retroperitoneal

masses (paragangliomas and neurogenic tumors) can rarely appear cystic.[4] Leiomyosarcomas occurring in the retroperitoneum can have large areas of cystic degeneration.[6]

The differential diagnosis of cysts in the retrorectal space is more limited. Developmental cysts are most common and include epidermoid and dermoid cysts and enteric and neurenteric cysts. Developmental cysts are most commonly seen in middle-aged women.[7] Enteric cysts can either be tailgut cysts (retrorectal cystic hamartoma) or cystic rectal duplications. With the exception of dermoid cysts, these do not have a specific appearance. Enteric cysts can have malignant degeneration.

Differential Diagnosis of Cystic Retroperitoneal Masses[4]

- All the etiologies of cystic peritoneal masses
- Lymphocele
- Urinoma
- Hematoma
- Cystic degeneration of solid neoplasms
- Bronchogenic cysts

Cystic Retrorectal Masses[7]

- Epidermoid cyst
- Dermoid cyst
- Tailgut cyst
- Cystic rectal duplication
- Cystic sacrococcygeal teratoma
- Anterior sacral meningocele

References

1. Levy AD, Cantisani V, Miettinen M. Abdominal lymphangiomas: imaging features with pathologic correlation. AJR Am J Roentgenol 2004;182:1485–1491
2. de Perrot M, Brundler M, Totsch M, Mentha G, Morel P. Mesenteric cysts. Toward less confusion? Dig Surg 2000;17:323–328
3. Stoupis C, Ros PR, Abbitt PL, Burton SS, Gauger J. Bubbles in the belly: imaging of cystic mesenteric or omental masses. Radiographics 1994;14:729–737
4. Yang DM, Jung DH, Kim H, et al. Retroperitoneal cystic masses: CT, clinical, and pathologic findings and literature review. Radiographics 2004;24:1353–1365
5. Yoo E, Kim MJ, Kim KW, Chung JJ, Kim SH, Choi JY. A case of mesenteric cystic lymphangioma: fat saturation

and chemical shift MR imaging. J Magn Reson Imaging 2006;23:77–80
6. Nishino M, Hayakawa K, Minami M, Yamamoto A, Ueda H, Takasu K. Primary retroperitoneal neoplasms: CT and MR imaging findings with anatomic and pathologic diagnostic clues. Radiographics 2003;23: 45–57
7. Dahan H, Arrive L, Wendum D. Docou le Pointe H, Djouhri H, Tubiana JM. Retrorectal developmental cysts in adults: clinical and radiologic-histopathologic review, differential diagnosis, and treatment. Radiographics 2001;21:575–584

106

Peritoneal Calcification

Peritoneal calcification could be metastatic or dystrophic in etiology. Metastatic calcification may secondary to a systemic imbalance (e.g., hyperparathyroidism); dystrophic calcification may be secondary to etiologies such as malignancy or local trauma.[1]

Types of Peritoneal Calcification[1]

- Common
  - Peritoneal dialysis
  - Prior peritonitis
  - Malignancy: Primary and secondary
- Rare
  - Meconium peritonitis
  - Peritoneal tuberculosis
  - Hyperparathyroidism
  - Postsurgical heterotopic ossification
  - Pneumocystis carinii infection
  - Amyloidosis

Benign versus Malignant Peritoneal Calcification[1]

- Benign calcification: Sheetlike appearance
- Malignant calcification: Associated nodal calcification

References

1. Agarwal A, Yeh BM, Breiman RS, Qayyum A, Coakley FV. Peritoneal calcification: causes and distinguishing features on CT. AJR Am J Roentgenol 2004;182: 441–445

107

Retroperitoneal Fibrosis

In cases of potential retroperitoneal fibrosis, it may be difficult to differentiate between confluent retroperitoneal adenopathy (e.g., from lymphoma) and retroperitoneal fibrosis. It may also be difficult to differentiate idiopathic retroperitoneal fibrosis and fibrosis secondary to small retroperitoneal metastatic implants. Other diseases that can mimic retroperitoneal fibrosis are fibromatosis involving the retroperitoneum (usually associated with Gardner's syndrome) and inflammatory pseudotumor, which is usually seen in children.[1]

Retroperitoneal Adenopathy versus Idiopathic Fibrosis

Retroperitoneal adenopathy is usually easily distinguished by its lobular contour. Substantial elevation of aorta from the spine is seen with adenopathy and not idiopathic fibrosis,[2] although a mild degree of aortic elevation has been reported with idiopathic fibrosis.[3]

Idiopathic Fibrosis versus Malignant Retroperitoneal Fibrosis

Malignant retroperitoneal fibrosis may displace the aorta anteriorly and the ureters laterally, whereas idiopathic fibrosis usually displaces the ureters medially and does not displace the aorta.[1] Malignant idiopathic retroperitoneal fibrosis has heterogeneous high T2-weighted signal on magnetic resonance imaging (T2WI) with ill-defined margins. Idiopathic retroperitoneal fibrosis has homogeneous low T2WI signal with well-defined margins.[4]

References

1. Vaglio A, Salvarani C, Buzio C, et al. Retroperitoneal fibrosis. Lancet 2006;367:241–251
2. Degesys GE, Dunnick NR, Silverman PM, Cohan RH, Illescas FF, Castagno A. Retroperitoneal fibrosis: use of CT in distinguishing among possible causes. AJR Am J Roentgenol 1986;146:57–60
3. Brooks AP, Reznek RH, Webb JA. Aortic displacement on computed tomography of idiopathic retroperitoneal fibrosis. Clin Radiol 1989;40:51–52
4. Arrive L, Hricak H, Tavares NJ, Miller TR. Malignant verus nonmalignant retroperitoneal fibrosis: differentiation with MR imaging. Radiology 1989;172:139–143

V Pelvis

108

The Differential Diagnosis of Leiomyomas

Leiomyomas are sometimes difficult to differentiate from ovarian lesions (see Chapter 112), or other uterine abnormalities such as leiomyosarcomas or adenomyomas.

Leiomyoma versus Adenomyoma

Differentiation of leiomyoma and adenomyoma (**Table 108.1**) is important as leiomyomas can be treated with a myomectomy, but adenomyomas require a hysterectomy. Submucosal leiomyomas in particular may be difficult to differentiate from adenomyoma.

Leiomyoma versus Leiomyosarcoma

Leiomyomas and leiomyosarcomas usually cannot be differentiated unless metastases are present, but the features that are suggestive of leiomyosarcoma are featured below.

Features of Leiomyosarcomas[1–3]

- Ill-defined, irregular margins
- >50% high signal on T2-weighted magnetic resonance imaging (MRI)
- High signal intensity areas on T1-weighted MRI
- Contrast-enhanced characteristics
  - Small well-defined non-enhanced areas
  - Early contrast enhancement (at 1 min)

Table 108.1 Leiomyoma versus Adenomyoma[4, 5]

	Leiomyoma	Adenomyoma
Poorly defined border	–	+
Minimal mass effect relative to size of lesion	–	+
Configuration paralleling the endometrium	rounded	Elliptical
Irregular endometrial interface with lesion	–	±
Dilated vessels at myometrial interface	+	–
Areas of high T2WI signal intensity	Prominent in large lesions	Sparse
Hyperintense linear striations radiating from the endometrium to the myometrium	–	+

Abbreviations: T2WI, T2-weighted magnetic resonance imaging.

References

1. Goto A, Takeuchi S, Sugimura K, Maruo T. Usefulness of Gd-DTPA contrast-enhanced dynamic MRI and serum determination of LDH and its isozymes in the differential diagnosis of leiomyosarcoma from degenerated leiomyoma of the uterus. Int J Gynecol Cancer 2002;12:354–361
2. Tanaka YO, Nishida M, Tsunoda H, Okamoto Y, Yoshikawa H. Smooth muscle tumors of uncertain malignant potential and leiomyosarcomas of the uterus: MR findings. J Magn Reson Imaging 2004;20:998–1007
3. Schwartz LB, Zawin M, Carcangiu ML, Lange R, McCarthy S. Does pelvic magnetic resonance imaging differentiate among the histologic subtypes of uterine leiomyomata? Fertil Steril 1998;70:580–587
4. Reinhold C, Tafazoli F, Mehio A, Wang L, Atri M, Siegelman ES, Rohoman L. Uterine adenomyosis: endovaginal US and MR imaging features with histopathologic correlation. Radiographics 1999;19:S147–S160
5. Togashi K, Ozasa H, Konishi I, et al. Enlarged uterus: differentiation between adenomyosis and leiomyoma with MR imaging. Radiology 1989;171:531–534

109

Uterine Sarcomas

Uterine sarcomas constitute 1 to 3% of malignant uterine tumors. The most common sarcomas are mixed mullerian sarcoma (also known as carcinosarcoma), leiomyosarcomas, and endometrial stromal sarcomas. Mixed mullerian tumors (MMT) are the most common (40 to 70%) followed by leiomyosarcoma (40 to 50%). Endometrial stromal sarcomas (ESS) are more rare (10%).[1] Low-grade endometrial stromal sarcomas usually are seen in a younger age group (premenopausal) than mixed mullerian sarcomas or high-grade endometrial stromal sarcomas (postmenopausal).[2,3]

Imaging features can be helpful in distinguishing the uterine sarcomas from each other as well as from other lesions such as endometrial carcinoma, leiomyoma (see Chapter 108), and adenomyosis.

1. Leiomyosarcomas tend to present as large myometrial masses.
2. MMT and ESS present as invasive endometrial masses.[1]

Features of Endometrial Stromal Sarcoma

- Presents as endometrial thickening or polypoid mass with extensive myometrial involvement
- Bands of low T2-weighted magnetic resonance imaging (T2WI) signal intensity in the area of myometrial invasion.
- Contiguous extension of lesion along fallopian tubes, uterine ligaments and ovaries. IV leiomyomatosis can also have this pattern of spread.

Differential Diagnosis of Endometrial Stromal Sarcoma

Endometrial Stromal Sarcomas versus Endometrial Carcinoma

Unlike endometrial carcinoma with myometrial invasion, the myometrial component usually predominates in ESS. ESS usually presents as a larger mass, with more irregular margins. There are often nodular lesions at the tumor margin, and nodular intramyometrial extension. In addition, ESS usually enhances more than the myometrium, which is a rare finding in endometrial carcinoma.[4]

Endometrial Stromal Sarcomas versus Leiomyoma

Leiomyomas with endometrial involvement could potentially mimic ESS, but ESS usually has infiltrative margins in contrast to the well-defined margin of a leiomyoma.

Endometrial Stromal Sarcomas versus Adenomyosis

Although adenomyosis may have poorly defined margins like ESS, adenomyosis is hypointense on T2WI unlike ESS, which is hyperintense.

Features of Mixed Mullerian Tumors

Mixed mullerian tumors are usually nonspecific in appearance. They usually present as endometrial masses invading the myometrium. Clues to the diagnosis include the large size of the mass and rapid growth of metastatic disease (usually local, lymphatic, and intraperitoneal).[5,6]

References

1. Sahdev A, Sohaib SA, Jacobs I, Shepherd JH, Oram DH, Reznek RH. MR imaging of uterine sarcomas. AJR Am J Roentgenol 2001;177:1307–1311
2. Koyama T, Togashi K, Konishi I, et al. MR imaging of endometrial stromal sarcoma: correlation with pathologic findings. AJR Am J Roentgenol 1999;173:767–772
3. Takeuchi M, Matsuzaki K, Uehara H, Yoshida S, Nishitani H, Shimazu H. Pathologies of the uterine endometrial cavity: usual and unusual manifestations and pitfalls on magnetic resonance imaging. Eur Radiol 2005;15: 2244–2255
4. Ueda M, Otsuka M, Hatakenaka M, et al. MR imaging findings of uterine endometrial stromal sarcoma: differentiation from endometrial carcinoma. Eur Radiol 2001;11:28–33
5. Shapeero LG, Hricak H. Mixed mullerian sarcoma of the uterus: MR imaging findings. AJR Am J Roentgenol 1989;153:317–319
6. Smith T, Moy L, Runowicz C. Mullerian mixed tumors: CT characteristics with clinical and pathologic observations. AJR Am J Roentgenol 1997;169: 531–535

110

Endometrial Carcinoma versus Polyp

Endometrial polyps and endometrial carcinoma are both causes of endometrial thickening. There are several features on magnetic resonance imaging (MRI) that favor endometrial polyp over carcinoma, but these are not accurate enough to obviate biopsy. Endometrial polyps and endometrial carcinoma do not differ in enhancement characteristics.[1]

Features of Endometrial Polyp on Magnetic Resonance Imaging[1]

- Central fibrous core (low T2-weighted MRI signal)
- Intratumoral cysts
- Lack of myometrial invasion

References

1. Grasel RP, Outwater EK, Siegelman ES, Capuzzi D, Parker L, Hussain SM. Endometrial polyps: MR imaging features and distinction from endometrial carcinoma. Radiology 2000;214:47–52

111

Septate versus Bicornuate Uterus

A septate uterus is the most common mullerian duct abnormality and is associated with the poorest reproductive outcomes. It is important to differentiate a septate from bicornuate uterus as a septate uterus is often treated with hysteroscopic resection of the septum, whereas a bicornuate uterus usually does not require surgery.[1]

Several imaging findings can be seen in a bicornuate uterus, but not a septate uterus. The fundal cleft in the external uterine contour is the most useful finding to differentiate a bicornuate from septate uterus. Tissue separating the horns is identical to myometrium in signal intensity in a bicornuate uterus. However, the septum in a septate uterus can also have myometrial signal intensity. In a septate uterus, the fundal portion of the septum has myometrial signal intensity, but a complete septum (extending to cervical os) has low T2-weighted magnetic resonance imaging signal (fibrous tissue) in the mid and inferior portions. A partial septum will more likely have myometrial signal intensity throughout the septum.[1] The intercornual distance may not be as useful as a fundal cleft for distinguishing a bicornuate from septate uterus, as the intercornual distance in a septate uterus can be increased if a leiomyoma or adenomyosis involves the septum.[1]

Features of Bicornuate Uterus

- Fundal cleft >1 cm in depth
- Intercornual distance >4 cm
- Tissue separating the horns is myometrial signal intensity (can be seen in partial septate uterus)

References

1. Troiano RN, McCarthy SM. Mullerian duct anomalies: imaging and clinical issues. Radiology 2004;233:19–34

112

Ovarian versus Uterine Origin of a Pelvic Mass

It is sometimes difficult to determine whether a pelvic mass is of uterine or ovarian origin.

Findings Suggestive of Ovarian Origin

An ovarian origin is highly likely if the suspensory ligament[1] or ovarian vein[2] can be tracked to the mass. The gonadal veins often course along the lateral and dorsal border of an ovarian mass, with the branches wrapping around the mass. With uterine masses, the gonadal veins often show abrupt interruption at the lateral margin of the mass.[3]

Findings Suggestive of Uterine Origin

Uterine subserosal leiomyomas usually have vessels between the uterus and leiomyoma that are rarely seen in extrauterine tumors.[4] In addition, leiomyomas occasionally have a high T2-weighted magnetic resonance imaging signal intensity rim.[5]

References

1. Saksouk FA, Johnson SC. Recognition of the ovaries and ovarian origin of pelvic masses with CT. Radiographics 2004;24:S133–S146
2. Lee JH, Jeong YK, Park JK, Hwang JC. "Ovarian vascular pedicle" sign revealing organ of origin of a pelvic mass lesion on helical CT. AJR Am J Roentgenol 2003;181: 131–137
3. Asayama Y, Yoshimitsu K, Aibe H, et al. MDCT of the gonadal veins in females with large pelvic masses: value in differentiating ovarian versus uterine origin. AJR Am J Roentgenol 2006;186:440–448
4. Kim SH, Sim JS, Seong CK. Interface vessels on color-power Doppler US and MRI: a clue to differentiate subserosal uterine myomas from extrauterine tumors. J Comput Assist Tomogr 2001;25:36–42
5. Mittl RL Jr, Yeh IT, Kressel HY. High-signal-intensity rim surrounding uterine leiomyomas on MR images: pathologic correlation. Radiology 1991;180:81–83

113

Benign versus Malignant Ovarian Mass

Features of Malignancy

The findings most predictive of malignancy in an ovarian lesion studied with contrast-enhanced magnetic resonance imaging (MRI) are[1,2]

- Necrosis in a solid lesion
- Vegetations in a cystic lesion
- Ascites

Borderline versus Stage I Neoplasms

Borderline malignant ovarian neoplasms cannot be reliably distinguished from Stage I early invasive neoplasms by computed tomography (CT) or MRI. However, invasive stage I tumors tend to have thicker septations and size of solid components.[3] Septations >3 mm in thickness are more worrisome for malignancy.[4]

Primary versus Secondary Ovarian Neoplasm

It is difficult to distinguish primary ovarian neoplasm from secondary neoplasm. Multilocularity detected by MRI imaging favors the diagnosis of primary ovarian malignancy.[5]

References

1. Hricak H, Chen M, Coakley FV, et al. Complex adnexal masses: detection and characterization with MR imaging – multivariate analysis. Radiology 2000;214: 39–46
2. Sohaib SA, Sahdev A, Van Trappen P, Jacobs IJ, Reznek RH. Characterization of adenexal masses on MR imaging. AJR Am J Roentgenol 2003;180:1297–1304
3. deSouza NM, O'Neill R, McIndoe GA, Dina R, Soutter WP. Borderline tumors of the ovary: CT and MRI features and tumor markers in differentiation from stage I disease. AJR Am J Roentgenol 2005;184:999–1003
4. Imaoka I, Wada A, Kaji Y, et al. Developing a MR imaging strategy for diagnosis of ovarian masses. Radiographics 2006;26:1431–1448
5. Brown DL, Zou KH, Tempany CM, et al. Primary versus secondary ovarian malignancy: imaging findings of adnexal masses in the Radiology Diagnostic Oncology Group Study. Radiology 2001;219:213–218

Ovarian Lesions with Hyperintensity on T1-Weighted Magnetic Resonance Imaging

The differential diagnosis of ovarian lesions with hyperintensity on T1-weighted magnetic resonance imaging (T1WI) is limited. Teratomas are the only lesions that have T1WI hyperintensity secondary to fat and are easily differentiated with fat-saturated images. Endometriomas are sometimes difficult to differentiate from hemorrhagic cysts. Certain imaging features may be helpful (**Table 114.1**). The types of T1WI hyperintense ovarian lesions include[1]

- Teratoma
- Endometrioma
- Hemorrhagic cyst
- Hemorrhagic neoplasm
- Mucinous lesions: Rare, in high viscosity lesions

Table 114.1 Features of Endometrioma versus Hemorrhagic Cyst[1–3]

	Endometrioma	Hemorrhagic cyst
T1WI	Hyperintense – Diffuse	Hyperintense – Diffuse or peripheral
T2WI	Hypointense	Hyperintense
Number	Multiple, bilateral	Single
Associated Findings	Cul-de-sac lesions	None
	Dilated fallopian tubes with high T1WI	
	Adhesion to surrounding organs	
Wall Thickness	Thicker, hypointense on T2WI	Thin
Follow-up	Persist	Regress

Abbreviations: T1WI, T1-weighted magnetic resonance imaging; T2WI, T2-weighted magnetic resonance imaging.

References

1. Siegelman ES, Outwater EK. Tissue characterization in the female pelvis by means of MR imaging. Radiology 1999;212:5–18
2. Jeong YY, Outwater EK, Kang HK. Imaging evaluation of ovarian masses. Radiographics 2000;20:1445–1470
3. Imaoka I, Wada A, Kaji Y, et al. Developing a MR imaging strategy for diagnosis of ovarian masses. Radiographics 2006;26:1431–1448

115

Ovarian Lesions with Hypointensity on T2-Weighted Magnetic Resonance Imaging

Low T2-weighted signal on magnetic resonance imaging (T2WI) in a solid ovarian lesion is usually secondary to fibrous tissue or blood products. It is usually a sign of benignity. The exception is a Krukenberg tumor. Bilaterality and prominent enhancement would suggest a Krukenberg tumor.[1] Endometriomas are characteristically hypointense on T2. Other ovarian lesions that are hypointense on T2WI are Brenner tumors, fibromas, and fibrothecomas, and cystadenofibromas.

A Brenner tumor is a benign transitional cell tumor. Brenner tumors are associated with an epithelial ovarian neoplasm (often mucinous cystadenoma) of the ipsilateral or contralateral ovary in 30% of cases. The Brenner tumor appears as a solid nodule. Cystic components are rare; when cysts are seen, they are likely related to the associated cystadenomas. Calcification is common.[1,2]

Fibromas, fibrothecomas, and thecomas are subtypes of sex-cord stromal tumors, with fibromas being the most common. There is a spectrum extending from lipid-rich thecomas with estrogenic activity and little fibrosis to fibromas with no theca cells. Thecomas are unlikely to have areas of T2WI hypointensity. Fibromas may present with Meigs syndrome (ascites and pleural effusions). Calcifications can be seen.[3]

Cystadenofibromas are not related to fibromas. Cystadenofibromas have an epithelial component unlike fibromas. These lesions appear as multilocular cystic masses with a solid fibrotic component.[4]

Ovarian Lesions with Hypointensity on T2-Weighted Magnetic Resonance Imaging[2,5]

- Endometrioma
- Brenner tumor
- Fibroma
- Fibrothecoma
- Cystadenofibroma
- Krukenberg tumor

References

1. Togashi K. MR imaging of the ovaries: normal appearance and benign disease. Radiol Clin North Am 2003; 41:799–811
2. Siegelman ES, Outwater EK. Tissue characterization in the female pelvis by means of MR imaging. Radiology 1999;212:5–18
3. Sala EJ, Atri M. Magnetic resonance imaging of benign adnexal disease. Top Magn Reson Imaging 2003;14: 305–327
4. Jeong YY, Outwater EK, Kang HK. Imaging evaluation of ovarian masses. Radiographics 2000;20:1445–1470
5. Ha HK, Baek SY, Kim SH, Kim HH, Chung EC, Yeon KM. Krukenberg's tumor of the ovary: MR imaging features. AJR Am J Roentgenol 1995;164:1435–1439

116

Periurethral and Vaginal Cysts

Periurethral cysts could be related to the urethra or vagina. Vaginal cysts, although they can occur near the urethral region, can usually be differentiated from other periurethral cysts such as urethral diverticula. This distinction is necessary for differential diagnosis.

Vaginal Cysts

Vaginal cysts should be distinguishable from other periurethral cysts because they arise from the vagina. Mesonephric (e.g., Gartner's duct) cysts are usually vaginal and Bartholin's cysts are vulvar. Epidermal inclusion cysts could be vaginal or vulvar in location.[1] Vaginal cysts can be divided into four types:[2]

1. Epidermal inclusion cysts: These are lined by stratified squamous epithelium and are located in the lower lateral or posterior vaginal wall and related to prior surgery or trauma (e.g., episiotomy repair).
2. Gartner's duct cysts: These are of mesonephric origin and are usually located in the anterolateral vaginal wall following the route of the mesonephric duct.
3. Mullerian cysts: These are of mullerian origin and are not grossly distinguishable from Gartner's duct cysts.
4. Bartholin's cysts: These arise from Bartholin's glands, which are located at the posterolateral vaginal introitus. These glands secrete lubricating mucus during sexual arousal. Bartholin's cysts are at or below the level of the symphysis pubis. This differentiates them from Gartner's duct cysts, which are above the level of the inferior symphysis pubis.[3]

Other Periurethral Cysts

A periurethral cyst not arising from the vagina could represent a urethral diverticulum, submucosal urethral cyst, or Skene's gland cyst or abscess. A urethral diverticulum communicates with the urethra; however this may not be identified in all cases. If a communication cannot be identified, the cyst could represent a submucosal cyst or diverticulum. Skene's glands are also known as the lesser vestibular or paraurethral glands and are homologous to the male prostate. Skene's gland cysts or abscesses can be identified by their location just lateral to the external urethral meatus.[3]

Types of Periurethral and Vaginal Cysts[1–3]

- Vaginal
- Epidermal inclusion cyst
- Gartner's duct cyst
- Mullerian cyst
- Bartholin's cyst
- Periurethral
- Urethral diverticulum
- Submucosal urethral cyst
- Skene's gland cyst or abscess

References

1. Moulopoulos LA, Varma DG, Charnsangavej C, Wallace S. Magnetic resonance imaging and computed tomography appearance of asymptomatic paravaginal cysts. Clin Imaging 1993;17:126–132
2. Prasad SR, Menias CO, Narra VR, et al. Cross-sectional imaging of the female urethra: technique and results. Radiographics 2005;25:749–761
3. Hahn WY, Israel GM, Lee VS. MRI of female urethral and periurethral disorders. AJR Am J Roentgenol 2004;182: 677–682

117

Prostatic Cysts

The differential diagnosis of prostatic cysts can be approached by first considering whether the cyst is midline or lateral in location. Midline cysts include utricle, mullerian duct, ejaculatory duct, and vas deferens cysts.

Midline Prostatic Cysts

Utricle Cysts

Utricle cysts (**Table 117.1**) are the most common congenital cysts and are usually diagnosed in childhood due to the association with genitourinary abnormalities such as hypospadias and cryptorchidism. Utricle cysts are due to dilatation of the prostatic utricle, a potential space that drains into the prostatic urethra at the level of the verumontanum.

Mullerian Duct Cysts

Mullerian duct cysts (**Table 117.1**) arise from remnants of the Mullerian duct. They are typically larger than utricle cysts and extend above the prostate, potentially presenting as a pelvic mass. There is no association with external genitalia abnormalities, although there is a rare association with renal agenesis. If aspirated, neither type of cyst contains sperm. Carcinoma is a rare complication in both types of cysts.

Paramedian Cysts

Paramedian cysts located close to the midline include ejaculatory duct and vas deferens cysts. Unlike Mullerian duct and utricle cysts, these cysts contain spermatozoa. If large they can be difficult to distinguish from Mullerian duct and utricle cysts. Ejaculatory duct cysts are usually

Table 117.1 Mullerian versus Utricle Cysts[1,3]

	Mullerian Duct Cysts	Utricle Cysts
Size	Large	<10 mm
Location	Extend cephalad to prostate	Do not extend above prostate
	Usually midline, rarely could be slightly lateral	Always midline
Age	3rd and 4th decades	1st and 2nd decades
Associations	Renal agenesis (rare)	Hypospadias, cryptorchidism, renal agenesis
Urethral communication	No	Yes
Calcification	Possible	No

acquired, resulting from obstruction. They may contain calculi. Ejaculatory duct and vas deferens cysts can be distinguished by their location. Ejaculatory duct cysts are intraprostatic, seen along the course of the ejaculatory duct. They are lateral to the midline at the prostatic base and midline at the verumontanum level. Vas deferens cysts are supraprostatic.[1]

Types of Midline Prostatic Cysts[1,2]

- Prostatic utricle cyst
- Mullerian duct cyst
- Cystadenoma

- Simple cyst
- Ejaculatory duct cyst
- Vas deferens cyst
- Transurethral resection of prostate (TURP) defect

Types of Lateral Prostatic Cysts[1]

- Benign prostatic hyperplasia with cystic degeneration
- Retention cyst
- Abscess
- Seminal vesicle cyst

References

1. Nghiem HT, Kellman GM, Sanberg SA, Craig BM. Cystic lesions of the prostate. Radiographics 1990;10:635–650
2. Yasumoto R, Kawano M, Tsujino T, Shindow K, Nishisaka N, Kishimoto T. Is a cystic lesion located at the midline of the prostate a mullerian duct cyst? Analysis of aspirated fluid and histopathological study of the cyst wall. Eur Urol 1997;31:187–189
3. McDermott VG, Meakam TJ, Stolpen AH, Schnall MD. Prostatic and periprostatic cysts: findings on MR imaging. AJR Am J Roentgenol 1995;164:123–127

VI   Musculoskeletal

118

Bone Lesions with Low Hypointensity on T2-Weighted Magnetic Resonance Imaging

Numerous bone lesions can have hypointense areas on T2-weighted magnetic resonance imaging (T2WI) secondary to sclerosis, calcification, or fibrosis. Primary lymphoma of bone is sometimes hypointense on T2WI.[1]

Most lesions that are hypointense on T2WI are sclerotic. Less commonly, osteolytic lesions can have foci of low T2WI signal. A rare tumor that demonstrates this finding is desmoplastic fibroma, which is the osseus counterpart of soft tissue fibromatoses. It is most commonly seen in the third and fourth decades of life and may have a slight male predominance. The most common sites are the mandible, pelvis, and femur, with a predilection for the metaphyses.[2]

Osteolytic Bone Lesions with Low Signal Intensity on T2-Weighted Magnetic Resonance Imaging[1-6]

- Fibrous dysplasia
- Giant-cell tumor
- Lymphoma
- Leiomyosarcoma
- Hemophilic pseudotumor
- Desmoplastic fibroma (desmoid tumor of bone)

References

1. White LM, Schweitzer ME, Khalili K, Howarth DJ, Wunder JS, Bell RS. MR imaging of primary lymphoma of bone: variability of T2-weighted signal intensity. AJR Am J Roentgenol 1998;170:1243–1247
2. Frick MA, Sundaram M, Unni KK, et al. Imaging findings in desmoplastic fibroma of bone: distinctive T2 characteristics. AJR Am J Roentgenol 2005;184:1762–1767
3. Sundaram M, Akduman I, White LM, McDonald DJ, Kandel R, Janney C. Primary leiomyosarcoma of bone. AJR Am J Roentgenol 1999;172:771–776
4. Park JS, Ryu KN. Hemophilic pseudotumor involving the musculoskeletal system: spectrum of radiologic findings. AJR Am J Roentgenol 2004;183:55–61
5. Norris MA, Kaplan PA, Pathria M, Greenway G. Fibrous dysplasia: magnetic resonance imaging appearance at 1.5 tesla. Clin Imaging 1990;14:211–215
6. Aoki J, Tanikawa H, Ishii K, et al. MR findings indicative of hemosiderin in giant-cell tumor of bone: frequency, cause, and diagnostic significance. AJR Am J Roentgenol 1996;166:145–148

119

Benign Bone Lesions with Surrounding Edema

Marrow and soft tissue edema is often seen in malignant bone lesions. However, marrow and soft tissue edema can sometimes be seen surrounding the following benign bone lesions:[1,2]

- Chondroblastoma
- Osteoid osteoma
- Osteoblastoma
- Brodie's abscess
- Eosinophilic granuloma

References

1. Kroon HM, Bloem JL, Holscher HC, et al. MR imaging of edema accompanying benign and malignant bone tumors. Skeletal Radiol 1994;23:261–269

2. Beltran J, Aparisi F, Bonmati LM, et al. Eosinophilic granuloma: MRI manifestations. Skeletal Radiol 1993; 22:157–161

120

Bone Lesions with Fluid-Fluid Levels

The finding of fluid-fluid levels in a bone lesion has been most frequently described in aneurysmal bone cysts, but is a nonspecific finding usually related to prior hemorrhage. The finding is seen in both benign and malignant lesions, but the greater the proportion of the lesion containing fluid-fluid levels, the more likely the lesion is benign.[1]

Types of Bone Lesions with Fluid-Fluid Levels[1–8]

- Aneurysmal bone cyst
- Telangiectatic osteosarcoma
- Classic osteosarcoma
- Chondroblastoma
- Giant cell tumor
- Fibrous dysplasia
- Simple bone cyst
- Malignant fibrous histiocytoma of bone
- Fibrosarcoma
- Metastasis
- Plasmacytoma
- Ossifying fibroma
- Brown tumor
- Osteoblastoma
- Clear cell chondrosarcoma
- Langerhans cell histiocytosis
- Intraosseous ganglion
- Intraosseous lipoma

References

1. O'Donnell P, Saifuddin A. The prevalence and diagnostic significance of fluid-fluid levels in focal lesions of bone. Skeletal Radiol 2004;33:330–336
2. Ishida T, Yamamoto M, Goto T, Kawano H, Yamamoto A, Machinami R. Clear cell chondrosarcoma of the pelvis in a skeletally immature patient. Skeletal Radiol 1999;28:290–293
3. Davies AM, Evans N, Mangham DC, Grimer RJ. MR imaging of brown tumour with fluid-fluid levels: a report of three cases. Eur Radiol 2001;11:1445–1449
4. Kickuth R, Laufer U, Pannek J, Adamietz IA, Liermann D, Adams S. Magnetic resonance imaging of bone marrow metastasis with fluid-fluid levels from small cell neuroendocrine carcinoma of the urinary bladder. Magn Reson Imaging 2002;20:691–694
5. Kendi AT, Kara S, Altinok D, Keskil S. Sinonasal ossifying fibroma with fluid-fluid levels on MR images. AJNR Am J Neuroradiol 2003;24:1639–1641
6. Harter SB, Nokes SR. Plasmacytoma of the sacrum: fluid-fluid levels on MR images. AJR Am J Roentgenol 1995;165:741–742
7. Hindman BW, Thomas RD, Young LW, Yu L. Langerhans cell histiocytosis: unusual skeletal manifestations observed in thirty-four cases. Skeletal Radiol 1998;27:177–181
8. Vilanova JC, Dolz JL, Maestro de Leon JL, Aparicio A, Aldoma J, Capdevila A. MR imaging of a malignant schwannoma and an osteoblastoma with fluid-fluid levels. Report of two new cases. Eur Radiol 1998;8:1359–1362

121

Enchondroma versus Chondrosarcoma

Enchondromas and low-grade chondrosarcomas may be difficult to differentiate by imaging (**Table 121.1**). The presence of pain related to the lesion is helpful as almost all chondrosarcoma patients present with pain. However, enchondromas can be seen as an incidental finding on imaging in patients with musculoskeletal pain from other etiologies. Location is very helpful as chondroid lesions in the axial skeleton are highly likely to be malignant and lesions in the hands and feet are unlikely to be malignant. Usually, lesions in the long tubular bones are difficult to differentiate.[1]

Table 121.1 Features of Enchondroma versus Chondrosarcoma[2–5]

	Enchondroma	Chondrosarcoma
Size > 5 cm	−	+
Deep endosteal scalloping ($> {}^2/_3$ cortical thickness)	−	+
Extensive endosteal scalloping (associated with entire length of lesion)	−	+
Cortical destruction	−	+
Soft tissue mass	−	+
Perilesional edema	−	+
Early and exponential enhancement*	−	+

* Enchondromas may have delayed enhancement

References

1. Flemming DJ, Murphey MD. Enchondroma and chondrosarcoma. Semin Musculoskelet Radiol 2000;4:59–71
2. Geirnaerdt MJ, Hogendoorn PC, Bloem JL, Taminiau AH, van der Woude HJ. Cartilaginous tumors: fast contrast-enhanced MR imaging. Radiology 2000;214:539–546
3. Murphey MD, Flemming DJ, Boyea SR, Bojescul JA, Sweet DE, Temple HT. Enchondroma versus chondrosarcoma in the appendicular skeleton: differentiating features. Radiographics 1998;18:1213–1237
4. Geirnaerdt MJ, Hermans J, Bloem JL, et al. Usefulness of radiography in differentiating enchondroma from central grade 1 chondrosarcoma. AJR Am J Roentgenol 1997;169:1097–1104
5. Janzen L, Logan PM, O'Connell JX, Connell DG, Munk PL. Intramedullary chondroid tumors of bone: correlation of abnormal peritumoral marrow and soft-tissue MRI signal with tumor type. Skeletal Radiol 1997;26:100–106

122

Osteochondroma versus Chondrosarcoma

Malignant transformation to chondrosarcoma is seen in 1% of patients with solitary osteochondromas and 3 to 5% of patients with hereditary multiple exostoses.[1] Osteochondromas that grow or cause pain after skeletal maturity should be suspected of malignant degeneration.

Features that can be used to diagnose malignant degeneration by computed tomography (CT) or magnetic resonance imaging (MRI) in a skeletally mature patient are thickness of the cartilage cap and enhancement.

1. Cartilage cap thickness: Cartilage cap thickness >1.5 cm is worrisome for malignancy.[1]
2. Enhancement: Early (≤10 s) and exponential enhancement is seen in chondrosarcoma. Osteochondromas in skeletally mature patients will not show early enhancement, but some will have delayed enhancement and all will enhance in the equilibrium phase.[2]

Note that these criteria differ in a skeletally immature patient. In a skeletally immature patient, the cartilage cap can be expected to be thicker normally due to continued growth and physeal vessels in unfused growth plates may cause early enhancement.[2] Thus, in a skeletally immature patient, the enhancement pattern cannot be used to differentiate osteochondroma from chondrosarcoma, and cartilage cap thickness >3 cm should be used instead of 1.5 cm as a criterion for malignancy. However, malignant degeneration of osteochondromas in skeletally immature patients is very rare.

References

1. Murphey MD, Choi JJ, Kransdorf MJ, Flemming DJ, Gannon FH. Imaging of osteochondroma: variants and complications with radiologic-pathologic correlation. Radiographics 2000;20:1407–1437

2. Geirnaerdt MJ, Hogendoorn PC, Bloem JL, Taminiau AH, van der Woude HJ. Cartilaginous tumors: fast contrast-enhanced MR imaging. Radiology 2000;214: 539–546

123

Malignant versus Benign Soft Tissue Lesions

Magnetic resonance imaging (MRI) may be helpful in differentiating benign from malignant soft tissue lesions, although there is conflicting evidence in the literature. In published prospective studies, the sensitivity ranges from 78 to 100%, and the specificity from 17 to 89%.[1]

Specific diagnoses are sometimes possible based on signal intensity (lipoma, fibrous lesions), or signal intensity and lack of enhancement (cyst, ganglion). Vascular lesions such as soft tissue hemangiomas (lobulation, septation, and low-signal intensity dots)[2] can often be definitively diagnosed.

Note that, unlike malignant bone tumors, malignant soft tissue masses may have well-defined margins; thus, lesion margins are usually not a helpful differentiating factor.[3] In particular, synovial sarcomas are often small with well-defined margins.[4]

Characteristics of Malignant Soft Tissue Masses[1,3,5]

- Size > 5 cm
- Deep location
- Heterogeneous T1-weighted MRI (T1WI) signal intensity
- High T2-weighted MRI (T2WI) signal intensity
- Increased T2WI signal in surrounding muscle: Only useful in patients who have not had previous surgery or radiation, and when there is no suspicion of an inflammatory mass.[6]
- Earlier onset of enhancement
- Early enhancement followed by plateau or washout
- Higher maximum enhancement
- Greater rate of enhancement
- Peripheral or inhomogeneous enhancement
- Necrosis
- Intralesional hemorrhage
- Bone involvement
- Neurovascular involvement

References

1. Gielen JL, De Schepper AM, Vanhoenacker F, et. al. Accuracy of MRI in characterization of soft tissue tumors and tumor-like lesions. A prospective study in 548 patients. Eur Radiol 2004;14:2320–2330
2. Teo EL, Strouse PJ, Hernandez RJ. MR imaging differentiation of soft-tissue hemangiomas from malignant soft-tissue masses. AJR Am J Roentgenol 2000;174:1623–1628
3. Kransdorf MJ, Murphey MD. Radiologic evaluation of soft-tissue masses: a current perspective. AJR Am J Roentgenol 2000;175:575–587
4. Ma LD, McCarthy EF, Bluemke DA, Frassica FJ. Differentiation of benign from malignant musculoskeletal lesions using MR imaging: pitfalls in MR evaluation of lesions with a cystic appearance. AJR Am J Roentgenol 1998;170:1251–1258
5. van Rijswijk CS, Geirnaerdt MJ, Hogendoorn PC, et. al. Soft-tissue tumors: value of static and dynamic gadopentetate dimeglumine-enhanced MR imaging in prediction of malignancy. Radiology 2004;233:493–502
6. Beltran J, Simon DC, Katz W, Weis LD. Increased MR signal intensity in skeletal muscle adjacent to malignant tumors: pathologic correlation and clinical relevance. Radiology 1987;162:251–255

124

Cystic-Appearing Soft Tissue Masses

Noncystic or partially cystic soft tissue masses can occasionally mimic true cystic lesions such as synovial cysts, bursa, or ganglia. If this is suspected, contrast can be given to determine whether the lesion is truly cystic.

The most common lesions that need to be differentiated from cysts are nerve sheath tumors and intramuscular myxomas. Both of these lesions can have homogeneous high T2-weighted magnetic resonance imaging (T2WI) signal comparable to fluid. Contrast can easily differentiate these lesions from cysts. Nerve sheath tumors may have a specific morphologic appearance (see Chapter 127). Myxomas are intramuscular (as opposed to the intermuscular location of most cysts), and often have a thin surrounding rim of fat.[1]

Malignant lesions with cystic or cystic-appearing areas can usually be differentiated from completely cystic lesions by their heterogeneity.

Differential Diagnosis of Cystic-Appearing Soft Tissue Masses[2]

- Nerve sheath tumor
- Intramuscular myxoma
- Metastases
- Myxoid malignancy
- Synovial sarcoma
- Chondrosarcoma

References

1. Murphey MD, McRae GA, Fanburg-Smith JC, Temple HT, Levine AM, Aboulafia AJ. Imaging of soft-tissue myxoma with emphasis on CT and MR and comparison of radiologic and pathologic findings. Radiology 2002;225:215–224

2. Ma LD, McCarthy EF, Bluemke DA, Frassica FJ. Differentiation of benign from malignant musculoskeletal lesions using MR imaging: pitfalls in MR evaluation of lesions with a cystic appearance. AJR Am J Roentgenol 1998;170:1251–1258

125

Soft Tissue Lesions with Fluid-Fluid Levels

In soft tissue lesions, a fluid-fluid level is a nonspecific finding usually related to prior hemorrhage. Soft tissue hematomas can have fluid-fluid levels. A rare lesion containing fluid-fluid levels is angiomatoid fibrous histiocytoma,[1] which is a low-grade neoplasm affecting children and young adults. This is usually superficial, and most common in the extremities followed by the trunk.

Differential Diagnosis of Soft Tissue Lesions with Fluid-Fluid Levels[1-6]

- Cavernous hemangioma
- Synovial sarcoma
- Hematoma
- Malignant fibrous histiocytoma
- Schwannoma
- Myositis ossificans
- Synovial hemangioma
- Angiomatoid fibrous histiocytoma

References

1. Li CS, Chan WP, Chen WT, et al. MRI of angiomatoid fibrous histiocytoma. Skeletal Radiol 2004;33:604–608
2. Mendez JC, Saucedo G, Melendez B. Cystic trigeminal schwannoma with fluid-fluid levels. Eur Radiol 2004;14:1941–1943
3. Hatano H, Morita T, Kobayashi H, Ito T, Segawa H. MR imaging findings of an unusual case of myositis ossificans presenting as a progressive mass with features of fluid-fluid level. J Orthop Sci 2004;9:399–403
4. Tsai JC, Dalinka MK, Fallon MD, Zlatkin MB, Kressel HY. Fluid-fluid level: a nonspecific finding in tumors of bone and soft tissue. Radiology 1990;175: 779–782
5. Greenspan A, Azouz EM, Matthews J, Decarie JC. Synovial hemangioma: imaging features in eight histologically proven cases, review of the literature, and differential diagnosis. Skeletal Radiol 1995;24: 583–590
6. Keenan S, Bui-Mansfield LT. Musculoskeletal lesions with fluid-fluid level: a pictorial essay. J Comput Assist Tomogr 2006;30(3):517–524

126

Lipoma versus Liposarcoma

Magnetic resonance imaging (MRI) is useful in distinguishing simple lipomas from liposarcomas (**Table 126.1**). MRI is very specific in diagnosing simple lipomas. However, many lesions thought to represent well-differentiated liposarcoma are benign lipoma variants such as necrotic lipoma and chondroid lipoma.[1]

Table 126.1 Differentiating Features between Lipoma and Liposarcoma[1–4]

	Lipoma	Liposarcoma
Homogeneous fat signal	+	−
Completely irregular margins (interdigitation with surrounding muscle)	+	−
Older patients	±	+
Male sex predilection	−	+
Thickened or nodular septa	−	+
Associated nonadipose mass-like areas	−	+
Calcification	Less common	More common
Size >10 cm	−	+
< 75% Fat	−	+
Septal enhancement	±	+
Prominent foci of high T2WI signal	−	+

Abbreviations: T2WI, T2-weighted magnetic resonance imaging.

References

1. Gaskin CM, Helms CA. Lipomas, lipoma variants, and well-differentiated liposarcomas (atypical lipomas): results of MRI evaluations of 126 consecutive fatty masses. AJR Am J Roentgenol 2004;182: 733–739
2. Kransdorf MJ, Bancroft LW, Peterson JJ, Murphey MD, Foster WC, Temple HT. Imaging of fatty tumors: distinction of lipoma and well-differentiated liposarcoma. Radiology 2002;224:99–104
3. Ohguri T, Aoki T, Hisaoka M, et al. Differential diagnosis of benign peripheral lipoma from well-differentiated liposarcoma on MR imaging: is comparison of margins and internal characteristics useful? AJR Am J Roentgenol 2003;180:1689–1694
4. Murphey MD, Carroll JF, Flemming DJ, Pope TL, Gannon FH, Kransdorf MJ. From the archives of the AFIP: benign musculoskeletal lipomatous lesions. Radiographics 2004;24:1433–1466

127

Nerve Sheath Tumors

Neurofibroma versus Schwannoma

Neurofibromas and schwannomas often cannot be differentiated by imaging. The features listed in **Table 127.1** can be helpful in differentiating between these two nerve sheath tumors. The most accurate differentiating signs are the target sign, pattern of enhancement, fascicular appearance, and a hyperintense rim.[1]

Benign versus Malignant Nerve Sheath Tumors

It is usually not possible to differentiate benign from malignant nerve sheath tumors. The following findings suggest malignancy:[2]

• Heterogeneity
• Infiltrative margins
• Prominent enhancement
• Rapid growth
• Large size (>5 cm)

Table 127.1 Differentiating Features between Schwannomas and Neurofibromas[1,3,4]

	Schwannoma	Neurofibroma
Relation to nerve	Eccentric	Central
Heterogeneity*	+	−
Target sign**	−	+
Central enhancement	−	+
Diffuse enhancement	+	−
Fascicular appearance	+	−
Thin T2WI hyperintense rim	+	−

Abbreviations: T2WI, T2-weighted magnetic resonance imaging.

* Secondary to degeneration, cystic change

** The target sign consists of a peripheral hyperintensity and central hypointensity on T2WI

References

1. Jee WH, Oh SN, McCauley T, et al. Extraaxial neurofibromas versus neurilemmomas: discrimination with MRI. AJR Am J Roentgenol 2004;183:629–633
2. Murphey MD, Smith WS, Smith SE, Kransdorf MJ, Temple HT. From the archives of the AFIP: Imaging of musculoskeletal neurogenic tumors: radiologic-pathologic correlation. Radiographics 1999;19:1253–1280
3. Cerofolini E, Landi A, DeSantis G, Maiorana A, Canossi G, Romagnoli R. MR of benign peripheral nerve sheath tumors. J Comput Assist Tomogr 1991;15:593–597
4. Lin J, Martel W. Cross-sectional imaging of peripheral nerve sheath tumors: characteristic signs on CT, MR imaging, and sonography. AJR Am J Roentgenol 2001;176:75–82

128

Osteomyelitis versus Neuropathic Arthropathy in the Diabetic Foot

Differentiation of osteomyelitis and neuropathic arthropathy in the diabetic foot is difficult by imaging. Nevertheless, several imaging features are helpful in differential diagnosis (**Table 128.1**). The location of the abnormality is often the most useful differentiating feature.

Table 128.1 Differentiating Features between Osteomyelitis and Neuropathic Arthropathy in the Diabetic Foot[1–3]

	Osteomyelitis	Neuropathic Arthropathy
Location	Pressure points Bony prominences*	Midfoot†
Multiple joints	+	−
Ulceration	+	−
Cellulitis (replacement of soft tissue fat)	+	−
Sinus tract	+	−
Subchondral cysts	−	+
Marrow signal abnormality	More extensive	Less extensive
Soft tissue fluid collections	+	−
Thick rim enhancement of soft tissue fluid collection	+	−
Diffuse joint fluid enhancement	+	−
Joint erosion	+	−
Intraarticular loose bodies	−	+

* Metatarsal heads, interphalangeal joints, calcaneus, malleoli

† The cuboid is the only bone in the midfoot commonly involved with osteomyelitis.

References

1. Chatha DS, Cunningham PM, Schweitzer ME. MR imaging of the diabetic foot: diagnostic challenges. Radiol Clin North Am 2005;43:747–757
2. Gil HC, Morrison WB. MR imaging of diabetic foot infection. Semin Musculoskelet Radiol 2004;8:189–198
3. Ahmadi ME, Morrison WB, Carrino JA, et al. Neuropathic arthropathy of the foot with and without superimposed osteomyelitis: MR imaging characteristics. Radiology 2006;238:622–631

129

Subchondral Bone Marrow Edema

The differential diagnosis of subchondral bone marrow edema is broad, but can be narrowed with clinical history and associated findings. Potential trauma or infection can be evaluated by history and a tumor should have an associated focal lesion. After these have been excluded, a cartilage defect or diffuse cartilage thinning associated with the abnormal bone marrow signal should be sought for as osteoarthritis is a common cause of abnormal subchondral signal. Tendon abnormalities (e.g., epicondylitis) often result in abnormal signal in the subjacent bone, although this is usually not subchondral in location.

Subchondral Insufficiency Fracture versus Osteonecrosis with Subchondral Fracture

If a subchondral fracture is seen the differential diagnosis in the knee is subchondral insufficiency fracture versus spontaneous osteonecrosis of the knee (SONK) and a subchondral insufficiency fracture versus subchondral fracture associated with osteonecrosis in the hip. Several imaging findings are helpful in differentiating these entities.

1. Articular surface involvement: The subchondral fracture associated with osteonecrosis is adjacent to the articular surface and may be associated with a contour deformity, whereas a subchondral fracture associated with

insufficiency fracture is at some distance from the articular surface.[1] However, mechanical etiologies of osteonecrosis (such as SONK) may have accompanying subchondral insufficiency fractures. The size of the subchondral abnormality is also helpful in determining reversibility. Subchondral lesions thicker than 4 mm and longer than 12.5 mm in the hip and 14 mm in the knee are associated with osteonecrosis.[2,3]

2. Fracture signal: Although the fracture lines in both osteonecrosis and insufficiency fractures can be hypointense on T2-weighted magnetic resonance images (T2WI), the fracture line in osteonecrosis can sometimes be hyperintense on T2WI, particularly in the hip.[1,4]

3. Marrow edema: In the hip, there is little surrounding T2WI hyperintense edema around a subchondral fracture from osteonecrosis, as the bone is mostly necrotic at this stage. A subchondral insufficiency fracture will usually have a substantial amount of surrounding T2WI hyperintense edema.[5]

Early Osteonecrosis versus Transient Osteoporosis

Early osteonecrosis can have bone marrow edema without a geographic or subchondral abnormality and resemble transient osteoporosis. Transient osteoporosis usually presents in pregnant women in the third trimester and in middle-aged men, without risk factors for osteonecrosis.

The pattern of bone marrow edema in the hip can differ. Osteonecrosis usually has more limited edema, sometimes confined to the femoral head. Transient osteoporosis usually has more extensive edema, extending into the femoral neck and intertrochanteric region. The edema in transient osteoporosis may have a straight lateral margin. In approximately one out of five cases, the bone marrow edema in transient osteoporosis will spare the subchondral region.[6]

Differential Diagnosis of Subchondral Bone Marrow Edema

- Osteoarthritis
- Microfracture or macrofracture: traumatic
- Subchondral stress or insufficiency fracture
- Stress reaction
- Early avascular necrosis: hip
- Spontaneous osteonecrosis of the knee
- Transient osteoporosis
- Reflex sympathetic dystrophy
- Infection
- Tumor
- Tendon abnormalities (usually not subchondral)

References

1. Lecouvet FE, Malghem J, Maldague BE, Vande Berg BC. MR imaging of epiphyseal lesions of the knee: current concepts, challenges, and controversies. Radiol Clin North Am 2005;43:655–672
2. Vande Berg BC, Malghem JJ, Lecouvet FE, Jamart J, Maldague BE. Idiopathic bone marrow edema lesions of the femoral head: predictive value of MR imaging findings. Radiology 1999;212:527–535
3. Lecouvet FE, van de Berg BC, Maldague BE, et al. Early irreversible osteonecrosis versus transient lesions of the femoral condyles: prognostic value of subchondral bone and marrow changes on MR imaging. AJR Am J Roentgenol 1998;170:71–77
4. Stevens K, Tao C, Lee SU, et al. Subchondral fractures in osteonecrosis of the femoral head: comparison of radiography, CT, and MR imaging. AJR Am J Roentgenol 2003;180:363–368
5. Watson RM, Roach NA, Dalinka MK. Avascular necrosis and bone marrow edema syndrome. Radiol Clin North Am 2004;42:207–219
6. Malizos KN, Zibis AH, Dailiana Z, Hantes M, Karachalios T, Karantanas AH. MR imaging findings in transient osteoporosis of the hip. Eur J Radiol 2004; 50:238–244

130

Synovial Chondromatosis versus Rice Bodies

Loose bodies from synovial chondromatosis may sometimes be difficult to differentiate[1] from rice bodies. Rice bodies are most commonly seen in rheumatoid arthritis. They are of unknown etiology, but could be related to synovial microinfarction and shedding.

The loose bodies in synovial chondromatosis will vary in signal intensity depending upon their composition. Nonmineralized loose bodies will be intermediate to slightly high in signal intensity on T1-weighted magnetic resonance images (T1WI) and high in signal intensity on T2-weighted magnetic resonance images (T1WI). Calcified bodies will be low in signal intensity on both T1WI and T2WI. Ossified bodies will have the signal characteristics of bone.

Rice bodies are smaller and more uniform in size than the loose bodies in chondromatosis. Rice bodies tend to be lower in signal intensity than nonmineralized loose bodies in chondromatosis on both T1WI and T2WI. Thus, rice bodies will be difficult to visualize on T1WI and more easily seen on T2WI, whereas nonmineralized loose bodies in chondromatosis may be easier to see on T1WI and harder to see on T2WI (they may be similar in intensity to fluid on T2WI).[1,2]

Erosions can be seen in conjunction with both loose bodies and synovial osteochondromatosis, but the erosions in synovial osteochondromatosis are typically larger and more sharply defined.

References

1. Morrison JL, Kaplan PA. Water on the knee: cysts, bursae, and recesses. Magn Reson Imaging Clin N Am 2000;8:349–370

2. Chen A, Wong LY, Sheu CY, Chen BF. Distinguishing multiple rice body formation in chronic subacromial-subdeltoid bursitis from synovial chondromatosis. Skeletal Radiol 2002;31:119–121

131

Hypointense Synovium on T2-Weighted Magnetic Resonance Imaging

Causes of intraarticular hypointensity on T2-weighted magnetic resonance imaging (T2WI) can be divided into diffuse and focal manifestations. Of the diffuse manifestations, amyloid and fibrous pannus do not have a paramagnetic effect on gradient echo images, which is helpful in distinguishing these etiologies from those with T2WI hypointensity secondary to bleeding and hemosiderin deposition. Paramagnetic effect in gouty tophi is variable, depending on whether there is hemosiderin deposition in the tophus.[1]

A cause of focal intraarticular T2WI hypointensity is localized nodular synovitis. Localized nodular synovitis is similar histologically to pigmented villonodular synovitis (PVNS), but has a different clinical presentation and response to treatment. It can be treated by simple excision and does not typically recur, whereas PVNS requires extensive synovectomy. The most common location is the infrapatellar fat pad. Compared with PVNS, it involves a smaller portion of synovium, has smooth margin, has less hemosiderin, and is not associated with a hemorrhagic effusion.[2]

Another cause of focal intraarticular T2 hypointensity is the cyclops lesion. The cyclops lesion is a focal arthrofibrosis in Hoffa's fat pad near the tibial insertion of a reconstructed anterior cruciate ligament.

Differential Diagnoses Related to Diffuse Intraarticular Hypointensity on T2-Weighted Magnetic Resonance Imaging[3,4]

- Pigmented villonodular synovitis
- Hemophilic arthropathy
- Siderotic synovitis: secondary to chronic hemarthrosis
- Chronic rheumatoid arthritis: secondary to fibrous pannus
- Synovial osteochondromatosis: if the loose bodies are calcified they are usually hypointense on T2WI
- Gout
- Amyloid arthropathy

Differential Diagnoses Related to Focal Intraarticular Hypointensity on T2-Weighted Magnetic Resonance Imaging

- Localized nodular synovitis
- Cyclops lesion

References

1. Gentili A. Advanced imaging of gout. Semin Musculoskelet Radiol 2003;7:165–167
2. Huang GS, Lee CH, Chan WP, Chen CY, Yu JS, Resnick D. Localized nodular synovitis of the knee: MR imaging appearance and clinical correlated in 21 patients. AJR Am J Roentgenol 2003;181:539–543
3. Narvaez JA, Narvaez J, Ortega R, De Lama E, Roca Y, Vidal N. Hypointense synovial lesions on T2-weighted images: differential diagnosis with pathologic correlation. AJR Am J Roentgenol 2003;181:761–769
4. Sheldon PJ, Forrester DM, Learch TJ. Imaging of intraarticular masses. Radiographics 2005;25:105–119

132

Increased Meniscal Signal Not Related to Tear

Meniscal signal not related to tear is usually secondary to degeneration. In addition, there are numerous interpretive pitfalls related to normal variants, which have been well described.[1] A common artifact is the magic angle effect on intermediate and T1-weighted magnetic resonance images (T1WI). This usually involves the posterior horn lateral meniscus, is ill-defined, does not extend to an articular surface, and is not seen on T2-weighted magnetic resonance images (T2WI).

Less common causes of increased meniscal signal not related to a tear are

- Meniscal cysts
- Meniscal ossicles
- Chondrocalcinosis
- Meniscal contusion
- Meniscal vascularity
- Postoperative meniscus

Meniscal Cysts

Meniscal cysts are associated with a meniscal tear. An intrasubstance meniscal cyst is usually less intense than fluid on T2WI. It resembles intrasubstance degeneration, but the meniscus is swollen.[2]

Meniscal Ossicles

On magnetic resonance imaging (MRI), a meniscal ossicle should not be confused with a tear as an ossicle is rounded and has bone signal intensity (high on T1WI and low on T2WI).[3]

Chondrocalcinosis

Radiographic correlation is necessary to diagnose chondrocalcinosis. It is difficult to differentiate from a tear based on MRI alone. Chondrocalcinosis tends to be less linear than a tear. Unlike the majority of meniscal tears, chondrocalcinosis is also hyperintense on T2WI and short T1-weighted inversion time (STIR) images.[4]

Meniscal Contusion

A meniscal contusion manifests as high signal intensity extending to an articular surface, but unlike a tear the signal is amorphous. There are usually adjacent bone contusions and often an anterior cruciate ligament tear.[5]

Meniscal Vascularity

High signal intensity not related to a tear is more prevalent in children (seen in 60% under age 13). This may be related to meniscal vascularity and is most prevalent in the posterior horn medial meniscus. Meniscal high signal intensity in children that equivocally extends to an articular surface usually does not represent a tear, although unequivocal articular surface extension does indicate a tear.[6]

Postoperative Meniscus

Meniscal tears that have been treated conservatively or with surgical repair will continue to show increased signal on T1WI and proton density weighted images for an indeterminate period.[7] The presence of increased T2WI signal or gadolinium is necessary to diagnose a recurrent tear or a tear that has not healed. Note that the signal intensity of gadolinium in a tear may be slightly less intense than that of the gadolinium in the joint space.[8]

Intrameniscal signal that does not extend to an articular surface preoperatively may appear to extend to an articular surface after partial meniscectomy and thus mimic a meniscal tear.

Differential Diagnoses Related to Increased Meniscal Signal Not Secondary to Tear[1-8]

- Degeneration
- Normal variant
- Artifact
- Intrasubstance meniscal cyst
- Chondrocalcinosis
- Meniscal ossicle
- Meniscal contusion
- Meniscal vascularity
- Postoperative meniscus

References

1. Rubin DA, Paletta GA Jr. Current concepts and controversies in meniscal imaging. Magn Reson Imaging Clin N Am 2000;8:243–270
2. Helms CA. The meniscus: recent advances in MR imaging of the knee. AJR Am J Roentgenol 2002;179:1115–1122
3. Schnarkowski P, Tirman PF, Fuchigami KD, Crues JV, Butler MG, Genant HK. Meniscal ossicle: radiographic and MR imaging findings. Radiology 1995;196:47–50
4. Kaushik S, Erickson JK, Palmer WE, Winalski CS, Kilpatrick SJ, Weissman BN. Effect of chondrocalcinosis on the MR imaging of knee menisci. AJR Am J Roentgenol 2001;177:905–909
5. Cothran RL Jr, Major NM, Helms CA, Higgins LD. MR imaging of meniscal contusion in the knee. AJR Am J Roentgenol 2001;177:1189–1192
6. Takeda Y, Ikata T, Yoshida S, Takai H, Kashiwaguchi S. MRI high-signal intensity in the menisci of asymptomatic children. J Bone Joint Surg Br 1998;80:463–467
7. Totty WG, Matava MJ. Imaging the postoperative meniscus. Magn Reson Imaging Clin N Am 2000;8:271–283
8. De Smet AA, Horak DM, Davis KW, Choi JJ. Intensity of signal contacting meniscal surface in recurrent tears on MR arthrography compared to that of contrast material. AJR Am J Roentgenol 2006;187:W565–8

133

Meniscal Tear without Signal Extending to the Articular Surface

The majority of meniscal tears are associated with increased signal extending to an articular surface on magnetic resonance imaging (MRI). However, some tears can be associated with meniscal signal not extending to an articular surface.

A grade 2C signal refers to an extensive central wedge-shaped meniscal signal that does not extend to an articular surface. If symptoms can be traced to the site of the grade 2C signal, there will be a meniscal tear in ~50% of cases.[1]

A meniscal tear should be diagnosed if a discrete meniscal signal is seen associated with a parameniscal cyst, even if the signal does not extend to an articular surface.

Intrasubstance signal in a lateral discoid meniscus is more clinically significant than the same finding in a nondiscoid meniscus. This finding can be associated with symptomatic intrasubstance tears.[2]

Differential Diagnoses Related to Meniscal Tears without Signal Extending to the Articular Surface[1,2]

- Grade 2C intrasubstance signal
- Discoid meniscus intrasubstance signal
- Parameniscal cyst

References

1. McCauley TR, Jee WH, Galloway MT, Lynch K, Jokl P. Grade 2C signal in the meniscus on MR imaging of the knee. AJR Am J Roentgenol 2002;179:645–648

2. Ryu KN, Kim IS, Kim EJ, et al. MR imaging of tears of discoid lateral menisci. AJR Am J Roentgenol 1998;171:963–967

134

Absent Bow-Tie Sign

The body of the meniscus resembles a bow tie on sagittal magnetic resonance imaging (MRI). As the body of the meniscus averages 9 to 12 mm in width, on a sequential sagittal MRI done with 4 to 5 mm slice thickness, two bow ties should be seen in both the medial and lateral menisci.[1] The absent bow-tie sign refers to the visualization of less than two bow ties. The most common cause of the absent bow-tie sign is a bucket handle meniscal tear, but other etiologies are possible.

Another type of tear that can result in an absent bow-tie sign is a radial tear. There is no displaced fragment in a radial tear. In a radial tear the gap in the bow tie is small. A bucket handle tear will result in a larger gap in the bow tie. The free edge is truncated in a radial tear, which distinguishes it from partial volume averaging.

Differential Diagnoses Related to Absent Bow Tie Sign[1]

- Bucket handle meniscal tear
- Osteoarthritis
- Small menisci (children, small adults)
- Radial tears
- Prior meniscectomy

References

1. Helms CA, Laorr A, Cannon WD Jr. The absent bow tie sign in bucket-handle tears of the menisci in the knee. AJR Am J Roentgenol 1998;170:57–61

135

Meniscal Extrusion

Meniscal extrusion refers to the extension of the meniscus beyond the tibial margin. A significant degree of extrusion has been defined as >25% of meniscal width and >3 mm.[1,2] The medial meniscus may be more prone to extrusion as it is more firmly attached to the joint capsule (by the deep medial collateral ligament) than the lateral meniscus, and thus would sublux when the medial capsule is displaced by an effusion or osteophyte.[3] Absence of the meniscofemoral ligament(s) is associated with lateral meniscal extrusion when a lateral meniscal root tear occurs.[4] Meniscal extrusion has been associated with numerous abnormalities

Findings Associated with Meniscal Extrusion[1-6]

- Osteoarthritis
- Meniscal tear (large radial tear, extensive tear, complex tear, tear involving meniscal root)
- Meniscal degeneration–severe
- Joint effusion (usually in athletes)
- Anterior cruciate ligament insufficiency (usually in athletes)
- Normal variant: Related to anterior insertion of the anterior horn

References

1. Costa CR, Morrison WB, Carrino JA. Medial meniscus extrusion on knee MRI: is extent associated with severity of degeneration or type of tear? AJR Am J Roentgenol 2004;183:17–23
2. Miller TT, Staron RB, Feldman F, Cepel E. Meniscal position on routine MR imaging of the knee. Skeletal Radiol 1997;26:424–427
3. Rennie WJ, Finlay DB. Meniscal extrusion in young athletes: associated knee joint abnormalities. AJR Am J Roentgenol 2006;186:791–794
4. Brody JM, Lin HM, Hulstyn MJ, Tung GA. Lateral meniscus root tear and meniscus extrusion with anterior cruciate ligament tear. Radiology 2006;239:805–810
5. Gale DR, Chaisson CE, Totterman SM, Schwartz RK, Gale ME, Felson D. Meniscal subluxation: association with osteoarthritis and joint space narrowing. Osteoarthritis Cartilage 1999;7:526–532
6. Puig L, Monllau JC, Corrales M, Pelfort X, Melendo E, Caceres E. Factors affecting meniscal extrusion: correlation with MRI, clinical, and arthroscopic findings. Knee Surg Sports Traumatol Arthrosc 2006;14:394–398

Medial Fluid Collections around the Knee

The numerous etiologies of medial fluid collections around the knee can be initially differentiated by the location relative to the joint line and the medial collateral ligament bursa.[1,2]

The Joint Line

A Baker's cyst is superior to the joint line and fluid in the pes anserinus bursa is inferior to the joint line. Ganglion cysts are variable in location. The remaining fluid collections are centered at the joint line.

The Medial Collateral Ligament (MCL Bursa)

If a collection is at the level of the joint line, the next question is the location relative to the MCL bursa. The MCL itself can be involved with tears or bursitis. Semimembranous-tibial collateral ligament bursal fluid is posterior to the MCL and comma-shaped. Meniscocapsular separation and meniscal cysts are usually posterior to the MCL bursa, involving the region of the posterior horn medial meniscus.

Fluid Collections Outside the Medial Collateral Ligament Bursa

The fluid collections outside the MCL bursa are usually easily diagnosed. The following features are helpful for differentiating the fluid collections near or involving the MCL bursa:

- *MCL bursitis* In contrast to a MCL tear, the deep layer of the MCL is intact in bursitis.
- *MCL tear* A complete tear is easily diagnosed. Occasionally a partial tear of the deep layer can result in fluid deep to the intact superficial MCL layer, mimicking MCL bursitis.[2] Increased signal involving the deep MCL layer can differentiate this from MCL bursitis.
- *Meniscal cyst* A meniscal cyst is associated with a meniscal tear. It is usually posterior to the MCL bursa at the level of the posterior meniscus. Although meniscocapsular separation also occurs at this level, the signal intensity in meniscocapsular separation is usually ill defined.
- *Meniscocapsular separation* Meniscocapsular separation usually results in a more ill-defined signal than the entities above. In addition, there can be associated findings including meniscal displacement, meniscal corner tears, irregular meniscal outline, and extension to the meniscal fascicles.[3]

Differential Diagnosis Related to Medial Fluid Collections around the Knee

- Baker's (popliteal) cyst
- Ganglion cyst
- Medial (tibial) collateral ligament bursitis
- Pes anserinus bursitis
- Semimembranosus-tibial collateral ligament bursitis
- Meniscal cyst
- Medial collateral ligament tear
- Meniscocapsular separation

References

1. De Maeseneer M, Shahabpour M, Van Roy F, et al. MR imaging of medial collateral ligament bursa: findings in patients and anatomic data derived from cadavers. AJR Am J Roentgenol 2001;177:911–917
2. Morrison JL, Kaplan PA. Water on the knee: cysts, bursae, and recesses. Magn Reson Imaging Clin N Am 2000;8:349–370
3. De Maeseneer M, Shahabpour M, Vanderdood K, Van Roy F, Osteaux M. Medial meniscocapsular separation: MR imaging criteria and diagnostic pitfalls. Eur J Radiol 2002;41(3):242–252

137

Fluid Collections around the Posterior Cruciate Ligament

Fluid collections behind the posterior cruciate ligament (PCL) are often ganglion cysts. However, there are two other fluid collections that can mimic a PCL ganglion cyst: a pericruciate meniscal cyst (related to a posterior horn medial meniscus tear) and fluid in the PCL recess.[1,2]

Features of a Pericruciate Meniscal Cyst[2]

- Communicates with tear of posterior horn medial meniscus
- Centered on PCL: a ganglion cyst is usually at the femoral or tibial PCL insertion
- May surround PCL

Features of a Posterior Cruciate Ligament Recess

The PCL recess is a common recess posterior to the PCL. This does not usually contain fluid unless there is a substantial amount of fluid in the joint. The following features are seen with fluid in the PCL recess:[1]

- Communicates with medial joint compartment
- Absence of joint capsule around recess
- Lack of contact with proximal one third of PCL
- Intimate contact with posterior meniscofemoral ligament (ligament of Wrisberg): the ligament is at the posterosuperior aspect of the PCL recess

Differential Diagnosis Related to Fluid Collections around the Posterior Cruciate Ligament[1,2]

- Ganglion cyst
- Pericruciate meniscal cyst
- Posterior cruciate ligament recess fluid

References

1. de Abreu MR, Kim HJ, Chung CB, et al. Posterior cruciate ligament recess and normal posterior capsular insertional anatomy: MR imaging of cadaveric knees. Radiology 2005;236:968–973
2. Lektrakul N, Skaf A, Yeh L, et al. Pericruciate meniscal cysts arising from tears of the posterior horn of the medial meniscus: MR imaging features that simulate posterior cruciate ganglion cysts. AJR Am J Roentgenol 1999;172:1575–1579

138

Increased Signal in the Rotator Cuff Not Related to Full-Thickness Tear

There are numerous etiologies of increased signal in the rotator cuff on magnetic resonance imaging (MRI) not related to a full-thickness tear.

Increased signal (isointense to muscle) can be seen in the supraspinatus tendon in asymptomatic individuals on short echo time (TE) images. On long TE images, this signal resolves or remains isointense to muscle. This can be distinguished by its characteristic location and appearance. It occurs 5–10 mm proximal to the greater tuberosity insertion, is round or oval and ~8 mm in diameter.[1] This may be multifactorial in origin, and contributing factors include magic angle effect, partial volume averaging, and early degeneration in a vascular watershed region.[2–4]

Tendinosis can be difficult to distinguish from normal variant increased signal. Normal variant increased signal has a characteristic location and appearance as described above. Both tendinosis and normal variant increased signal are seen best on low TE images and should decrease in signal intensity on long TE images. If the signal resolves completely on long TE images it is likely a normal variant related to magic angle effect. Unlike normal variant increased signal, tendinosis sometimes thickens the cuff.

Interstitial partial tears can sometimes be difficult to distinguish from tendinosis (articular and bursal surface tears have discontinuity in their respective surfaces). Tears have higher (fluid) signal intensity and are usually associated with tendon thinning rather than thickening.

Recent joint injections can cause increased signal on long TE images mimicking a tear.[5] Rotator cuff repairs utilizing tendon-to-tendon anastomoses result in increased tendon signal on both proton density and T2-weighted MR images (T2WI).[6] However, the signal is less intense than fluid on T2WI.

Findings Related to Rotator Cuff Signal Not Related to a Full-Thickness Tear[1,5,6]

- Normal variant
- Tendinosis
- Partial thickness tear
- Recent joint injection
- Rotator cuff surgery

References

1. Tsao LY, Mirowitz SA. MR imaging of the shoulder. Imaging techniques, diagnostic pitfalls, and normal variants. Magn Reson Imaging Clin N Am 1997;5:683–704
2. Mirowitz SA. Normal rotator cuff: MR imaging with conventional and fat-suppression techniques. Radiology 1991;180:735–740
3. Davis SJ, Teresi LM, Bradley WG, Ressler JA, Eto RT. Effect of arm rotation on MR imaging of the rotator cuff. Radiology 1991;181:265–268
4. Erickson SJ, Cox IH, Hyde JS, Carrera GF, Strandt JA, Estkowski LD. Effect of tendon orientation on MR imaging signal intensity: a manifestation of the "magic angle" phenomenon. Radiology 1991;181:389–392
5. Hodler J, Kursunoglu-Brahme S, Snyder SJ, et al. Rotator cuff disease: assessment with MR arthrography versus standard MR imaging in 36 patients with arthroscopic confirmation. Radiology 1992;182:431–436
6. Owen RS, Iannotti JP, Kneeland JB, Dalinka MK, Deren JA, Oleaga L. Shoulder after surgery: MR imaging with surgical validation. Radiology 1993;186:443–447

139

Superior Labral Anterior-Posterior Tear versus Sublabral Recess

There are numerous variants in the anterior-superior labrum. Variants such as the Buford complex (absent anterior-superior labrum and hypertrophied middle glenohumeral ligament) and sublabral foramen can usually be differentiated from superior labral anterior to posterior (SLAP) tears as these variants occur anterior (in the 1 to 3 o'clock position) to the typical location of SLAP tears. SLAP tears are often difficult to differentiate from a normal variant sublabral recess. These are both seen at the 11 to 1 o'clock position of the glenoid labrum in the region of the biceps anchor. The type II tears (stripping of the superior labrum and attached biceps tendon from the glenoid cartilage) are the most common and also the most easily confused with a sublabral recess. Although in some cases, there is an overlap in appearance and these entities cannot be distinguished, the following findings are usually seen in SLAP tears rather than in a sublabral recess.[1,2]

Features of SLAP Tears

- Signal intensity extends posterior to the biceps anchor, into the posterior third of the superior glenoid. However, this can be seen in normal patients and has poor specificity for a SLAP tear.[3]
- Anteroposterior extension of signal intensity on axial fat-saturated T1-weighted magnetic resonance images (MRI) is usually seen in SLAP tears. The absence of this finding is helpful for excluding a SLAP tear. However, this can also be be seen in 61% of sublabral recesses.[4]
- Laterally curved signal intensity
- Irregular signal intensity
- There are two lines of high signal intensity. This is the "double Oreo cookie" sign: one line is the tear, the other the recess.
- A wide separation (>2 mm on MRI or 2.5 mm on MR arthrography) can be seen between the labrum and glenoid. However, a sublabral recess can be > 2 mm in normal cases.[3,5]
- A concomitant anterosuperior labral tear is much more commonly seen with a SLAP tear than a sublabral recess.[4]

References

1. De Maeseneer M, Van Roy F, Lenchik L, et al. CT and MR arthrography of the normal and pathologic anterosuperior labrum and labral-bicipital complex. Radiographics 2000;20:S67–S81

2. Tuite MJ, Cirillo RL, De Smet AA, Orwin JF. Superior labrum anterior-posterior (SLAP) tears: evaluation of three MR signs on T2-weighted images. Radiology 2000;215:841–845

3. Tuite MJ, Rutkowski A, Enright T, Kaplan L, Fine JP, Orwin J. Width of high signal and extension posterior to biceps tendon as signs of superior labrum anterior to posterior tears on MRI and MR arthography. AJR Am J Roentgenol 2005;185:1422–1428

4. Jin W, Kyung NR, Se HK, et al. MR arthrography in the differential diagnosis of Type II superior labral antero-posterior lesion and sublabral recess. AJR Am J Roentgenol 2006;187:887–893

5. Smith DK, Chopp TM, Aufdemorte TB, Witkowski EG, Jones RC. Sublabral recess of the superior glenoid labrum: study of cadavers with conventional nonenhanced MR imaging, MR arthrography, anatomic dissection and limited histologic examination. Radiology 1996;201:251–256

Abnormal Signal in the Rotator Cuff Muscles

Abnormal signal in the rotator cuff musculature on magnetic resonance imaging (MRI) can be secondary to a rotator cuff tear or nerve abnormality. A rotator cuff tear will result in muscular atrophy and increased T1-weighted MRI signal secondary to fatty infiltration. Denervation will in first result in neurogenic edema (bright on T2-weighted MRI), followed by atrophy.

The pattern of muscle involvement is helpful in differentiating these etiologies of abnormal muscle signal (**Table 140.1**).

Muscular atrophy secondary to rotator cuff tear is easily diagnosed. However, infraspinatus muscle atrophy can occur without an infraspinatus tendon tear. Infraspinatus muscle atrophy is usually associated with an anterior (supraspinatus and/or subscapularis) tendon tear.[1] Even with a supraspinatus tear, infraspinatus atrophy is sometimes seen without accompanying supraspinatus atrophy. Thus, isolated infraspinatus atrophy can be secondary to an anterior tendon tear, infraspinatus tear, spinoglenoid notch mass, or nerve injury.

In quadrilateral space syndrome, the axillary nerve is usually compressed by a mass or by fibrous bands. However, isolated teres minor atrophy has been seen in patients without clinical suspicion of quadrilateral space syndrome or visualized mass in the quadrilateral space, and this finding may sometimes be secondary to nerve injury or other shoulder abnormality.[2,3]

A cause of abnormal signal in multiple muscles is Parsonage–Turner syndrome, which is an acute brachial neuritis, possibly viral in etiology.

Findings Related to Abnormal Signal in the Rotator Cuff Muscles

- Rotator cuff tear
- Nerve compression
- Nerve injury
- Nerve inflammation

Table 140.1 Patterns of Abnormal Signal Intensity in the Rotator Cuff[1,4,5]

	Supraspinatus	Infraspinatus	Teres Minor	Deltoid
Suprascapular Notch Compression	+	+	−	−
Spinoglenoid Notch Compression	−	+	−	−
Quadrilateral Space Syndrome	−	−	+	±
Parsonage–Turner	±	±	−	±
Supraspinatus Tear	±	±	−	−
Infraspinatus Tear	−	±	−	−

References

1. Yao L, Mehta U. Infraspinatus muscle atrophy: implications? Radiology 2003;226:161–164
2. Cothran RL Jr, Helms C. Quadrilateral space syndrome: incidence of imaging findings in a population referred for MRI of the shoulder. AJR Am J Roentgenol 2005;184: 989–992
3. Sofka CM, Lin J, Feinberg J, Potter HG. Teres minor denervation on routine magnetic resonance imaging of the shoulder. Skeletal Radiol 2004;33:514–518
4. Linker CS, Helms CA, Fritz RC. Quadrilateral space syndrome: findings at MR imaging. Radiology 1993;188: 675–676
5. Helms CA, Martinez S, Speer KP. Acute brachial neuritis (Parsonage-Turner syndrome): MR imaging appearance—report of three cases. Radiology 1998;207: 255–259

VII   Spine

Focal Vertebral Lesions

Focal vertebral lesions can be benign or malignant. Focal benign lesions include hemangiomas, focal fatty marrow, focal red marrow, bone islands and can also be the result of hematopoietic growth factors. Focal lesions can also occur as the result of treatment of aplastic anemia with transplant or immunosuppressive therapy and following bone marrow transplant for malignancy; however, the findings will be more diffuse. The main concern when encountering a focal lesion is malignancy, which can be metastatic or less commonly, primary. Metastases can be solitary, multiple, or diffuse. Many times, biopsy, bone scan, or additional follow-up studies will be required to separate malignant lesions from benign; nevertheless, there are some differentiating features between metastases and the relatively common, benign vertebral hemangioma (**Table 141.1**).

Hemangiomas

The appearance of hemangiomas on magnetic resonance imaging (MRI) can be variable, with lesions with more adipocytes being hyperintense on T1-weighted MR images (T1WI) and intermediate on T2-weighted MR images (T2WI), and lesions with high vascularity/interstitial edema are intermediate signal on T1WI

Table 141.1 Differentiating Features between Vertebral Hemangiomas and Metastases

	Vertebral Hemangioma	Metastasis
Signal Intensity on T1WI	Intermediate to high	Low
Signal Intensity on T2WI	Intermediate to high	Variable, may depend on degree of sclerosis Generally hyperintense
Enhancement on MRI	Variable	Generally enhance, although may be variable due to degree of sclerosis
CT	Prominent trabeculae may have fat density "Polka dot" pattern	Sclerotic lesions with well- or ill-defined margins, or lytic destructive pattern
Multiple	About $^1/_3$ of cases	Often
Comments	Look for "polka dot" pattern on CT and high signal on T1WI	DWI – variable; more commonly hyperintense; may be a combination of T2WI-shine through and restricted diffusion

Abbreviations: CT, computed tomography; DWI, diffusion weighted imaging; MRI, magnetic resonance imaging; T1WI, T1-weighted MR images; T2WI, T2-weighted MR images.

and T2 hyperintense. Hemangiomas can also have varying degrees of heterogeneity reflecting their histology. Occasionally, hemangiomas can be hypointense and enhance significantly and then can be confused with malignant lesions. On computed tomography (CT) and x-rays, hemangiomas have a characteristic appearance (**Table 141.1**). In addition, hemangiomas can be symptomatic occasionally, and have an associated paraspinal or epidural mass that can lead to compression of neural structures. These hemangiomas are vascular, can be associated with prominent paraspinal vessels, and are sharply marginated. However, they are seldom associated with vertebral body collapse and almost entirely occur in the thoracic region. These less common lesions do not usually have the characteristic hyperintensity on T1WI, and they may not have the characteristic CT appearance, but it should be sought.

Bone Metastases

Bone metastases are seen in 5 to 10% of patients with cancer, and in ~70% of patients with metastatic disease. The spine is the most common site of skeletal metastases, and most are spread hematogenously. Metastases are best seen in patients with fatty marrow as hypointense lesions on T1WI. In patients with abundant red marrow (such as children), their detection on T1WI may be more difficult. T1WI alone may not show all metastases even in adults. Therefore, additional sequences such as T1WI with contrast and fat-saturation, T2WI with fat-saturation or STIR (short tau inversion recovery) or IRFSE (fast spin-echo inversion recovery), and GRE (gradient echo) chemical shift imaging have been advocated to improve detection (also see Chapters 142 and 144).

Additional Readings

1. Baudrez V, Galant C, Vande Berg BC. Benign vertebral hemangioma: MR-histological correlation. Skeletal Radiol 2001;30(8):442–446
2. Friedman DP. Symptomatic vertebral hemangiomas: MR findings. AJR Am J Roentgenol 1996;167(2): 359–364
3. Lien HH, Blomlie V, Blystad AK, Holte H, Langholm R, Kvaloy S. Bone-marrow MR imaging before and after autologous marrow transplantation in lymphoma patients without known bone-marrow involvement. Acta Radiol 1997;38(5):896–902
4. Taoka T, Mayr NA, Lee HJ, et al. Factors influencing visualization of vertebral metastases on MR imaging versus bone scintigraphy. AJR Am J Roentgenol 2001; 176(6):1525–1530
5. Vande Berg BC, Lecouvet FE, Galant C, Maldague BE, Malghem J. Normal variants and frequent marrow alterations that simulate bone marrow lesions at MR imaging. Radiol Clin North Am 2005;43(4):761–770 ix.
6. Vanel D, Dromain C, Tardivon A. MRI of bone marrow disorders. Eur Radiol 2000;10(2):224–229

142

Diffusely Abnormal Marrow Signal on Magnetic Resonance Imaging

Magnetic resonance imaging (MRI) can provide sensitive evaluation of neoplastic lesions or other pathologic conditions affecting the bone marrow. There is a gradual conversion of hematopoietic marrow to fatty marrow throughout the skeleton, reaching the adult appearance by 25 years of age. Lesions such as fractures will be evident on MRI due to the replacement of normal fatty elements by edema or blood; neoplastic processes will be evident due to the replacement of marrow elements with neoplastic cells.

Nonmalignant Marrow Signal Changes

There are nonneoplastic conditions that can also change the appearance of normal marrow. These include the administration of hematopoietic growth factors in healthy stem cell donors, anemia, low oxygen tension, and cigarette smoking, all of which create an appearance of greater hematopoietic marrow (i.e., less fatty marrow), which can simulate neoplastic involvement. In addition, children, young women, and athletes have marrow that is more hematopoietic.

Neoplastic and Therapy-Related Marrow Changes

Malignancies that can result in diffuse marrow signal abnormality include hematopoietic malignancies such as leukemia, myeloma, and lymphoma, as well as diffuse marrow infiltration from carcinoma. Chemotherapy, radiation, and bone marrow transplantation also can alter marrow signal. Bone marrow signal can decrease on T1-weighted MRI (T1WI) initially following chemotherapy or radiation therapy. A decrease in marrow signal intensity on T1WI following the preparatory regimen has been described. Within three months of transplantation a characteristic "band pattern" of hyperintensity centrally and an intermediate signal peripherally on T1WI with hyperintensity peripherally and central low signal on STIR images appears. In the longer term following bone marrow transplantation, the marrow develops a greater component of fatty marrow signal on T1WI and short T1 inversion time (STIR) sequences (although it can remain heterogeneous). There can also be persistent focal areas of lower signal on the T1WI (barely evident on STIR images), which are thought to represent focal areas of bone marrow regeneration rather than tumor. In patients who have had radiation therapy, the marrow often becomes quite hyperintense on the T1WI due to fatty replacement of marrow elements. This appearance can occur as early as 2 months following therapy, although it is generally seen after a longer time interval (see also Chapter 24 for a more detailed discussion including myeloma and Paget's disease).

Processes that Can Cause Abnormal Marrow Signal (Replacement of Normal Adult Fatty Marrow)

- Neoplastic:
  - Hematopoietic malignancies (leukemia, lymphoma, myeloma)
  - Diffuse carcinoma metastases
  - Myelofibrosis and other myelodysplastic syndromes
- Benign:
  - Anemia
  - Iron overload (siderosis, hemochromatosis)

- Hematopoietic growth factors
- Low oxygen tension
- Acquired immune deficiency syndrome (AIDS)
- Chronic renal disease
- Other factors or conditions:
  - Cigarette smoking
  - Being an athlete
  - Obesity in middle-aged women
  - Increased percentage of red marrow due to young age

Additional Readings

1. Mitchell MJ, Logan PM. Radiation-induced changes in bone. Radiographics 1998;18(5):1125–1136 quiz 1242–3
2. Plecha DM. Imaging of bone marrow disease in the spine. Semin Musculoskelet Radiol 2000;4(3):321–327
3. Restrepo CS, Lemos DF, Gordillo H, et al. Imaging findings in musculoskeletal complications of AIDS. Radiographics 2004;24(4):1029–1049
4. Stevens SK, Moore SG, Amylon MD. Repopulation of marrow after transplantation: MR imaging with pathologic correlation. Radiology 1990;175(1):213–218
5. Vande Berg BC, Lecouvet FE, Galant C, Maldague BE, Malghem J. Normal variants and frequent marrow alterations that simulate bone marrow lesions at MR imaging. Radiol Clin North Am 2005;43(4):761–770 ix.

143

Benign versus Pathologic (Neoplastic) Fracture

Thoracic and lumbar compression fractures are common in patients with senile, steroid-induced or other etiologies of osteoporosis. Metastatic disease also commonly affects the spine and can also result in compression fractures. Some findings on conventional imaging have been shown to be useful discriminating features in differentiating benign from malignant compression fractures (**Table 143.1**). Signal intensity on T1- or T2-weighted magnetic resonance images (T1WI,

Table 143.1 Differentiating Features between Metastatic and Benign Compression Fractures

	Malignant	Benign
Vertebral Body Posterior Border	Convex posterior border	Retropulsed posterior bone fragment
Epidural Mass	May be large (particularly if encasing dural sac)	May be present
Paraspinal Mass	May be large (a useful feature, particularly if focal)	Often present
CT Findings	Destruction of cancellous or cortical bone	Cortical fracture involving the anterolateral aspect of the vertebral body
	Focal paraspinal or epidural mass	Cortical fracture of the posterior aspect of the vertebral body with bony retropulsion
		Generally no destruction of cancellous bone
		Intravertebral vacuum phenomenon
		Well-defined linear or circumferential fracture lines in the cancellous bone
Distribution of Abnormal Marrow Signal/ Enhancement on MRI	Abnormal signal in pedicle or posterior elements	Spared normal bone marrow signal in portions of the vertebral body
	Near complete replacement of body marrow signal	Hypointense band on T1WI and T2WI
Diffusion Weighted Imaging	Hyperintense with decreased ADC*	Hypointense with increased ADC
Additional Findings	Additional metastases	Multiple compression fractures
		Hyperintense "fluid signal" focus adjacent to fractured endplate

Abbreviations: ADC, apparent diffusion coefficient; CT, computed tomography; MRI, magnetic resonance imaging; T1WI, T1-weighted MR images; T2WI, T2-weighted MR images.

*Variable signal intensities and ADCs have been described for pathologic fractures in different series.

T2WI) or enhancement characteristics have not been shown to be useful. Benign and metastatic compression fractures can have diffuse paraspinal masses, but a focal paraspinal mass is more common in metastatic compression fractures. Likewise, an epidural mass that encases the dural sac is more common in metastatic disease.

Diffusion weighted images may help characterize fractures, with restricted diffusion a feature of some pathologic fractures secondary to the presence of densely packed tumor cells.

The finding of a "fluid sign," a linear focus adjacent to the fractured endplate with intensity similar to cerebrospinal fluid on the T2WI, is seen most commonly in benign fractures and only rarely in malignant ones. This is thought to be due to edema and osteonecrosis. Although several findings can lead one to favor one etiology over the other, there is significant overlap and no finding or combination of findings can reliably discriminate between benign and malignant compression fractures. Often, follow-up studies, multiple correlative studies, or biopsies are needed to establish the diagnosis.

Additional Readings

1. Baur A, Stabler A, Arbogast S, Duerr HR, Bartl R, Reiser M. Acute osteoporotic and neoplastic vertebral compression fractures: fluid sign at MR imaging. Radiology 2002;225(3):730–735
2. Herneth AM, Philipp MO, Naude J, et al. Vertebral metastases: assessment with apparent diffusion coefficient. Radiology 2002;225(3):889–894
3. Jung HS, Jee WH, McCauley TR, Ha KY, Choi KH. Discrimination of metastatic from acute osteoporotic compression spinal fractures with MR imaging. Radiographics 2003;23(1):179–187
4. Laredo JD, Lakhdari K, Bellaiche L, Hamze B, Janklewicz P, Tubiana JM. Acute vertebral collapse: CT findings in benign and malignant nontraumatic cases. Radiology 1995;194(1):41–48
5. Spuentrup E, Buecker A, Adam G, van Vaals JJ, Guenther RW. Diffusion-weighted MR imaging for differentiation of benign fracture edema and tumor infiltration of the vertebral body. AJR Am J Roentgenol 2001;176(2):351–358
6. Yuh WT, Mayr NA, Petropoulou K, Beall DP. MR fluid sign in osteoporotic vertebral fracture. Radiology 2003;227(3):905

Posterior Element Lesions

There are a few tumors that preferentially involve the posterior elements. These include

- Common:
  - Osteoid osteoma
  - Osteoblastoma
  - Aneurysmal bone cyst
  - Metastases
  - Chondrosarcoma
  - Hemangioma
  - Paget's disease
- Rare:
  - Unicameral (simple) bone cyst – more commonly found at the metaphysis of long bones
  - Osteochondroma – more common in long bones and appendicular skeleton (incidence in spine in multiple hereditary exostoses is 3%)
  - Osteosarcoma

Of these, osteoblastoma and osteoid osteoma are considered similar lesions, and are differentiated by size (generally, osteoid osteomas are up to 1.5 cm, 2.0 cm by some authors) with osteoblastomas larger. Although they are considered as similar lesions, they do have differences in their appearances other than just size (**Table 144.1**). The etiology of aneurysmal bone cysts is unclear, and the presence of a soft

Table 144.1 Differentiating Features between Osteoid Osteoma, Osteoblastoma, and Aneurysmal Bone Cyst

	Osteoid Osteoma	Osteoblastoma	Aneurysmal Bone Cyst
Size	≤ 1.5 – 2.0 cm	> 1.5 – 2.0 cm	Any
CT	Nidus with surrounding sclerosis Nidus can be lytic (~30%), lytic with central calcification (~50%), or rarely sclerotic May induce cortical thickening, sclerotic pedicle	Typical appearance: 　Expansile osteolytic lesion with osteogenic matrix mineralizations or a thin shell-like periosteal reaction or sclerotic rim May appear similar to osteoid osteoma with central lucency and surrounding sclerosis May have a more aggressive appearance with expansion, bone destruction, and soft tissue infiltration	Expansile Fluid/fluid levels (better demonstrated with MRI) Marked thinning of cortex

(Continued on page 302)

Table 144.1 *(Continued)* Differentiating Features between Osteoid Osteoma, Osteoblastoma, and Aneurysmal Bone Cyst

	Osteoid Osteoma	Osteoblastoma	Aneurysmal Bone Cyst
MRI	Nidus – variable depending on degree of mineralization T1WI: Hypointense to isointense T2WI: Hyperintense to hypointense	Variable signal depending on amount of osteoid matrix production T1WI: Hypointense to isointense T2WI: Hyperintense to hypointense	Expansile lesion Multiple cavities with fluid/fluid levels due to layering blood products Hypointense surrounding rim due to fibrous tissue
	Surrounding edema	May have low signal rim Reactive edema usually present and may involve adjacent soft tissues and adjacent vertebrae	Edema of adjacent soft tissues
Enhancement	Yes, dynamic imaging may be helpful. Hypervascular nidus MRI: Enhancement of nidus as well as perinidal edema	Yes Tumor as well as adjacent marrow and soft tissue edema may enhance	Yes Wall and septa
Comments	10–20% in the spine Most patients <25 years old Series 1: Thoracic = Lumbar > Cervical Series 2: Lumbar > Cervical > Thoracic Almost always increased uptake on Tc99 MDP Bone scan	32–46% in the spine 90% diagnosed in 2nd–3rd decade. May have soft tissue mass which is inflammatory or neoplastic Neurologic deficits 25–50% Thoracic and lumbar spine > cervical MRI may overestimate the extent of the lesion due to extensive reaction and adjacent soft tissue masses, which may be inflammatory	Most common in 1st two decades Thoracic spine most common spinal site May look like telangiectatic osteosarcoma May be associated with other lesions

Abbreviations: CT, computed tomography; MRI, magnetic resonance imaging; T1WI, T1-weighted MR images; T2WI, T2-weighted MR images; Tc99 MDP, technetium-99 methylene diphosphonate.

tissue component should raise concern for other underlying bone lesions, including a telangiectatic osteosarcoma. Of the less common lesions, chondrosarcoma arises in the spine in 3 to 12% of cases. It is in the posterior elements 40% of the time and in both the body and posterior elements 45% of the time. Metastases are common lesions of the spine, and the spine is the most common site of bony metastases; however, the vertebral bodies (80%) are more commonly involved than the posterior elements.

Additional Readings

1. Harish S, Saifuddin A. Imaging features of spinal osteoid osteoma with emphasis on MRI findings. Eur Radiol 2005;15(12):2396–2403
2. Murphey MD, Andrews CL, Flemming DJ, Temple HT, Smith WS, Smirniotopoulos JG. From the archives of the AFIP. Primary tumors of the spine: radiologic pathologic correlation. Radiographics 1996;16(5):1131–1158
3. Shaikh MI, Saifuddin A, Pringle J, Natali C, Sherazi Z. Spinal osteoblastoma: CT and MR imaging with pathological correlation. Skeletal Radiol 1999;28(1): 33–40
4. Woertler K. Benign bone tumors and tumor-like lesions: value of cross-sectional imaging. Eur Radiol 2003;13(8):1820–1835
5. Zileli M, Cagli S, Basdemir G, Ersahin Y. Osteoid osteomas and osteoblastomas of the spine. Neurosurg Focus 2003;15(5):E5

145

Posterior Vertebral Body Scalloping

A variety of conditions can result in increased concavity of the posterior margin of a vertebral body (vertebral scalloping). Slow growing or congenital intraspinal masses, dural ectasia, chronically elevated intraspinal pressure, connective tissue disorders, acromegaly, neurofibromatosis type I (NF-1), or congenital skeletal disorders can all be associated with posterior vertebral scalloping. Dural ectasia is seen in diseases/syndromes such as Marfan syndrome, Ehlers–Danlos syndrome, NF-1, and ankylosing spondylitis. Bony effects are greater in the caudal spines of patients with dural ectasia due to greater pressure effects. In Marfan syndrome, thinning of the pedicles and lamina has also been described. In NF-1, the causes of vertebral scalloping are unknown and may be due to dural ectasia, erosion from adjacent neurofibroma, or primary mesodermal dysplasia of the meninges.

Causes of Posterior Vertebral Scalloping

Syndromes/Systemic Diseases

- Marfan syndrome
- Neurofibromatosis
- Proteus syndrome
- Achondroplasia
- Ehlers–Danlos syndrome
- Ankylosing spondylitis
- Mucopolysaccharidoses (Morquio, Hurler's)
- Posterior meningocele
- Acromegaly

Slow-growing/Congenital Masses

- Myxopapillary ependymoma
- Ganglioglioma
- Meningioma
- Neurofibroma
- Cyst
- Lipoma

Miscellaneous

- Normal variant (usually only mild)
- Long-standing hydrocephalus

Additional Readings

1. Kumar R, Guinto FC Jr, Madewell JE, Swischuk LE, David R. The vertebral body: radiographic configurations in various congenital and acquired disorders. Radiographics 1988;8(3):455–485
2. Stuber JL, Palacios E. Vertebral scalloping in acromegaly. Am J Roentgenol Radium Ther Nucl Med 1971;112(2):397–400
3. Wakely SL. The posterior vertebral scalloping sign. Radiology 2006;239(2):607–609

146

Lesions within the Spinal Canal

Classically, lesions involving the spinal canal have been approached by location. The division into extradural (outside the dural sac), intradural-extramedullary (within the dural sac, but outside the spinal cord) and intramedullary (within the spinal cord or filum terminale) has been the classic radiologic grouping. Extradural neoplasia is most common, and are often due to metastases involving the vertebrae, being followed by intradural-extramedullary tumors, with nerve sheath tumors and meningiomas being the most common, and lastly by the intramedullary tumors, which are predominantly astrocytomas and ependymomas.

Epidural Lesions

Degenerative etiologies, including disc bulges, herniations, migratory fragments, facet arthorpathy, and ligamentum flavum redundancy, are the most common epidural lesions, exerting extrinsic compression on the thecal sac and nerve roots (see **Chapter 149**). Purely spinal epidural infections or neoplasms are relatively uncommon. Most of the primary neoplasms arising within the spinal epidural space are lymphomas, nerve sheath tumors, and rarely meningiomas (3.5% of spinal meningiomas are purely epidural). There have been reports of other neoplasms rarely involving the epidural space without bony involvement such as cavernous hemangiomas and extraskeletal Ewing's sarcoma. Hodgkin's or non-Hodgkin's lymphoma can occur in the spinal epidural space without bony involvement, rarely. Lymphomas may involve the epidural space by either extension from mediastinal or retroperitoneal adenopathy, hematogenous spread, or less frequently from the vertebral body. Metastatic disease can involve the epidural space without bony involvement, especially metastases from prostate, breast, and lung cancer, as well as lymphoma and leukemic infiltration. Rarely hematomas can have associated enhancement and mimic tumors, and in acute epidural hematomas the enhancement may be peripheral, septated, or within the hematoma. When within the hematoma, it has been postulated to represent extravasation and an "active" lesion. Epidural hematomas are usually from venous bleeding and occur more commonly dorsally.

Causes of Epidural Lesions

- Neoplasms
  - Primary (lymphoma, nerve sheath tumors, rarely meningiomas, others)
  - Metastatic/direct extension (lymphoma, leukemia, prostate, lung, breast, others)
  - Lymphoproliferative disorder
  - Myeloma
- Hematoma
- Infection (phlegmon, abscess)
- Extramedullary hematopoiesis
- Epidural lipomatosis
- Amyloidoma

Additional Readings

1. Chang FC, Lirng JF, Chen SS, et al. Contrast enhancement patterns of acute spinal epidural hematomas: a report of two cases. AJNR Am J Neuroradiol 2003; 24(3):366–369
2. Fukui MB, Swarnkar AS, Williams RL. Acute spontaneous spinal epidural hematomas. AJNR Am J Neuroradiol 1999;20(7):1365–1372
3. Lyons MK, O'Neill BP, Marsh WR, Kurtin PJ. Primary spinal epidural non-Hodgkin's lymphoma: report of eight patients and review of the literature. Neurosurgery 1992;30(5):675–680
4. Sharif HS. Role of MR imaging in the management of spinal infections. AJR Am J Roentgenol 1992;158(6): 1333–1345
5. Shin JH, Lee HK, Rhim SC, Cho KJ, Choi CG, Suh DC. Spinal epidural extraskeletal Ewing sarcoma: MR findings in two cases. AJNR Am J Neuroradiol 2001;22(4): 795–798
6. Shin JH, Lee HK, Rhim SC, Park SH, Choi CG, Suh DC. Spinal epidural cavernous hemangioma: MR findings. J Comput Assist Tomogr 2001;25(2):257–261

147

Intradural Extramedullary Lesions

Meningiomas and nerve sheath tumors are the most common intraspinal tumors, with meningiomas representing approximately 25 to 40% and nerve sheath tumors representing 16 to 30% of adult intraspinal tumors, with some series reporting nerve sheath tumors as the most frequent intraspinal mass. Because they both commonly arise somewhat laterally in the spinal canal in the intradural extramedullary space (with the nerve sheath tumors most commonly arising from the dorsal sensory roots), they are sometimes difficult to differentiate. Tumors in this space should compress and displace the spinal cord, should expand the cerebrospinal fluid space above and below, and compress the epidural fat.

Nerve Sheath Tumors

Nerve sheath tumors include neurofibromas and schwannomas, which have been variably called neurinomas, neurolemmomas, and neuromas. Despite several attempts, no technique can reliably distinguish these neoplasms by imaging. Magnetic resonance imaging (MRI) features of nerve sheath tumors reflect their variable histology and growth pattern (**Table 147.1**).

Table 147.1 Differentiating Features between Meningiomas and Nerve Sheath Tumors

	Meningioma	Nerve Sheath Tumor
Unenhanced CT	May have calcifications May be hyperdense to spinal cord	May remodel bone/expand neural foramen
CT/Myelography	Compress and displace the spinal cord and epidural fat Expand the CSF space above and below*	Compress and displace the spinal cord and epidural fat Expand the CSF space above and below*
Unenhanced T1WI	Homogeneous, isointense to mildly hypointense to cord	Heterogeneous, hypointense to isointense, with or without blood products
Enhanced T1WI	Homogeneous enhancement	Heterogeneous or peripheral ring enhancement
T2WI	Homogeneously isointense to mildly hyperintense to cord Similar affect on cord and subarachnoid space as seen on CT myelography*	Variably hyperintense and heterogeneous, with foci of greater hyperintensity Similar affect on cord and subarachnoid space as seen on CT myelography*

(Continued on page 308)

Table 147.1 *(Continued)* Differentiating Features between Meningiomas and Nerve Sheath Tumors

	Meningioma	Nerve Sheath Tumor
Broad Dural Attachment	Yes	No
Dural Tail	Frequent	No
Cystic Areas	Rare	Common
Additional Distinguishing Features	More likely to have calcifications May be psammomatous	Foci of hyperintensity, hypointensity or cystic components on T2WI Central loss of enhancement Blood products and hyperintense foci on T1WI "Dumbbell" configuration (Lesion has a component inside and outside the canal with "waist" at the foramen.)

Abbreviations: CSF, cerebrospinal fluid; CT, computed tomography; T1WI, T1-weighted magnetic resonance imaging; T2WI, T2-weighted magnetic resonance imaging.

*It is often easiest to localize these lesions within the spinal canal at their superior or inferior margins.

Meningiomas

Meningiomas are most common in the thoracic spine (up to 80%) followed by the cervical spine (15 to 17%) with few reported in the lumbar spine. Approximately 90% are intradural with the next most common presentation having an extradural component, with intramedullary lesions very rare. Tumors with mixed presentations tend to have more variable imaging characteristics. Like nerve sheath tumors, they are discrete, well circumscribed, round or oval masses (**Table 147.1**).

Other Lesions

Free disk fragments tend to occur in the lumbar spine, at L3 to L4 and L4 to L5, distinguishing them from meningiomas by location. They have variable MRI appearances, but demonstrate thin peripheral enhancement of surrounding granulation tissue. Sarcoidosis presents most frequently in the cervical and thoracic regions, often without a known history of systemic disease. Together with enhancing intradural masses, sarcoidosis tends to present with synchronous parenchymal and leptomeningeal foci of signal abnormality and abnormal enhancement. Intradural extramedullary tuberculoma is another rare presentation of a common disease, appearing as a nodular enhancing mass. The less common vascular tumors such as hemangioblastomas, capillary hemangiomas and paragangliomas can be differentiated from the more common tumors by the presence of associated draining veins, which may be seen within the subarachnoid space and along the cord surface. Capillary hemangiomas appear as isointense on T1-weighted MRI (T1WI), hyperintense on T2-weighted MRI (T2WI), and have pronounced enhancement, although reports have also described them as only mildly hyperintense on T2WI, heterogeneous, and with areas of hyperintensity on T1WI.

Magnetic Resonance Spectroscopy

MR spectroscopy has been suggested to successfully characterize these lesions. Tumors such as meningiomas and schwannomas had elevated choline levels, consistent with increased cellular proliferation. Schwannomas have elevated myoinositol levels, and meningiomas have increased alanine.

Differential Diagnosis of Intradural Extramedullary Lesions

- Nerve sheath tumors
  - Schwannoma (neurinomas)
  - Neurofibroma
  - Malignant nerve sheath tumor
  - Ganglioneuroma (rare)
- Meningioma
- Drop metastases
- Lymphoma
- Hemangioblastoma
- Paraganglioma
- Ependymoma (rare)
- Capillary hemangioma (rare; may have "dural tail")
- Cavernous hemangioma
- Hemangioendothelioma
- Arteriovenous malformation (AVM)
- Sarcoidosis
- Tuberculosis

Additional Readings

1. Abdullah, D.C., Raghuram, K., Phillips, C.D., Jane, J.A., Jr., and Miller, B., Thoracic intradural extramedullary capillary hemangioma. AJNR Am J Neuroradiol, 2004. 25(7): p. 1294-6.
2. Choi, B.Y., Chang, K.H., Choe, G., Han, M.H., Park, S.W., Yu, I.K., et. al. Spinal intradural extramedullary capillary hemangioma: MR imaging findings. AJNR Am J Neuroradiol, 2001. 22(4): p. 799-802.
3. Isoda, H., Takahashi, M., Mochizuki, T., Ramsey, R.G., Masui, T., Takehara, Y., et. al. MRI of dumbbell-shaped spinal tumors. J Comput Assist Tomogr, 1996. 20(4): p. 573-82.
4. Li, M.H., Holtas, S. and Larsson, E.M., MR imaging of intradural extramedullary tumors. Acta Radiol, 1992. 33(3): p. 207-12.
5. Van Goethem, J.W., van den Hauwe, L., Ozsarlak, O., De Schepper, A.M., and Parizel, P.M., Spinal tumors. Eur J Radiol, 2004. 50(2): p. 159-76.

Intramedullary Spinal Cord Lesions

About 5% of spinal tumors are intramedullary. In children, astrocytomas predominate, whereas in adults ependymomas predominate, with astrocytoma next in frequency, and hemangioblastomas a distant third. Tumors cannot be definitively differentiated, but may have features suggestive of a particular diagnosis (**Table 148.1**). Most spinal cord tumors enhance, and those that do not are usually astrocytomas. Ependymomas tend to be well circumscribed and more easily resected than astrocytomas; hence they can be surgically cured. A specific type of ependymoma, the myxopapillary type, constitutes 30% and occurs almost exclusively in the conus and filum terminale. Cysts may be associated with many intramedullary tumors,

Table 148.1 Differentiating Features between Ependymomas, Astrocytomas, and Hemangioblastomas

	Ependymoma	Astrocytoma	Hemangioblastoma
Incidence	60% of adults 4th and 5th decade peak	24–30% of adults Up to 90% of children 3rd and 4th decades for adults	Up to 5.8% of adults 30–40 years, younger in VHL
Edema	60%	23%	Extensive
Location	Cervical, conus, filum terminale (MP)	Thoracic (most say cervicothoracic, 50% in upper thoracic)	Thoracic, cervical
Location in Cord	Central	Eccentric	Superficial, peripheral, frequently posterior
Enhancement	Homogeneous, may be only mild to moderate	Heterogeneous, mild to moderate, partial	Intense
Borders	Well defined	Ill defined	Well defined
Cysts/Syrinx	Commonly has satellite cysts or syrinxes May have rostral cysts that extend into dorsal medulla or to floor of 4th ventricle	More commonly intratumoral cysts than satellite cysts May have associated syrinx	Syrinx in 40–64%
MRI Signal	T1WI: Hypointense (except MP which can be hyperintense) T2WI: Hyperintense (mild)	T1WI: Hypointense to isointense T2WI: Hyperintense (mild)	T1WI: Hypointense to isointense T2WI: Isointense to hyperintense

Table 148.1 *(Continued)* Differentiating Features between Ependymomas, Astrocytomas, and Hemangioblastomas

	Ependymoma	Astrocytoma	Hemangioblastoma
Distinguishing Features	Associated hemosiderin - "cap sign"- hemosiderin on either end due to chronic hemorrhage	May be large and infiltrating	Hydrosyringomyelia or edema Up to 33% assoc with VHL May be multiple in VHL Associated flow voids or pial enhancement
Mean Height	3–4 vertebrae	5–6 vertebrae	1 vertebra (occasionally large)

Abbreviations: MP, myxopapillary ependymoma; T1WI, T1-weighted magnetic resonance imaging; T2WI, T2-weighted magnetic resonance imaging; VHL, Von Hippel–Lindau syndrome.

uncommon with metastases, and more commonly with ependymomas, where large cervical cysts can extend into the medulla and elevate the fourth ventricle. Hemangioblastomas can occur as isolated tumors, or in association with Von Hippel–Lindau syndrome, where they may be multiple. Gangliogliomas are reported to be rare; however, it has been suggested they are underdiagnosed and should be considered in young patients with long tumors (average eight segments), which have patchy enhancement that extends to the surface, mixed signal on T1-weighted precontrast magnetic resonance images, bone remodeling, and/or scoliosis, tumor cyst (with peripheral enhancement), and absence of edema.

Differential Diagnosis of Intramedullary Spinal Cord Lesions

- Common:
  - Astrocytoma (more common in children than adults)
  - Ependymoma (most common intramedullary tumor in adults)
- Uncommon:
  - Hemangioblastoma
  - Metastasis
- Rare:
  - Cavernous malformations
  - Lymphoma
  - Lipoma
  - Ganglioglioma
  - Oligodendroglioma
- Nonneoplastic:
  - Multiple sclerosis (MS)
  - Transverse myelitis
  - Infarct
  - Granuloma
  - Abscess
  - Sarcoidosis

Additional Readings

1. Baleriaux DL. Spinal cord tumors. Eur Radiol 1999; 9(7):1252–1258
2. Patel U, Pinto RS, Miller DC, et al. MR of spinal cord ganglioglioma. AJNR Am J Neuroradiol 1998;19(5): 879–887
3. Sun B, Wang C, Wang J, Liu A. MRI features of intramedullary spinal cord ependymomas. J Neuroimaging 2003;13(4):346–351
4. Van Goethem JW, van den Hauwe L, Ozsarlak O, De Schepper AM, Parizel PM. Spinal tumors. Eur J Radiol 2004;50(2):159–176

149

Diskitis/Osteomyelitis, Degenerative Disease, and Scar

Both degenerative changes and infection can result in marrow and disk signal changes, as well as enhancement. Differentiation can be difficult at times, as chronic infections can often have indolent presentations. There are findings that can be used to help differentiate infection from degenerative changes (**Table 149.1**). (For a discussion about neoplastic processes involving the vertebral bodies, please see Chapter 143.) These features can include patterns of enhancement, associated epidural or paraspinal tissue or fluid collections, disk signal changes, and endplate signal changes.

Table 149.1 Differentiating Features between Diskitis/Osteomyelitis and Degenerative Changes

	Diskitis / Osteomyelitis	Degenerative
Disk Signal	Increased on T2WI Loss of normal hypointense intranuclear cleft	Generally decreased on T2WI (Disks can occasionally develop cystic degeneration that is hyperintense on T2WI.)
T1WI Marrow Signal	Decreased	Normal, decreased, increased
T2WI Marrow Signal	Increased	Normal, decreased, increased
Enhancement	Common in areas of signal abnormality	Occasionally, but less common and less extensive
Paraspinal Tissue/ Inflammatory Changes	Generally, yes	Generally, no
Epidural Enhancing Tissue/Fluid	Possibly	No
Vertebral Body Height	Eventual destruction, collapse on either side of disk space	Can develop some endplate irregularity or Schmorl's nodes, but not collapse or destruction
CT Endplate Changes	Osteolytic foci with endplate fragmentation	May have mild irregularity with sclerosis Generally, no fragmentation

Table 149.1 (*Continued*) Differentiating Features between Diskitis/Osteomyelitis and Degenerative Changes

	Diskitis / Osteomyelitis	**Degenerative**
Key Differentiating Features	The likelihood of infection increases as more findings are present with the constellation of enhancement of the intervertebral disk, adjacent vertebral bodies, increased signal on T2WI with loss of the low signal internuclear cleft, and paraspinal/epidural tissue being highly suggestive of infection.	

Abbreviations: CT, computed tomography; T1WI, T1-weighted magnetic resonance images; T2WI, T2-weighted magnetic resonance images.

Degenerative Marrow Changes

Vertebral body marrow signal changes adjacent to the endplates have been described in degenerative disk disease, and classified into type 1, type 2, and type 3 changes. Type 1 changes demonstrate "fluid like" features, with decreased signal to the marrow adjacent to the vertebral body endplate on T1-weighted magnetic resonance images (T1WI), and increased signal on the T2-weighted magnetic resonance images (T2WI). Type 2 changes demonstrate "fat like" features, with increased signal on T1WI and mildly increased to isointense signal on T2WI in the same areas. Type 3 changes consist of low signal on the T1WI and T2WI and correlate with sclerosis on plain radiographs. All of these marrow changes are associated with degenerative changes in the disk, including decreased signal on the T2WI due to desiccation, disk space narrowing, and "vacuum disk." Infection can show marrow signal similar to type 1 changes. However, the disk is generally hyperintense on T2WI, as opposed to the hypointense appearance more typical of degenerative changes. Although degenerative disks are generally hypointense on T2WI, high signal intensity on the T1WI has been shown to be related to mild to moderate calcification, while low signal intensity can be related to any degree of calcification or to vacuum phenomenon.

Spinal Infections

Spinal infections (diskitis/osteomyelitis/ infective spondylitis) can be caused by a variety of organisms, and present differently in children than adults largely due to different vascularization of the disks and endplates. In general, pediatric infections primarily involve the disk, whereas in adults bacteria usually seed the vertebral body near the endplates (particularly anteriorly, at the metaphysis), and then spread to the disk. Rarely, pyogenic organisms can cause an epidural abscess in the absence of detectable bone or disk disease. Patients on hemodialysis occasionally present with a rapidly progressive spondyloarthropathy that mimics the findings in infection.

Postoperative Spine

Postoperative patients are often imaged, and it is important to separate expected from unexpected, or pathologic, postoperative findings. Some morphologic features can help distinguish between residual/recurrent disks and scar (**Table 149.2**). The general rule is that scar enhances and disk does not. However, disk may enhance peripherally or on delayed (>30 minutes) imaging. Additionally, in the postoperative period

Table 149.2 Differentiating Features between Residual/Recurrent Disk Herniation and Scar

	Disk	Scar
Morphology	Smooth, polypoid, or lobulated margins	Irregular and indistinct margins
Contiguity with Disk	Yes (unless free fragment)	No
Mass Effect on Thecal Sac or Nerve Roots	Yes	Generally conforms to sac and surrounds roots, but can have mass effect
T2WI Signal	Low/intermediate, occasionally high when larger	Generally higher than disk
Enhancement	No, or peripheral*	Yes

Abbreviations: T2WI, T2-weighted magnetic resonance images.

*Occasionally, delayed enhancement is present.

up to 3 months, granulation tissue may impress on the ventral aspect of the dural sac and may have peripheral enhancement. Postoperative disk enhancement has a characteristic appearance with enhancement of the anulus at the site of surgery, with the majority having linear enhancement along the superior and inferior aspects of the disk, parallel to the endplates.

Hematoma and seroma may enhance peripherally and have an appearance indistinguishable from abscess, and can also be associated with postoperative soft tissue enhancement. Accelerated degenerative changes, such as endplate marrow signal changes (and enhancement) and disk height loss, can also develop in postoperative patients.

Additional Readings

1. Duda JJ Jr, Ross JS. The postoperative lumbar spine: imaging considerations. Semin Ultrasound CT MR 1993;14(6):425–436
2. Modic MT, Masaryk TJ, Ross JS, Carter JR. Imaging of degenerative disk disease. Radiology 1988;168(1):177–186
3. Modic MT, Steinberg PM, Ross JS, Masaryk TJ, Carter JR. Degenerative disk disease: assessment of changes in vertebral body marrow with MR imaging. Radiology 1988;166(1 Pt 1):193–199
4. Ross JS, Zepp R, Modic MT. The postoperative lumbar spine: enhanced MR evaluation of the intervertebral disk. AJNR Am J Neuroradiol 1996;17(2):323–331
5. Rothman MI, Zoarski GH. Imaging basis of disc space infection. Semin Ultrasound CT MR 1993;14(6):437–445
6. Sharif HS. Role of MR imaging in the management of spinal infections. AJR Am J Roentgenol 1992;158(6):1333–1345

Index